Obstetrics and Gynecology

THE CLINICAL CORE

OBSTETRICS
and
GYNECOLOGY

THE CLINICAL CORE

Ralph M. Wynn, M.D.

Director, Department of Obstetrics and Gynecology,
St. Joseph Mercy Hospital, Pontiac, Michigan
Professor of Obstetrics and Gynecology, Wayne State
University School of Medicine

FOURTH EDITION

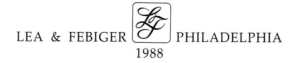

LEA & FEBIGER   PHILADELPHIA
1988

Lᴇᴀ & Fᴇʙɪɢᴇʀ
600 Washington Square
Philadelphia, Pa. 19106 U.S.A.
(215) 922-1330

First Edition 1974
Reprinted 1975
Second Edition 1979
Reprinted 1980, 1981, 1982
Third Edition 1983
Reprinted 1983, 1985
Fourth Edition 1988

Library of Congress Cataloging-in-Publication Data

Wynn, Ralph M.
    Obstetrics and gynecology.

    Includes bibliographies and index.
    1. Gynecology.   2. Obstetrics.   I. Title.
[DNLM: 1. Curriculum.   2. Genital Diseases, Female.
3. Obstetrics.   WQ W988o]
RG101.W96   1988   618   87-17292
ISBN 0-8121-1108-7

PRINTED IN THE UNITED STATES OF AMERICA

Print Number   4   3   2   1

TO

THE MEDICAL STUDENTS AND RESIDENTS
WHOM I HAVE HAD THE PRIVILEGE TO TEACH
DURING THE PAST THREE DECADES

The fourth edition of this textbook is dedicated to Leon C. Chesley, on the occasion of his eightieth birthday, in grateful recognition of his innumerable contributions to academic obstetrics and gynecology.

Preface

Education may be defined as planned change in behavior of the student over a period of time. Medical educators, in common with their colleagues in other fields, must therefore select experiences and teach them as rapidly and efficiently as possible to the level of performance described as acceptable behavior. The planning of medical curricula, including the process of selection, design, and sequential arrangement of instructional units, requires a rationale and thus cannot be left to chance.

A curriculum should be based on four educational principles: development of objectives, preparation of an entry test, construction of a set of learning activities, and formulation of procedures for evaluation of the results. A core curriculum defines the criteria for minimal competence required of all medical students. It provides at least three major advantages in the educational process. First, it reduces the amount of purely factual material to be learned. Second, it identifies the requisite knowledge and skill for all medical students. Third, it increases the time available for elective studies in the basic or clinical sciences.

The availability of a core curriculum that details the data base frees the teacher from the task of mere dissemination of information and allows him time for influencing attitudes and demonstrating skills. In a modern curriculum the student may proceed at his own rate to accomplish the educational objectives of the core and may devote more time to mastering areas of difficulty. The faster learner may pursue areas in depth or proceed to other areas. The construction of a core curriculum in obstetrics and gynecology is thus a step toward increased flexibility in the undergraduate medical curriculum. It spells out the minimal needs of every physician for knowledge and skills in obstetrics and gynecology and allows time for additional electives or special tracks for students who choose a career in this field.

A good textbook is probably the fastest means of transmitting a large body of knowledge. The skilled reader can control his rate of learning and can read the printed page more rapidly than any lecturer can deliver the same material intelligibly. As self-instructional media and synopses increase in quality and as retrieval of information from handbooks and other reference sources improves, the classic textbook, which struggles in vain to be both instructionally sound and encyclopedic, will gradually disappear. Quite different is the student text based on educational principles. It seldom presents new knowledge. Instead, it offers the available knowledge to the student in a selective, sequential, simplified presentation.

Although I have sought the advice of several colleagues in the preparation of this edition, the writing of the entire text is mine and I therefore accept full responsibility for the selection and arrangement in sequence of the material. I have attempted to make the definitions of terms in this text consistent with the recommendations of the Committee on Terminology of the American College of Obstetricians and Gynecologists wherever possible.

During preparation of this fourth edition, changes were made on virtually every page of the text. The most extensive revisions occurred in the sections on perinatal medicine, gynecologic infections, and control of reproduction. I have attempted to include all essential new information without substantially increasing the size of the book. Significant additions were made in the material dealing with basic reproductive biology. These additions reflect a trend to incorporate a brief course in basic human reproduction in the curricula of many American medical schools. Original anatomical drawings were expertly prepared by Dr. John E. Pauly in response to the requests of many medical students. Colleagues who provided valuable assistance in preparation of this edition are: Dr. Leon C. Chesley, who gave expert advise on preeclampsia and physiology and read the entire text; Dr. Iris Cosnow, who supplied the photomicrographs of serous cystadenocarcinoma of the ovary and lesions of the breast; Dr. Thomas V. Sedlacek, who supplied the illustrations of human papilloma virus infection of the cervix and again reviewed the material on gynecologic oncology; and Dr. Nancy Worthen, who skillfully prepared the material on sonography. The original new sonograms in this edition were included as an indication of the indispensability of ultrasound in modern obstetric and gynecologic diagnosis. I am especially indebted to Dr. John R. Marshall, who reviewed the entire text and made numerous editorial suggestions, most of which were incorporated, in each of the sections. As in the past, the timely appearance of this edition is due in large measure to the cooperation and efficiency of Mr. Thomas J. Colaiezzi of Lea & Febiger.

RALPH M. WYNN, M.D.
Pontiac, Michigan

Contents

Notes on the Use of
This Text

The importance of the material in each paragraph is indicated by the size of the type. The information contained in paragraphs set in large type is the clinical core. Because this is the minimal information in obstetrics and gynecology required of all medical students, it should be mastered in its entirety. The material within paragraphs set in smaller type contains additional important elements of the data base that may be included appropriately on undergraduate examinations in obstetrics and gynecology.

The core text defines only the data base required for minimal competence in the cognitive domain of obstetrics and gynecology. Detailed information, illustrative material, and references must be sought in standard textbooks, specialized treatises, and periodicals. Audiovisual aids, lectures, conferences, rounds, and clinical experiences with patients are required to achieve educational objectives in the affective and psychomotor (skills) domains. The basic reproductive biology included in this volume should provide the student with essential information for successful completion of an entry test to a clerkship in obstetrics and gynecology.

Obstetrics and Gynecology
THE CLINICAL CORE

I

History, Anatomy,
and Physical
Examination

The Gynecologic and Obstetric History

The patient's age is a most important factor in the evaluation of gynecologic signs and symptoms. For example, in the childbearing age the most important causes of uterine bleeding are associated with disorders of reproduction. In postmenopausal women, carcinomas of the genital tract figure prominently in differential diagnosis, whereas in adolescent girls the cause of abnormal uterine bleeding is much more likely to be endocrine.

Gravidity is synonymous with pregnancy and a gravida is a pregnant woman. A primigravida, or gravida 1, is a woman who is pregnant for the first time. A secundigravida is a woman in her second pregnancy. A multigravida is a pregnant woman who has been pregnant several times. The numeric designation of gravidity is not altered by plural gestation. For example, a patient who is pregnant for the first time with twins is gravida 1, and she becomes gravida 2 during her second pregnancy.

Parity is the state of having given birth to an infant weighing 500 g or more, alive or dead. When the weight of the infant is not known, an estimated gestational length of 20 weeks or more, calculated from the first day of the last menstrual period, may be used to establish parity. For purposes of defining parity, plural gestations are counted the same as singleton pregnancies.

A primipara is a woman who has given birth for the first time to an infant or infants, alive or dead, weighing 500 g or more. A primigravida is often incorrectly designated a primipara. A multipara is a woman who has given birth two or more times to an infant or infants weighing 500 g or more, alive or dead. The designation "grand" multipara is often applied to a woman who has given birth seven or more times to an infant or infants weighing 500 g or more.

There are two common methods of summarizing the obstetric history. The first identifies only gravidity, parity, and the number of abortions. For example, a woman who has had two term pregnancies, one of which was a twin pregnancy, and one abortion, and is now pregnant would be gravida 4, para 2, ab 1. Abortions should be recorded as spontaneous or induced (medically indicated or elective). The second uses four digits to indicate, respectively, the number of term pregnancies, premature deliveries, abortions, and living children. The history of the gravida 4, para 2, ab 1 just described would be abbreviated in the four-digit system as 2-0-1-3. A woman whose only pregnancy terminated in premature quintuplets, all of whom survived, would be designated gravida 1, para 1, ab 0 according to the first system, and 0-1-0-5 according to the second.

A parturient is a woman in the process of giving birth. A puerpera is a woman who has given birth during the preceding 42 days.

The chief complaint is the basic reason that the patient is seeking medical attention. In arriving at a diagnosis, it is often profitable to use the patient's own words in describing her chief complaint. Clinical acumen and experience are often required to discern the real reason behind the alleged chief complaint. For example, sexual incompatibility may often present as vulvar pruritus, or a fear of cancer may be expressed as concern over a trivial vaginal discharge.

The present illness should be described in detail. Listening to the patient carefully without undue direction of the questioning will usually provide most of the pertinent diagnostic information. In obtaining a gynecologic history, details of the following signs and symptoms should be elicited: changes or abnormalities in uterine bleeding; pain in the lower abdomen, flank, vagina, or external genitalia; a lesion on the external genitalia or a palpable mass in the pelvis; a change in the quality or quantity of vaginal discharge; changes in gastrointestinal or urinary habits; protrusion of the vaginal wall; and infertility.

When the major complaint involves a change or abnormality in uterine bleeding, a detailed menstrual history should be obtained at this point. When the chief complaint and present illness are not related primarily to vaginal bleeding, an abbreviated menstrual history should be recorded after the present illness.

The menstrual history should include the age of onset of menstrual periods (menarche), the interval between the periods, the duration of flow, the amount of flow as measured by the number of pads or tampons used, the date of the last normal menstrual period (LNMP), and the date of the preceding menstrual period (PMP). A formula for recording menarche, interval between periods in days, and duration of flow in days is exemplified by $14 \times 28 \times 4$, which indicates that menarche occurred at age 14, the first day of the period follows the first day of the preceding period by 28 days, and the duration of flow is 4 days. Dysmenorrhea (painful periods) and signs and symptoms of premenstrual tension should be recorded as part of the menstrual history.

Primary dysmenorrhea (essential, or functional, dysmenorrhea) is menstrual pain in the absence of a recognized pelvic lesion (p. 338). Secondary dysmenorrhea is menstrual pain caused by demonstrable pelvic disease.

Premenstrual tension is a condition characterized by increased nervousness, irritability, emotional instability, depression, frequent headaches, and edema. The syndrome may include painful swelling of the breasts, abdominal bloating, nausea, vomiting, fatigue, and a variety of other complaints. Premenstrual tension occurs during the 7 to 10 days preceding menstruation and usually disappears a few hours after the onset of menstrual flow (p. 339).

In older women, the date of the last menstrual period (menopause) and a history of associated symptoms such as hot flashes and sweating should be elicited. The menopause strictly refers to the cessation of menstrual function, whereas the climacteric is the period of a woman's life characterized by cessation of menses as well as vasomotor changes and a variety of endocrine, somatic, and psychic readjustments (p. 331).

In an adult woman the relation of changes in uterine bleeding to use of exogenous hormones including oral contraceptives and postmenopausal replacement should be clarified. Changes in menstrual patterns should be distinguished from uterine bleeding unrelated to the menses.

Menorrhagia is excessive (hypermenorrhea) or prolonged menstrual bleeding, whereas metrorrhagia is irregular acyclic uterine bleeding. Menometrorrhagia is irregular or excessive uterine bleeding during menstruation as well as between menstrual periods. Menometrorrhagia may be a sign of a variety of diseases and is not a diagnostic entity.

Hypomenorrhea is a diminution in the amount of flow or a shortening of the duration of menstruation. Oligomenorrhea is a reduction of the frequency of menstruation, in which the interval between the cycles is longer than 38 days but less than three months. The opposite of oligomenorrhea is polymenorrhea, which is abnormally frequent menstruation.

Abnormalities of bleeding confined to the menses are often of endocrine origin, whereas intermenstrual bleeding suggests other lesions including benign and malignant neoplasms. Bleeding after contact (intercourse or douching) should always suggest a malignant lesion, most often cervical cancer.

Pain should be described in terms of location, onset, and character. The history should note whether the pain is diffuse or localized, sharp or dull, constant or intermittent, mild or severe; whether it is abdominal, pelvic, vaginal, or lumbar; and whether it radiates to the thighs or is referred to the shoulder. Pain referred to the low back or buttocks is often associated with diseases of the cervix, urethra, or lower portions of the bladder and rectum. Pain localized to the lower abdomen may arise from the uterus or vagina. Adnexal pain is usually referred to the lower abdominal quadrants and often radiates down the medial aspect of the thigh. Dysmenorrhea and dyspareunia should be recorded at this point. The pain should be described as acute or chronic and its onset as sudden or gradual. If a precipitating event is ascertained, it should be recorded along with associated signs and symptoms of urinary tract or gastrointestinal disease, such as nausea, vomiting, dysuria, chills, and fever. The sequence of events preceding and following the onset of pain should be meticulously described and recorded chronologically. Any factors that ameliorate or aggravate the discomfort should be noted.

In the description of vaginal discharge, the relation to menses and coitus and the response to therapy should be noted. It must be recognized that vaginal discharge may stem from a primary lesion of the vulva, cervix, or corpus.

In obtaining a history of urinary incontinence it is necessary to differentiate stress incontinence (loss of urine upon increase in intraabdominal pressure, as in straining and coughing) from frequency and urgency with dribbling unrelated to stress and from total incontinence, which is a more or less constant loss of urine. In eliciting a history of fecal incontinence, the physician should document obstetric injuries and gynecologic procedures of possible etiologic importance.

Various complaints referable to pelvic relaxation are common in parous women. The history is of paramount importance in these patients because treatment is based more on symptoms than on purely anatomic defects.

Tables 1 through 3 are useful guides to recording the obstetric and gynecologic history and physical examination in institutions that employ this conventional method of obtaining these data. In institutions that use the problem-oriented record, the same information must be elicited but is generally recorded in the following four categories: objective data, subjective data, assessment, and plan.

Table 1. Gynecologic and Obstetric History

```
    I. Age, Parity, and Last Normal Menstrual Period
   II. Chief Complaint
  III. Present Illness
       A. Bleeding
          1. Change in interval, duration, and amount of menstrual
             bleeding
          2. Intermenstrual bleeding
          3. Contact bleeding
          4. Postmenopausal bleeding
          5. Relation to exogenous steroids
       B. Pain
          1. Location
          2. Relation to menses
```

Table 1. Continued

       3. Radiation
       4. Character
  C. Mass
       1. Location
       2. Time of onset
       3. Rate of growth
       4. Pain, discomfort, pruritus, discharge, or bleeding
       5. Relation to menses
  D. Vaginal discharge
       1. Color, odor, and consistency
       2. Onset, duration, and quantity
       3. Pain or pruritus
  E. Urinary and gastrointestinal symptoms
       1. Frequency, urgency, dysuria, urinary incontinence, and hematuria
       2. Diarrhea, constipation, tenesmus, fecal incontinence, and rectal bleeding
  F. Protrusion through the vagina
       1. Sensation of mass falling out
       2. Difficulty in emptying bowel
       3. Stress incontinence of urine
       4. Relaxed vaginal outlet
  G. Infertility
       1. Female factors (endometrial biopsy, hysterosalpingography)
       2. Male factors (semen analysis)
       3. Reproductive incompatibility (refer to specialist)
IV. Menstrual History
  A. Age of menarche
  B. Character of early cycles
  C. Interval between normal periods
  D. Amount and duration of normal periods
  E. Associated signs and symptoms
  F. Last normal menstrual period and previous normal menstrual period
  G. Premenstrual tension
  H. Abnormalities of uterine bleeding
  I. Hypomenorrhea or amenorrhea
  J. Relation to oral contraceptives
  K. Menopause
       1. Date of last menses
       2. Climacteric symptoms
V. Obstetric History
  A. Dates of deliveries
  B. Lengths of gestations
  C. Complications during pregnancy (bleeding, headache, edema)

Table 1. Continued

    D. Durations of labors
    E. Methods of deliveries (spontaneous, forceps, cesarean section)
    F. Weight, sex, and condition of infant at delivery
    G. Number and health of children now alive
    H. Postpartum complications
    I. Abortions
       1. Spontaneous
       2. Medically indicated
       3. Elective
  VI. Contraceptive History
    A. Type of contraceptive used
    B. Duration of use
    C. Reason for choice
    D. Satisfaction with method
    E. Effectiveness of method
    F. Undesirable side effects
  VII. Sexual History
    A. Regularity and type of sexual activity
    B. Libido, satisfaction, and orgasm
    C. Dyspareunia, frigidity, and other sexual problems such as premature ejaculation
  VIII. Medical History
    A. Diabetes
    B. Hypertension
    C. Cardiac disease
    D. Renal disease
    E. Syphilis
    F. Tuberculosis
    G. Epilepsy
    H. Exposure to rubella
    I. Allergies
    J. Present medications
  IX. Surgical History
    A. Dates of operations
    B. Surgeons and hospitals where performed
    C. Diagnoses
    D. Results
  X. Family History
    A. Twinning
    B. Hereditary diseases
  XI. Social History
    A. Tobacco
    B. Alcohol
    C. Drugs
    D. Occupation
    E. Hobbies and recreational activities

The Medical Record

Excellent medical records are invaluable in medicolegal defense. According to the Department of Professional Liability of the American College of Obstetricians and Gynecologists, good medical records must be accurate, objective, timely, comprehensive, legible, and unaltered. In addition, effective communication with the patient will serve to decrease the likelihood of legal action in the event of an unsuccessful outcome of treatment. Such communication involves: establishment of a healthy rapport with the patient and family; display of respect for the patient as a person; projection of the image of an ally; accurate reporting of the symptoms and history; disclosure of all relevant facts; explanation of any alternatives and reservations; assurance that the patient and family comprehend; answers to all questions; acquisition of valid consent; and provision of adequate follow-up.

Anatomy of the Female Pelvis and Perineum

The abdominopelvic cavity is a space enclosed by the bones, muscles, and fasciae of the abdominal and pelvic walls, from the diaphragm superiorly to the pelvic diaphragm inferiorly. The perineum is the outlet of the pelvis, specifically those structures inferior to the pelvic diaphragm. Knowledge of the bones, ligaments, and muscles that provide the boundaries and landmarks for this region is prerequisite to understanding the structures located in these areas.

The bony pelvis is composed of the right and left hip bones, sacrum, and coccyx (Fig. I-1). Each hip bone (os coxae) is composed of a pubis, ischium, and ilium. The two pubic bones are joined anteroinferiorly at the symphysis pubis. The two ischiopubic rami extend posterolaterally from the symphysis to the ischial tuberosities. The ischial spine is located superior to the ischial tuberosity; the concavity between these two structures is the lesser sciatic notch (Fig. I-2). The greater sciatic notch is directly superior to the ischial spine and is formed principally by the ilium. The greater and lesser sciatic notches are converted to foramina by the sacrospinous and sacrotuberous ligaments. Each ilium has an auricular facet for its articulation with the sacrum, and anterosuperior to the pelvic brim the bone forms a fan-shaped concavity called the iliac fossa. The obturator foramen is formed by the ischium and pubis. Except for a small opening anteriorly and superiorly called the obturator canal, the foramen is closed by the tough obturator membrane.

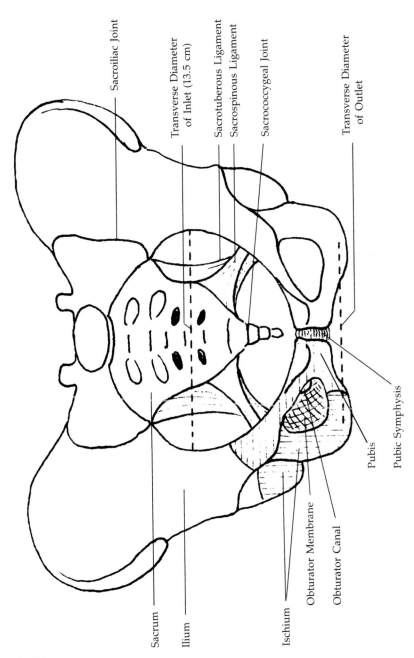

Sacroiliac Joint

Transverse Diameter of Inlet (13.5 cm)

Sacrotuberous Ligament

Sacrospinous Ligament

Sacrococcygeal Joint

Transverse Diameter of Outlet

Pubic Symphysis

Pubis

Obturator Membrane

Obturator Canal

Ischium

Sacrum

Ilium

FIG. I-1.

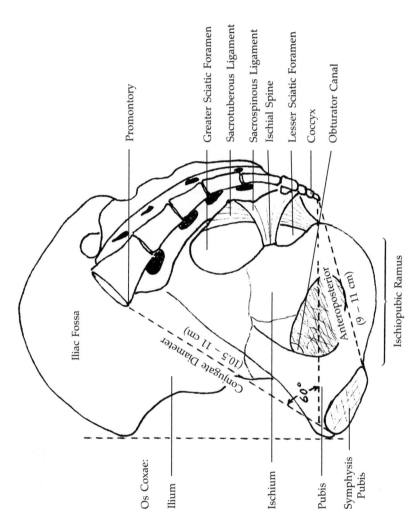

Fɪɢ. I-2.

The sacrum, composed of five fused vertebrae, has a concave pelvic, or anterior, surface. It is roughly triangular in shape. The base, formed by the body of the first sacral vertebra, has right and left alae that extend laterally to articulate with the ilia at the sacroiliac joints. The anterior border of the base is the promontory of the sacrum. There are four pairs of sacral foramina for the passage of spinal nerves from the vertebral canal.

The coccyx also is triangular in shape and is composed of 3 to 5 pieces. The first piece has prominent transverse processes that are joined to the sacrum by ligaments.

The pelvic brim is the boundary between the major and minor pelvis. From anteroinferior to posterosuperior the brim is composed of the symphysis pubis, the pubic crest, the iliopectineal line (the arcuate is the ilial part of this line), the anterior border of the ala, and the promontory (Fig. I-3). The major pelvis is superior to the pelvic brim and is formed by the iliac fossae and alae of the sacrum. The minor pelvis is inferior to the pelvic brim and is bound

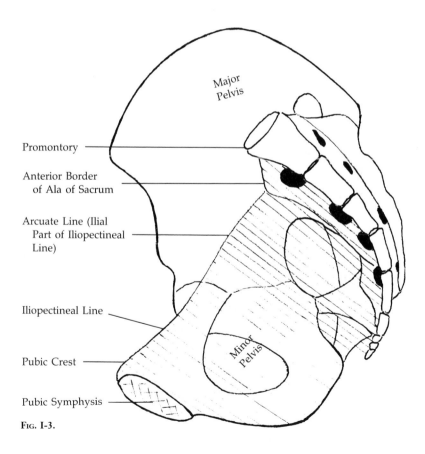

Fig. I-3.

by the inner surfaces of the sacrum, coccyx, ischium, pubis, and part of the ilium. In the minor pelvis are found the greater and lesser sciatic foramina, the obturator foramen with its obturator membrane, and the anterior sacral foramina.

In a living subject who is standing, the anterior superior iliac spines and the anterosuperior part of the symphysis pubis are in a vertical plane. The anterosuperior part of the symphysis pubis and the tip of the coccyx are in a horizontal plane.

There are four important articulations: the lumbosacral and sacrococcygeal, the sacroiliac joints, and the symphysis pubis. The lumbosacral joint has a thick intervertebral disc and a strong iliolumbar ligament extending from the transverse processes of L-5 to the iliac crest. The ligaments prevent axial rotation and keep L-5 from sliding anteriorly on the sacrum. The sacrococcygeal joint allows the coccyx to move posteriorly during defecation and parturition. The sacroiliac joints are large and involve the medial surface of the ilium posterior to the iliac fossa and the auricular facet of the sacrum. The joint is strengthened by the interosseous sacroiliac, dorsal sacral, and iliolumbar ligaments, which, along with the sacrotuberous and sacrospinous ligaments, resist anterior rotation of the sacrum when the weight of the body is imposed on the lumbosacral joint. The two hip bones are united anteriorly by fibrocartilage at the symphysis pubis.

In the female pelvis, as compared with the male, the bones are lighter, the joints smaller, the sacrum wider and shorter, the ischial tuberosities everted rather than inverted, the angle of the greater sciatic notch larger, the coccyx more posteriorly directed, the angle of the pubic arch greater (90° or more rather than about 60° for the male), and the pelvic diameters greater. The principal diameters of the inlet (pelvic brim) are the anteroposterior or conjugate between the superior end of the symphysis pubis and the promontory of the sacrum (10.5-11 cm) and the transverse, which is the greatest width across the inlet (13.5 cm). These diameters are about 0.5 cm greater in the female than in the male. The principal diameters of the outlet are the anteroposterior, from the inferior edge of the symphysis pubis to the tip of the coccyx (9-11 cm), and the transverse, between the two ischial tuberosities (11 cm). The diameters of the outlet are about 2.5 cm greater in the female than the male. There is an angle of about 60° between the conjugate line of the inlet and the horizontal plane, and one of about 15° between the anteroposterior line of the outlet and the horizontal plane in the female.

The abdominopelvic cavity is separated from the perineum by the pelvic diaphragm, which stretches across the pelvis like a hammock (Figs. I-4 and I-5). The pelvic diaphragm is formed by the

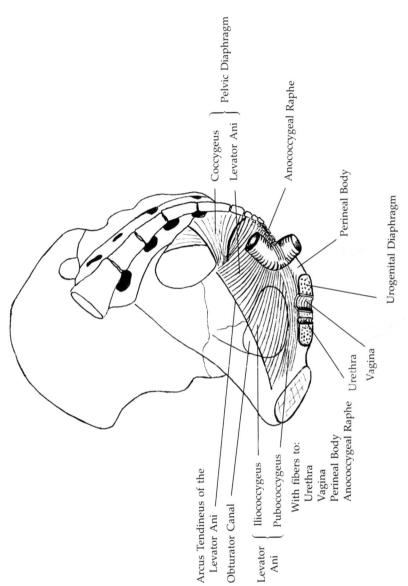

FIG. I-4.

levator ani and coccygeus from each half of the pelvis, which join in a continuous line posteriorly from the junction of the rectum and anal canal to the coccyx. Anteriorly the two sheets of muscle are separated by a space sometimes called the genital hiatus. The human coccygeus is unimportant, comprising merely a few strands of muscle coating the internal surface of the sacrospinous ligament. The levator ani, however, is very important and essential for the functional integrity of both the pelvis and perineum.

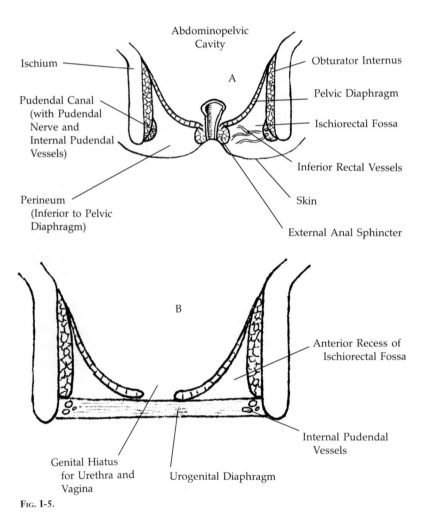

FIG. I-5.

The anterolateral walls of the minor pelvis are almost entirely covered by the obturator internus muscles, which originate from the obturator membrane and the pelvic surfaces of the pubis, ischium, and even part of the ilium (Fig. I-6). Its fibers converge on the lesser sciatic notch before making a right-angle turn to pass out of the pelvis into the gluteal region. The internal surface of this muscle is coated with the thick obturator fascia.

Each levator ani comprises a pubococcygeus and an iliococcygeus. The pubococcygeus originates from the posterior surface of the pubis along an oblique line extending from the lower border of the symphysis pubis to the obturator canal. Functionally it is two muscles, a medial part called the puborectalis and a lateral part called the pubococcygeus proper. The fibers of the puborectalis extend posteriorly; some insert into the side of the vagina (pubovaginalis), and others into the perineal body and the external anal sphincter; the remainder meet with their fellows from the opposite side posterior to the junction of the rectum and anal canal to form a rectal sling. This sling is responsible for the 90° angle between the ampulla of the rectum and the anal canal. Its integrity is important for both voluntary and involuntary control of the bowel. Fibers of the pubococcygeus interdigitate with those from the opposite side in a raphe extending from the junction of the rectum and anal canal to the coccyx.

The iliococcygeus is the second major component of the levator ani. It originates from a thickening of the obturator fascia that extends between the ischial spine posteriorly and the pubis, just anterior to the obturator canal. This thickened line is called the arcus tendineus, or tendinous arch of the levator ani. Fibers originating from the arch sweep posteriorly and medially to insert with those of the pubococcygeus in the anococcygeal raphe and coccyx. Some of the fibers of the iliococcygeus join the longitudinal coat of muscle around the anal canal. Although the pelvic diaphragm usually functions without conscious control, it is composed of striated muscle and is a voluntary muscle innervated by the anterior branches of the ventral rami of S-3 and S-4. Its principal function is to support the pelvic viscera and maintain the 90° angle at the junction between the rectum and anal canal.

The perineum is the outlet of the pelvis; it includes all structures inferior to the pelvic diaphragm. On the surface it is the floor of the groove between the thighs and buttocks and therefore includes the external genitalia and anus. When the thighs are spread and the skin removed, this surface becomes a diamond-shaped area bounded anteriorly by the symphysis pubis and arcuate pubic ligament, anterolaterally by the ischiopubic rami, laterally by the ischial tuberosities, posterolaterally by the sacrotuberous ligaments, and posteriorly by the tip of the coccyx (Fig. I-7). The perineum is a three-dimensional space bounded superomedially by the pelvic diaphragm, laterally by the obturator fascia, and inferiorly by the skin covering the diamond-shaped area previously described.

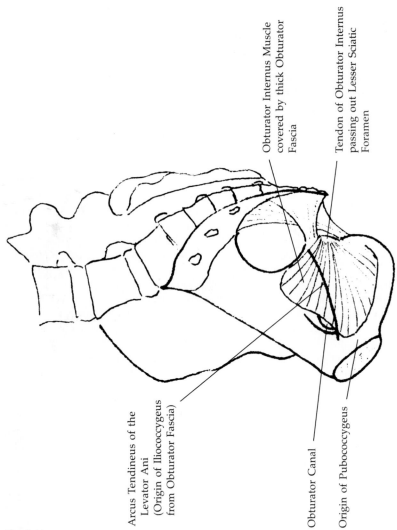

Obturator Internus Muscle
covered by thick Obturator
Fascia

Tendon of Obturator Internus
passing out Lesser Sciatic
Foramen

Arcus Tendineus of the
Levator Ani
(Origin of Iliococcygeus
from Obturator Fascia)

Obturator Canal

Origin of Pubococcygeus

Fig. I-6A.

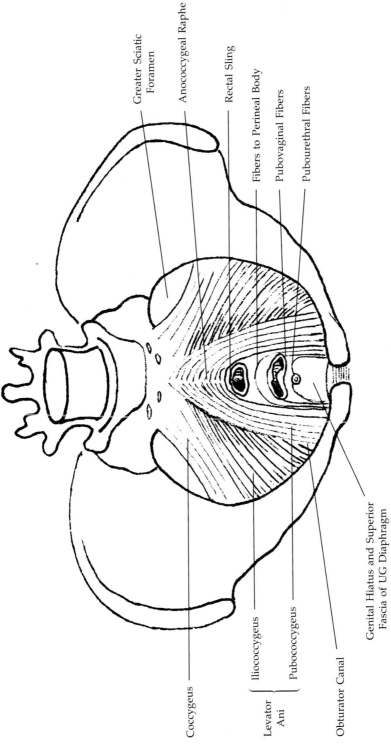

FIG. I-6B.

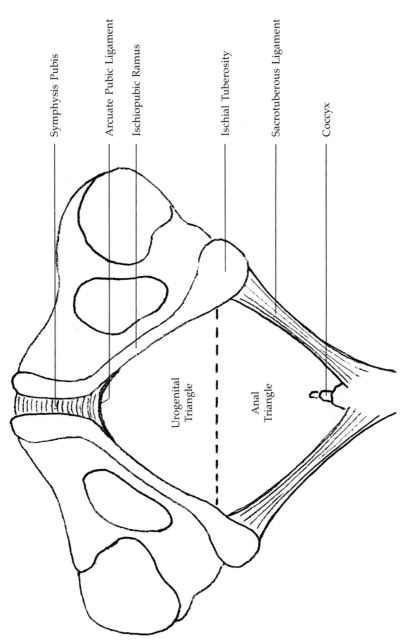

Symphysis Pubis

Arcuate Pubic Ligament

Ischiopubic Ramus

Ischial Tuberosity

Sacrotuberous Ligament

Coccyx

Urogenital Triangle

Anal Triangle

FIG. I-7.

The diamond-shaped perineum is divided into an anterior urogenital triangle and a posterior anal triangle by an arbitrary line drawn between the ischial tuberosities. The urogenital diaphragm is a thin sheet of muscle stretching between the two ischiopubic rami, covered on its superior and inferior surfaces with fascia. By definition, it is in the perineum, because it is just inferior to the pelvic diaphragm; it also is in the urogenital triangle, that is, anterior to the line between the ischial tuberosities. The anal triangle comprises the anus, external anal sphincter, ischiorectal fossae, and the vessels and nerves supplying them (Fig. I-8). These structures also are in the perineum, because they are inferior to the pelvic diaphragm.

There are three parts to the external anal sphincter: subcutaneous, superficial, and deep. The subcutaneous part, formed by a few circular fibers, causes the wrinkled appearance of the anal verge. The superficial part is fusiform, extending from the tip of the coccyx and anococcygeal raphe to the perineal body, which is a large mass of connective tissue interposed between the anus and anal canal posteriorly and the urogenital diaphragm and inferior part of the vagina anteriorly. The superficial part of the external anal sphincter is infiltrated by longitudinal fibers of the anal canal. The deep part of the sphincter comprises a thick, circular mass of fibers that mingle superiorly with the puborectalis portion of the levator ani. Anteriorly some of these fibers interdigitate with the superficial transverse perineus muscle. Like the pelvic diaphragm, the anal sphincter consists of voluntary muscle but functions without conscious control. The rectum and anal canal are coated by two layers of smooth muscle, an inner circular and an outer longitudinal. The circular layer is particularly thick at the end of the anal canal, where it forms the internal anal sphincter.

The ischiorectal fossae are fat-filled, wedge-shaped spaces located on either side of the anal canal and sphincter. The boundaries of the fossae are: anteriorly, the base of the urogenital diaphragm; laterally, the fascia covering the obturator internus muscle; mediosuperiorly, the levator ani of the pelvic diaphragm; inferiorly, the skin; and posteriorly, the sacrotuberous ligament.

Inferior rectal nerves and vessels course medially across each ischiorectal fossa from the pudendal canal in the lateral wall to the anal sphincter. They are branches of the pudendal nerve and internal pudendal vessels, which originate in the pelvis. To gain access to the perineum, they pass out of the pelvis into the gluteal area via the greater sciatic foramen, course around the ischial spine and sacrospinous ligament, and enter the perineum through the lesser sciatic foramen (Fig. I-9). From the lesser sciatic foramen posteriorly to the posterolateral corners of the urogenital diaphragm, the pudendal vessels and nerves lie in a canal formed by a split in the obturator fascia. The inferior rectal nerves and vessels are branches that pass through the wall of the pudendal canal to supply the fat of the ischiorectal fossa as well as the terminal part of the digestive tube

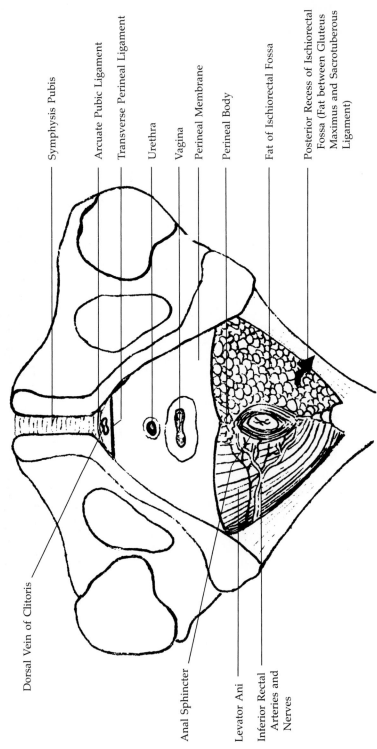

Symphysis Pubis

Arcuate Pubic Ligament

Transverse Perineal Ligament

Urethra

Vagina

Perineal Membrane

Perineal Body

Fat of Ischiorectal Fossa

Posterior Recess of Ischiorectal Fossa (Fat between Gluteus Maximus and Sacrotuberous Ligament)

Dorsal Vein of Clitoris

Anal Sphincter

Levator Ani

Inferior Rectal Arteries and Nerves

Fig. I-8.

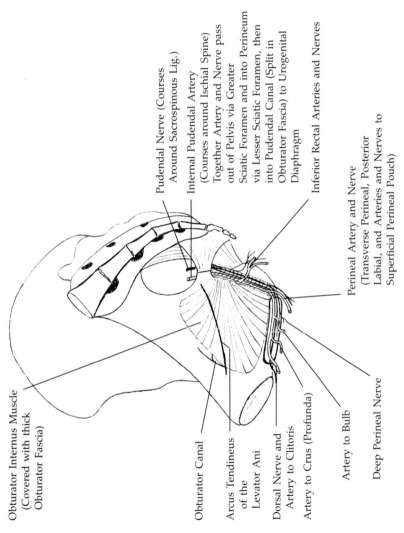

Obturator Internus Muscle
(Covered with thick
Obturator Fascia)

Obturator Canal

Arcus Tendineus
of the
Levator Ani

Dorsal Nerve and
Artery to Clitoris

Artery to Crus (Profunda)

Artery to Bulb

Deep Perineal Nerve

Pudendal Nerve (Courses
Around Sacrospinous Lig.)

Internal Pudendal Artery
(Courses around Ischial Spine)
Together Artery and Nerve pass
out of Pelvis via Greater
Sciatic Foramen and into Perineum
via Lesser Sciatic Foramen, then
into Pudendal Canal (Split in
Obturator Fascia) to Urogenital
Diaphragm

Inferior Rectal Arteries and Nerves

Perineal Artery and Nerve
(Transverse Perineal, Posterior
Labial, and Arteries and Nerves to
Superficial Perineal Pouch)

Fig. I-9.

with its sphincter. Because the pudendal canal follows a precise course, it is fairly easy to effect a perineal block by injecting an anesthetic agent into the area.

The external genital organs of the female (pudendum, or vulva) are located principally in the urogenital triangle but extend on to the lower abdominal wall (Fig. I-10). The mons pubis is a fatty fibrous pad of connective tissue anterior to the pubis; its skin is covered with hair after puberty. The labia majora begin at the mons, where their medial margins are united by a low ridge of skin, the anterior commissure. They diminish in size posteriorly and are joined again by a low ridge of skin anterior to the anus, the posterior commissure. The labia majora are sparsely covered with hair laterally, but their medial surfaces are smooth and moist. The pudendal cleft is the space separating the labia majora. The clitoris is the homologue of the penis; much of it is hidden behind the posteroinferior part of the mons in the anterior part of the pudendal cleft. The labia minora are a pair of thin folds of skin devoid of fat. In the nullipara they usually are hidden by the labia majora. Anteriorly each labium minus divides into a medial and lateral fold. The medial folds from the two sides join to form the frenulum, which connects to the glans of the clitoris. The lateral folds join to cover the surface of the clitoris and its glans as the prepuce. Posteriorly the labia minora pass on either side of the orifice of the vagina, diminish in size, and end by joining about 1 cm posterior to the vaginal orifice in a transverse ridge called the frenulum labiorum. The vestibule is the space between the labia minora; into it open the vagina, urethra, and ducts of the greater vestibular glands. The vaginal orifice opens in the middle of the vestibule, and the urethra terminates just anterior to it, about 2.5 cm posterior to the clitoris. The ducts of the greater vestibular glands empty into the vaginal orifice posterolaterally, just distal to the hymen. The vestibular fossa is the area between the vaginal orifice and the frenulum labiorum.

The superficial fascia of the urogenital triangle, with its superficial and deep perineal pouches, is continuous with Scarpa's fascia of the abdomen. The integument over the abdominal wall may be divided into skin and tela subcutanea. The skin is composed of the epidermis and dermis; the tela comprises the panniculus adiposus and a deeper membranous layer, the stratum fibrosum. In the lower, anterior abdominal wall, the panniculus adiposus is called Camper's fascia; the particularly well developed stratum fibrosum is called Scarpa's fascia. Inferiorly Scarpa's fascia attaches to the fascia lata of the thigh in a curved line from the two anterior superior iliac spines to the pubic tubercles. From the pubic tubercles, the lines of attach-

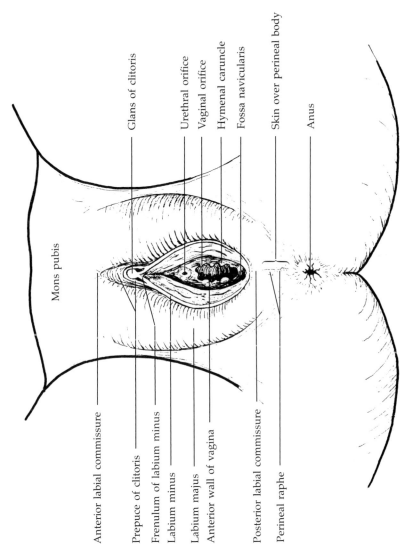

Glans of clitoris

Urethral orifice
Vaginal orifice
Hymenal caruncle
Fossa navicularis

Skin over perineal body

Anus

Mons pubis

Anterior labial commissure

Prepuce of clitoris
Frenulum of labium minus
Labium minus
Labium majus
Anterior wall of vagina

Posterior labial commissure
Perineal raphe

FIG. I-10.

ment follow the ischiopubic rami posterolaterally to the posterior border of the urogenital diaphragm, from which it doubles back anteriorly over its inferior surface as the perineal membrane. Scarpa's fascia of the abdominal wall changes its name to Colles' fascia of the perineum as it passes from the pubic tubercle to the ischiopubic ramus. Scarpa's fascia condenses in the midline over the anterior surface of the rectus sheath to form the fundiform ligament, which extends inferiorly to join the suspensory ligament of the clitoris, which arises directly from the symphysis pubis.

The perineal membrane is the superior boundary of the superficial perineal pouch. Colles' fascia limits this space inferiorly. The other boundaries are formed by the attachments of Colles' fascia laterally to the ischiopubic rami and posteriorly to the posterior border of the urogenital diaphragm (Fig. I-11). Medially the pouch is interrupted by the opening for the vagina; thus, Colles' fascia is continuous with the connective tissue that forms the core of the labia minora. Anteriorly the superficial perineal pouch (of the perineum) is continuous with the space just deep to Scarpa's fascia (of the abdominal wall). Openings between the two spaces occur on either side of the fundiform ligament through the so-called abdominolabial meatuses. These openings are bounded medially by the fundiform ligament, posteriorly by the pubic bones, laterally by the pubic tubercles, and anteriorly by the bridge of Scarpa's fascia between the pubic tubercles and fundiform ligament. The abdominolabial meatuses are filled by the digital processes of fat that extend from the superficial inguinal rings into the labia majora. Each process of fat is accompanied by minute blood vessels and the structures emerging from the inguinal canal, namely, the ilioinguinal nerve, which supplies the anterior part of the labium, and the round ligament of the uterus, which attaches to its skin.

The superficial perineal pouch is a potential space rather than a real space between the perineal membrane and the superficial perineal fascia (Colles'), because it is filled with the crura of the clitoris, the bulbs of the vestibule, the greater vestibular glands, three pairs of superficial perineal muscles, and the superficial perineal vessels and nerves. The crura are elongated, tapered columns of erectile tissue attached to the ischium and perineal membrane and are continuous anteriorly at the inferior part of the symphysis pubis with the corpora cavernosa of the clitoris. The bulbs of the vestibule are elongated, pyriform masses of erectile tissue attached to the perineal membrane on either side of the vaginal orifice. Anteriorly each bulb tapers and joins its fellow from the opposite side to form the slender anterior commissure of the bulbs. The greater vestibular glands are located posteriorly under the vestibular bulbs next to the perineal membrane. Their small ducts lead to the groove between the hymen and the labium minus. There are three pairs of superficial perineal muscles: the bulbospongiosus, the ischiocavernosus, and the superficial transverse perinei. Each bulbospongiosus attaches to the perineal body posteriorly and the perineal membrane anteriorly. Each ischiocavernosus muscle attaches to both the perineal membrane and the ischiopubic ramus. Its fibers cover the crus of the clitoris. The superficial transverse perinei muscles are very small and occasionally even absent. They originate from the

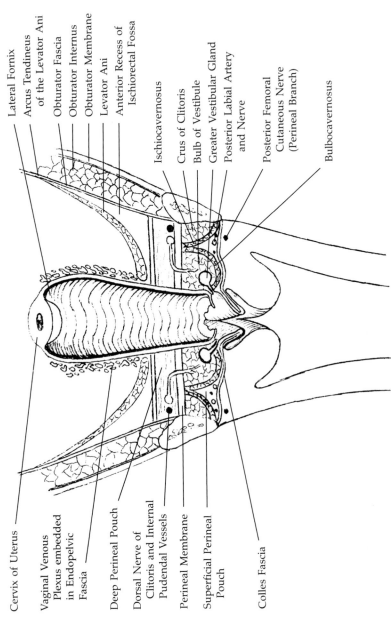

Lateral Fornix

Arcus Tendineus
of the Levator Ani

Obturator Fascia

Obturator Internus

Obturator Membrane

Levator Ani

Anterior Recess of
Ischiorectal Fossa

Ischiocavernosus

Crus of Clitoris

Bulb of Vestibule

Greater Vestibular Gland

Posterior Labial Artery
and Nerve

Posterior Femoral
Cutaneous Nerve
(Perineal Branch)

Bulbocavernosus

Cervix of Uterus

Vaginal Venous
Plexus embedded
in Endopelvic
Fascia

Deep Perineal Pouch

Dorsal Nerve of
Clitoris and Internal
Pudendal Vessels

Perineal Membrane

Superficial Perineal
Pouch

Colles Fascia

Fig. I-11.

ischial tuberosities and extend medially as narrow bands to insert in the anterior part of the perineal body and to interdigitate with the fibers of the bulbospongiosus muscle (Fig. I-12). The area is supplied by perineal branches of the internal pudendal vessels, which emerge from the anterior ends of the pudendal canals and divide into medial and lateral labial branches. Small transverse perineal arteries arise from the medial labial arteries and course toward the perineal body and posterior parts of the bulbs of the vestibule. Branches of the perineal nerves with the same names follow similar courses. The area is supplied in addition by the perineal branches of the two posterior femoral cutaneous nerves.

The deep perineal pouch is essentially the urogenital diaphragm with its fascias and the structures that pass through it. It is bounded inferiorly by the perineal membrane, which forms the superior boundary of the superficial perineal pouch, and superiorly by the fascia on the pelvic surface of the urogenital diaphragm. The contents of the deep perineal pouch include a segment of the vagina with the urethra partially embedded in its anterior wall, the sphincter urethrae and deep transverse perinei muscles, the dorsal nerves of the clitoris, the internal pudendal vessels, and the arteries to the bulb of the vagina. The sphincter urethrae is a thin layer of muscle fibers that encircle the urethra and extend between the two ischiopubic rami. The deep transverse perinei are thin bands of muscle stretching between the two ischial tuberosities; they parallel the superficial transverse perinei lying in the superficial perineal pouch (Fig. I-13). The dorsal nerves of the clitoris and the internal pudendal vessels enter the deep perineal pouch from the pudendal canals on each side. The dorsal nerves course along the sides of the ischiopubic rami, pierce the perineal membrane, and then lie on the dorsal surface of the crura and body of the clitoris all the way to its glans. The internal pudendal arteries also enter the deep perineal pouch from the pudendal canals and follow a course similar to that of the dorsal nerves of the clitoris. Each artery sends a branch, the artery to the bulb, medially to pierce the perineal membrane and enter the bulbs of the vagina on their deep surfaces. The internal pudendal arteries next send deep (profunda) branches through the perineal membrane to supply their respective crura. Finally the internal pudendal arteries themselves pierce the perineal membrane and parallel the dorsal nerves of the clitoris on the crura and body of the clitoris. These are the dorsal arteries of the clitoris.

Superior to the pelvic diaphragm are located the urinary bladder, the female internal genitalia, the rectum, and the nerves and vessels supplying both the pelvis and perineum. The urinary bladder (vesica urinaria) has four surfaces: one superior, two inferolateral, and one inferoposterior. The superior surface is roughly triangular and is located between the two ureters, which enter it posterolaterally, and the urachus, which is anterior in the midline. The sigmoid colon or ileum lies on the peritoneum covering the superior surface. The inferolateral surfaces of the bladder

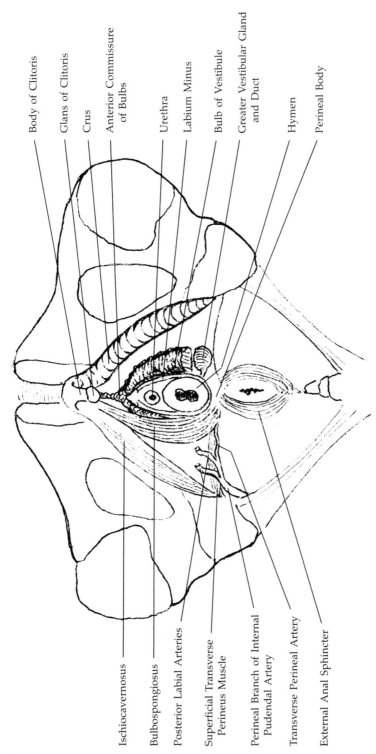

Body of Clitoris

Glans of Clitoris

Crus

Anterior Commissure of Bulbs

Urethra

Labium Minus

Bulb of Vestibule

Greater Vestibular Gland and Duct

Hymen

Perineal Body

Ischiocavernosus

Bulbospongiosus

Posterior Labial Arteries

Superficial Transverse Perineus Muscle

Perineal Branch of Internal Pudendal Artery

Transverse Perineal Artery

External Anal Sphincter

FIG. I-12.

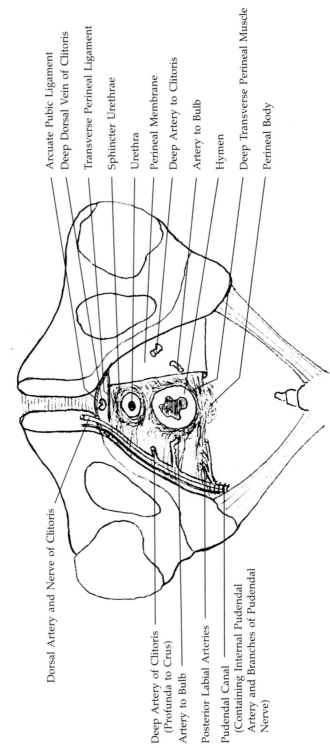

Arcuate Pubic Ligament

Deep Dorsal Vein of Clitoris

Transverse Perineal Ligament

Sphincter Urethrae

Urethra

Perineal Membrane

Deep Artery to Clitoris

Artery to Bulb

Hymen

Deep Transverse Perineal Muscle

Perineal Body

Dorsal Artery and Nerve of Clitoris

Deep Artery of Clitoris
(Profunda to Crus)

Artery to Bulb

Posterior Labial Arteries

Pudendal Canal
(Containing Internal Pudendal
Artery and Branches of Pudendal
Nerve)

FIG. I-13.

lie against the pubic bones, the obturator internus muscles, and the levator ani. The inferoposterior surface of the bladder (base) lies against the anterior wall of the vagina. The bladder is surrounded by vesical fascia, which is continuous with the extraperitoneal connective tissue. A well developed vesical plexus of veins lies in the fascia and separates the urinary bladder from the retropubic space.

Each ureter is about 25 cm long; half of it is in the abdomen and half in the pelvis (Fig. I-14). The ureter enters the pelvis at the bifurcation of the common iliac artery, descends anterior to the internal iliac artery, and crosses inferior to the uterine artery before entering the wall of the bladder. As the ureter passes inferior to the uterine artery, it frequently lies next to the lateral fornix of the vagina, but this anatomic relation may be only unilateral because the superior part of the vagina is often displaced considerably from the midline of the body.

The ureters do not go directly through the wall of the bladder; instead they angle from the point where they enter inferiorly and medially in an oblique fashion. Each ureter enters the lumen of the bladder about 2 cm posterolateral to the opening of the urethra and about 2 cm from the orifice of the other ureter. Thus a small triangle called the trigone of the bladder is formed by the openings of the three ducts. The surface of the mucosa over the trigone is relatively smooth, whereas it is wrinkled elsewhere when the bladder is empty. The interureteric fold is a prominent ridge between the openings of the two ureters.

The female urethra is only about 4 cm long. It passes from the neck of the bladder through the urogenital diaphragm to open in the vestibule just anterior to the vagina about 2.5 cm posterior to the glans of the clitoris. The distal end of the urethra is embedded in the anterior wall of the vagina. This relatively fixed relation is the reason it is occasionally injured during parturition or irritated by coitus.

The rectum is the part of the digestive tract between the sigmoid, or pelvic, colon and the anal canal. It begins where the sigmoid colon loses its mesentery, just anterior to the body of the third sacral vertebra. Although the word "rectum" means "straight," its 12-cm length follows the curvature of the sacrum and coccyx. The entire rectum may be considered a retroperitoneal structure, but peritoneum covers its proximal third on the anterior and lateral surfaces, and its middle third on the anterior surface. The distal third, where it dilates to form the ampulla, is inferior to the peritoneum. Where the peritoneum covers the anterior and lateral surfaces of the proximal part of the rectum, pararectal fossae are formed on both sides. In addition to the curvature caused by the concavity of the sacrum, the rectum has three lateral curvatures. A prominent indentation

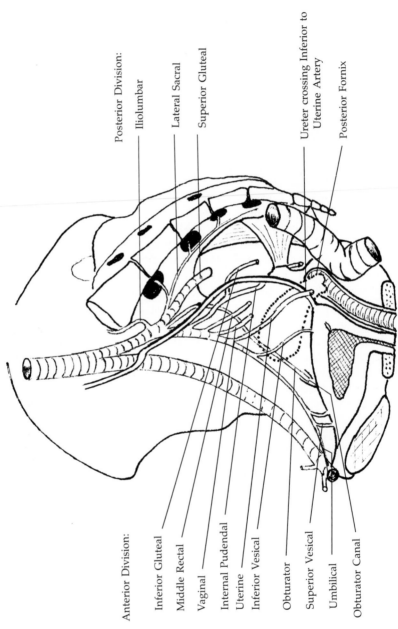

Posterior Division:
Iliolumbar
Lateral Sacral
Superior Gluteal

Ureter crossing Inferior to
Uterine Artery
Posterior Fornix

Anterior Division:
Inferior Gluteal
Middle Rectal
Vaginal
Internal Pudendal
Uterine
Inferior Vesical
Obturator
Superior Vesical
Umbilical
Obturator Canal

Fig. I-14.

of its right wall occurs at the bottom of the rectouterine pouch, and two smaller indentations of its left wall occur about 2 cm proximal and 2 cm distal to this point. These indentations produce the transverse folds (plicae transversales) or shelves that project into the lumen of the bowel. The large right plica may form a partial obstruction to the insertion of a proctoscope.

The rectum ends at its junction with the anal canal, about 4 cm anterior to the tip of the coccyx. There the digestive tube makes a 90° turn as a result of the pull of the puborectal portion of the levator ani. The anal canal is only about 2.5 to 3.5 cm long. Its superior part has 5 to 10 permanent longitudinal ridges called anal columns, which unite at their distal ends by semilunar folds, the anal valves. Together the ends of the anal columns and the anal valves form the circular, serrated pectinate line around the lumen. The pectinate line is an important landmark. Superior to it the epithelium is composed of columnar cells; its arterial supply and venous drainage are from the middle and superior rectal vessels, and the lymphatics drain to pelvic and lumbar nodes. The anal canal inferior to the pectinate line is composed of stratified squamous epithelium, is supplied by branches of the inferior rectal artery and vein (from the pudendal canals), and has a lymphatic drainage to the superficial and deep inguinal nodes. Superior to the pectinate line the bowel is fairly insensitive except to stretching, whereas inferior to the line, touch, pain, heat, and cold are perceived. The superior rectal artery and vein are continuations of the inferior mesenteric vessels. They divide into right and left branches, which descend in the submucosa of the rectum and anal canal down to the anal columns. Superior to the pectinate line they anastomose with the paired middle rectal vessels, and inferior to the line with the paired inferior rectal vessels. Dilation of the veins in the anal columns produces rectal hemorrhoids. When they remain superior to the pectinate line, they are called internal hemorrhoids. When they become large enough to project distal to the line, they are called external hemorrhoids. As the uterus enlarges during pregnancy, the venous return from the pelvis and perineum may be compromised. Anastomoses between the superior and middle rectal veins are sites where the portal and systemic circulations join. The increased venous pressure in this area during pregnancy may result in rectal hemorrhoids. Metastatic tumors superior to the pectinate line may remain undetected for a long time, because the area is moderately insensitive to pain and the lymphatic drainage is to pelvic nodes. Tumors or infections distal to the pectinate line, however, often are readily evident.

The anal canal is closed by the internal and external anal sphincters. The internal sphincter is merely a thickened portion of the circular coat of involuntary muscle surrounding the bowel. The external anal sphincter is under voluntary control.

The internal female genitalia consist of the ovaries, oviducts (uterine, or fallopian, tubes), uterus, and vagina (Fig. I-15).

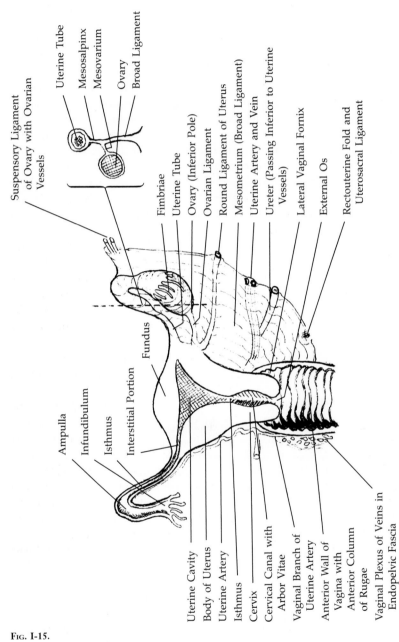

Fig. I-15.

The normal adult ovary measures 3 cm × 2 cm × 1.5 cm and weighs about 3 g. It is located on the side wall of the pelvis between the ureter and external iliac vein. The ovary is oriented so that its superior end projects toward the uterine tube and its inferior end toward the uterus. It is held by a short fold of peritoneum, the mesovarium, which is one of the parts of the broad ligament. The suspensory ligament of the ovary is continuous with the mesovarium and connects the tubal end of the gonad to the lateral pelvic wall. The suspensory ligament contains: the ovarian artery, which arises from the aorta just inferior to the renal artery; the ovarian veins, which drain into the inferior vena cava on the right side and into the left renal vein on the left; lymphatic vessels that drain to the lateral aortic and preaortic nodes (because they follow the ovarian veins superiorly); and a plexus of autonomic nerves. The ligament of the ovary extends from the uterine pole to the lateral margin of the uterus. It is about 2.5 cm long and raises a slight fold of peritoneum along the posterior surface of the broad ligament.

In the young nullipara, the ovary is smooth and pink; in elderly multiparas, it is gray and shrunken. Each ovary has a hilum, where the ovarian vessels and lymphatics enter and leave. The lateral surface of the ovary lies against the obturator internus muscle, the umbilical artery, and the obturator vessels and nerve. Its medial surface is partially covered by the lateral end of the uterine tube and by ileum or sigmoid colon.

The oviduct extends from the junction of the body and fundus of the uterus laterally, superiorly, and posteriorly towards the side wall of the pelvis. Each tube is about 11 cm long and may be divided into four parts: the infundibulum, ampulla, isthmus, and interstitial portion. The infundibulum is funnel-shaped and surrounded by fimbriae. One of them, the fimbria ovarica, is longer than the others and attaches to the ovary. The infundibulum contains the abdominal orifice of the uterine tube, which is about 2 to 3 mm in diameter. The ampulla of the uterine tube is long and irregularly dilated. It narrows to a short, straight isthmus, which connects to the uterus at the junction of its body and fundus. The intrauterine (interstitial) part of the uterine tube is about 1 cm long and extends through the myometrium to the uterine cavity. Most of the uterine tube lies in the free edge of the broad ligament, but its infundibulum emerges from it near the side of the pelvis to overlie the medial surface of the ovary. The part of the broad ligament that invests and is immediately adjacent to the uterine tube is called the mesosalpinx. In the male, the peritoneal cavity is a closed sac, but in the female it is open to the outer world via the vagina, uterus, and uterine tubes.

Several embryologic remnants are commonly encountered in the female genital tract. The epoophoron consists of a few minute tubules located in the mesovarium. These tubules course to the duct of the epoophoron, which lies horizontally in the broad ligament. The epoophoron and its duct are embryonic remnants of the mesonephric tubules and duct, respectively. The paroophoron consists of minute tubules lying in the broad ligament adjacent to the uterus. It is a remnant of the mesonephros. Vesicular appendices (hydatids) are small pedunculated cysts found in the broad ligament inferior to the infundibulum of the uterine tube. They form from the upper end of the mesonephric duct.

The uterus is a pear-shaped organ containing a flattened cavity; it lies between the rectum and bladder. It is about 8 cm long, 5 cm at its widest part, and 2.5 cm thick. Its walls are made of smooth muscle. The uterus often deviates from the midline, usually to the right. Its anterior, or vesical, surface is flattened against the bladder, and its posterior, or intestinal, surface is convex. The isthmus of each uterine tube enters the uterus at its widest part, the junction of the body and fundus. Peritoneum covers the fundus and part of the body and continues laterally as the broad ligament, which drapes over the outstretched uterine tubes. The utero-ovarian ligament attaches the ovary to the uterus just inferior to its junction with the uterine tube. The round ligament of the uterus begins anterior to the isthmic portion of the oviduct and extends laterally to the side wall of the pelvis, over the external iliac vessels to the deep inguinal ring, just lateral to the origin of the inferior epigastric artery. From there the ligament continues through the inguinal canal and the abdominolabial meatus to attach to the skin of the labium majus. Just as the utero-ovarian ligament (proper ligament of the ovary) raises a ridge of peritoneum on the posterior surface of the broad ligament, the round ligament raises a similar ridge on its anterior surface.

The cervix of the uterus is about 3 cm long and roughly cylindrical. It projects at a right angle into the vagina near its superior end. The cervical canal extends from the external os about 3 cm to the internal os. It is spindle-shaped, with anterior and posterior ridges, each with lateral branches. These two configurations are called plicae palmatae because of their resemblance to the branches of a palm tree. The cervical canal joins the triangular-shaped cavity of the uterus at the internal os. This triangle is formed by the openings of the two uterine tubes and the internal os of the cervical canal. The anterior and posterior walls of the uterus are apposed to each other. The cavity is lined with endometrium, which is surrounded by the thick, muscular myometrium. The uterus is frequently anteflexed and anteverted. Its body is slightly flexed where the flattened anterior surface lies against the bladder. The uterus lies at right angles to both the vagina and pelvic brim and therefore is anteverted when the bladder is empty. Retroversion occurs naturally when the bladder is full.

The parametrium is the fibroadipose tissue along the sides of the uterus; it supports the vessels and nerves supplying the organ. Because the end of the cervix projects into the vagina, the uterus is said to have intravaginal and supravaginal parts. The uterus is supplied by the uterine and ovarian arteries. The uterine artery, a branch of the internal iliac (hypogastric), courses medially in the cardinal ligament and divides into superior and inferior branches at the junction of the body and cervix. The uterus is innervated by branches of the sympathetic plexus around the arteries that supply it. These nerves arise from ganglia of the sympathetic chain located adjacent to vertebrae T10-L1 and S2-S4. Lymphatic vessels from the cervix travel to nodes alongside the rectum, on the pelvic surface of the sacrum, and associated with the iliac artery. Lymphatic vessels from the corpus of the uterus follow the ovarian vessels to nodes associated with the inferior vena cava and aorta, drain to nodes adjacent to the external iliac artery, and course along the round ligaments of the uterus through the inguinal canal, to the labia majora, and ultimately to the superficial inguinal nodes.

The vagina is a fibromuscular sheath located in the interior part of the pelvis and in the perineum. It extends from the external vaginal orifice in the vestibule through the urogenital diaphragm into the cavity of the pelvis. Its anterior wall is about 7.5 cm long and may be divided into three parts: an inferior third in contact with the urethra, a middle third in contact with the bladder, and a superior third that connects to the anterior part of the cervix. The posterior wall of the vagina is about 9 cm long and may be divided into three parts: the inferior segment contacts the perineal body, which separates it from the anal canal; the middle part is separated from the ampulla of the rectum by a heavy layer of connective tissue known as the rectovaginal septum; and the superior part connects to the posterior wall of the cervix and is covered by peritoneum of the rectouterine pouch (Fig. I-16). The attachment of the vagina to the anterior, lateral, and posterior walls of the cervix produces a continuous gutter around the cervix. The anterior part of this gutter is shallow and is called the anterior fornix. The posterior fornix is much deeper, and the lateral fornices are intermediate in depth.

The sides of the vagina are supported by endopelvic fascia; fibers from the puborectalis part of the levator ani insert into its side walls. These muscular fibers can act as a constrictor of the

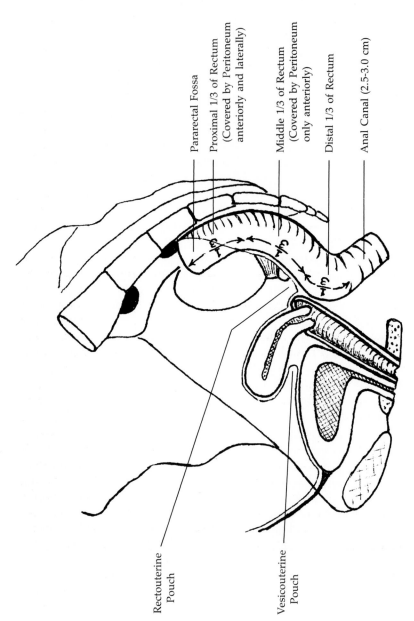

Pararectal Fossa

Proximal 1/3 of Rectum
(Covered by Peritoneum
anteriorly and laterally)

Middle 1/3 of Rectum
(Covered by Peritoneum
only anteriorly)

Distal 1/3 of Rectum

Anal Canal (2.5-3.0 cm)

Rectouterine
Pouch

Vesicouterine
Pouch

FIG. I-16.

vagina. More inferiorly the vagina passes through the urogenital diaphragm, where it receives some additional support. Finally, the bulbs of the vestibule and the bulbospongiosus muscle help to stabilize its distal portion. The anterior and posterior walls are in contact from a point just inferior to the cervix to the urogenital diaphragm and project into the lumen so that its cross section inferiorly resembles the letter "H." These projections into the lumen are known as anterior and posterior rugal columns; a series of raised ridges, or rugae, project from them laterally. The bulbs of the vestibule and their muscular covering tend to orient the introitus in an anterior-posterior direction. The hymen is a fold of mucous membrane inferior to the urogenital diaphragm at the introitus. After parturition, its remnants are called the carunculae hymenales (myrtiformes). The vagina is supplied by branches of the uterine, vaginal, middle rectal, and internal pudendal arteries and is surrounded by a very extensive venous plexus, which drains into veins of the same names. The vagina receives both sympathetic and parasympathetic nerves from the inferior hypogastric plexus as well as direct branches from the pelvic splanchnic nerves. Stimulation of the parasympathetic nerves produces an engorgement of the extensive perivaginal vascular plexus with subsequent production of vaginal lubricant, which is a serum-like transudate that passes from the vascular plexus through the vaginal wall. The vagina is devoid of glands, and neither those of the cervix nor those of the corpus have anything to do with production of this lubricant. The greater vestibular glands do not contribute to the normal vaginal lubrication.

Support of the pelvic viscera is accomplished by both muscles and connective tissue. The levator ani is particularly important. Its puborectal fibers pull the rectum anteriorly in such a manner that it provides considerable support for the vagina posteriorly. The urinary bladder lies against the vagina posteriorly and the pubic symphysis and levator ani anteriorly and inferiorly. The levator ani inserts into the sides of the vagina and the perineal body, and the urogenital diaphragm provides a floor anteriorly. The connective tissue of the pelvis is arranged loosely around the bladder (vesical fascia) and rectum (rectal fascia) and allows for their easy expansion, but the vesical and vaginal fascias are more closely attached, particularly inferiorly, where they form a vesicovaginal septum. The endopelvic fascia is further organized into pairs of suspensory "ligaments": the pubovesical, the lateral cervical, and the uterosacral ligaments. The pubovesical ligaments extend from the posterior part of the pubis just lateral to the symphysis to the neck of the bladder. The lateral cervical (transverse cervical, or cardinal) ligaments are condensations of endopelvic connective tissue around the uterine, vaginal, and vesical vessels and course from the sides of the pelvis to the junction of the cervix and vagina. Other parts of the ligament connect to the side of the bladder anteriorly and to the side of the rectum posteriorly. The uterosacral ligament is continuous with the lateral cervical ligament and projects from the junction of the body and cervix of the uterus to the middle of the sacrum. Thus, it lies in the rectouterine fold of peritoneum, which forms a boundary for the pararectal fossae. The round ligaments of the uterus provide little support for the uterus. They project anteriorly and laterally across the external iliac vessels to the deep inguinal ring, where they course through the inguinal canals to the labia majora.

The pelvic viscera are supplied by one paired and two unpaired arteries. The unpaired vessels are the median sacral and superior rectal arteries; the paired vessels are the internal iliacs. The median sacral artery is a very small vessel that arises at the level of L-4 from the dorsal wall of the aorta, crosses the body of L-5, and continues in the midline inferiorly on the pelvic surface of the sacrum. The superior rectal artery is a continuation of the inferior mesenteric as it crosses the pelvic brim. The vessel divides into right and left branches to supply the rectum and anastomose distally with the middle rectal arteries. The aorta branches into the two common iliac arteries at L-4, and they in turn divide into the internal and external iliac arteries. This division takes place about one third of the way along a line drawn from the origin of the common iliac arteries from the aorta to the midinguinal point, where the external iliacs pass into the thigh. The right common iliac artery crosses anterior to the left common iliac vein and lies at first medial and then anterior to the right common iliac vein. Both internal iliac arteries pass into the pelvis medial to the internal iliac veins.

The pattern of branching of the internal iliac arteries is quite variable, but generally each vessel divides into an anterior and posterior division. The anterior division of the internal iliac artery usually has the following branches: the umbilical, superior vesical, obturator, inferior vesical, uterine, vaginal, middle rectal, inferior gluteal, and internal pudendal.

The umbilical arteries are obliterated after birth, but their remnants can be seen extending along the side wall of the pelvis to the anterior abdominal wall. The superior vesical arteries supply the superior and lateral surfaces of the urinary bladder. The obturator artery is deep to all the other vessels; it arises from the internal iliac and hugs the side wall of the pelvis in its course anteriorly to exit through the obturator canal. There usually is an anastomosis between the obturator artery and the inferior epigastric. One or more inferior vesical arteries supply the urinary bladder. The uterine artery descends anterior to the ureter to the base of the broad ligament. It then crosses superior to the ureter near the lateral fornix of the vagina, where it divides into a descending vaginal branch and an ascending uterine branch. The ascending uterine takes a serpentine course up the side of the uterus before turning laterally to follow the uterine tube to anastomose with branches of the ovarian artery. A separate vaginal artery arises from the internal iliac and supplies the distal part of the vagina. It anastomoses with the vaginal branch of the uterine artery. The middle rectal artery is quite variable in size. It anastomoses superiorly with the superior rectal artery, a continuation of the inferior mesenteric; inferiorly it anastomoses with the inferior rectal artery, a branch of the internal pudendal, which supplies the ischiorectal fossa and anal canal inferior to the pelvic diaphragm. The last two branches of the anterior division of the internal iliac are the inferior gluteal and internal pudendal arteries, which leave the pelvis through the greater sciatic foramen inferior to the piriformis muscle. The internal pudendal artery hooks around the ischial spine to enter the pudendal canal inferior to the pelvic diaphragm in the perineum.

The posterior division of the internal iliac artery is smaller and usually has only three branches: the superior gluteal, the iliolumbar, and the lateral sacral. The superior gluteal artery is the largest branch; it passes superior to the piriformis muscle, out of the greater sciatic foramen, and into the gluteal region. The iliolumbar artery courses posterosuperiorly anterior to the ala of the sacrum. It gives rise to the ascending lumbar artery and a branch to the iliac fossa. The lateral sacral artery descends on the pelvic surface of the sacrum just anterior to the roots of the sacral plexus.

The veins of the pelvis are named the same as the arteries and generally follow a similar course but in the opposite direction. The internal iliacs join the external iliacs to form the common iliac veins. The vessels arise from a very extensive, thin-walled basketwork of veins around the urinary bladder, vagina, uterus, and rectum. They are easily torn during surgical manipulation and the resulting bleeding may be difficult to control. There are important anastomoses between the uterine and vaginal venous plexuses and the superior and inferior rectal veins as well as the lateral sacral veins.

The anastomosis with the superior rectal vein allows venous blood from the pelvis to enter the portal circulation via the inferior mesenteric vein. This connection between the systemic and portal circulations provides a means for cancer in the pelvic organs to metastasize to the liver. The connections between the lateral sacral veins and others in the pelvis are equally important, because the lateral sacral veins anastomose with those of the perivertebral plexus, a valveless system of veins that extends throughout the vertebral canal and connects with the venous sinuses of the brain. These anastomoses provide a route by which cancer may spread from the pelvic viscera directly to the brain without involving other areas of the body.

The pelvis is innervated by the lumbar, sacral, and coccygeal plexuses (Fig. I-17). The anterior rami of L-4 and L-5 join to form the lumbosacral trunk, which crosses the ala of the sacrum to join S-1 on the anterior surface of the piriformis muscle. The lumbosacral trunk is the contribution from the lumbar plexus. The sacral plexus is formed by L-4, L-5, and S-1 to S-4. Arising from the roots of the plexus are the nerve to the piriformis (S-1 and S-2), the pelvic splanchnic nerves (S-2, S-3, and S-4), and the nerves to the levator ani and coccygeus (S-3 and S-4). These nerves are distributed principally to the muscles and organs of the pelvis.

Other branches from the sacral plexus leave the pelvis through the greater sciatic foramen to innervate the lower extremity, the gluteal region, and the perineum: the sciatic (L-4, L-5, and S-1, S-2, and S-3), pudendal (S-2, S-3, and S-4), superior gluteal (L-4, L-5, and S-1), inferior gluteal (L-5, S-1, and S-2), nerve to the quadratus femoris (L-4, L-5, and S-1), nerve to the obturator internus (L-5, S-1, and S-2), and the posterior femoral cutaneous nerve (S-1, S-2, and S-3). Finally, there are two cutaneous branches that pass through the coccygeus muscle to innervate the skin around the coccyx: the perforating cutaneous branches of S-2 and S-3 and the perineal branch of S-4.

The pelvic splanchnic and pudendal nerves are particularly important, because they innervate the pelvis and perineum. The pudendal nerve leaves the pelvis through the greater sciatic foramen inferior to the piriformis muscle. It lies medial to the sciatic nerve and hooks around the sacrospinous ligament to enter the pudendal canal in the perineum. It is possible to effect a perineal block by injecting an anesthetic in the vicinity of the perineal nerves as they course around the sacrospinous ligaments. The tip of the ischial spine is palpated through the wall of the vagina and the needle is passed through the vaginal wall and the sacrospinous ligament just medial to the tip of the ischial spine. The internal pudendal vessels course around the ischial spine just lateral to the nerve but are protected by the bone.

The coccygeal plexus is formed by S-4, S-5, and C-1. It gives rise to dorsal and ventral rami, which supply the dorsum of the sacrum and the

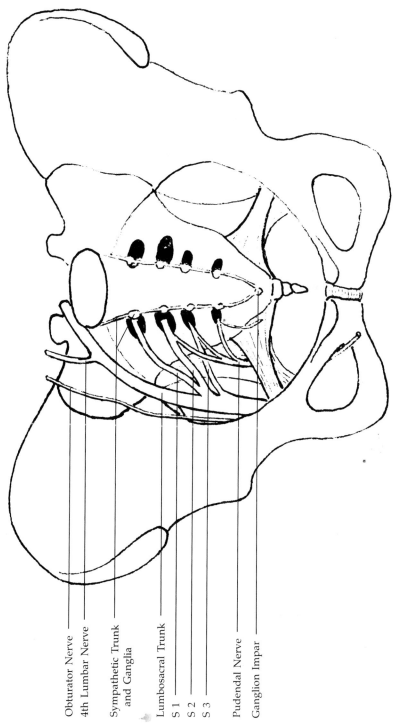

Obturator Nerve

4th Lumbar Nerve

Sympathetic Trunk
and Ganglia

Lumbosacral Trunk

S 1

S 2

S 3

Pudendal Nerve

Ganglion Impar

Fig. I-17.

skin around the coccyx. The organs of the pelvis and perineum receive a rich supply of autonomic nerve fibers from both the sympathetic and parasympathetic nervous systems. The sympathetic fibers arise directly from the sympathetic trunks in the pelvis or indirectly through the superior and inferior hypogastric plexuses. The parasympathetic nerves arise either directly from the pelvic splanchnic nerves or indirectly from the inferior hypogastric plexus.

The abdominal sympathetic trunks give rise to the preaortic (intermesenteric) plexus, which is joined by lumbar splanchnic nerves from L-3 and L-4 and extends inferior to the bifurcation of the aorta as the superior hypogastric plexus. This latter plexus divides into right and left hypogastric nerves, which descend into the pelvis. In the abdomen the sympathetic trunk lies on the bodies of the lumbar vertebrae. The two trunks pass deep to the common iliac vessels and enter the pelvis, where they lie medial to the sacral foramina. Along their course, four pairs of ganglia can be identified, and the trunks converge on a single ganglion impar just anterior to the coccyx. Gray rami communicantes from the ganglia pass laterally to join sacral and coccygeal nerves, and other visceral branches from these ganglia join the right and left hypogastric nerves and the inferior hypogastric plexus lying on either side of the rectum. The right and left hypogastric nerves (composed of fibers from the preaortic plexus, lumbar splanchnic nerves, and contributions from the sacral sympathetic chain) join the inferior hypogastric plexus, which then becomes a mixture of postganglionic sympathetic fibers and preganglionic parasympathetic fibers from the pelvic splanchnic nerves (S-2, S-3, and S-4). Pelvic splanchnic nerves also send fibers superiorly across the common iliac vessels to the inferior mesenteric artery, where they are distributed to the transverse, descending, and sigmoid portions of the colon. In general, the parasympathetic fibers, which originate from the pelvic splanchnic nerves (S-2, S-3, and S-4) and are distributed either directly or through the inferior hypogastric plexus to the viscera, cause the muscle of the bladder and bowel to contract but their sphincters to relax. They dilate the vessels supplying the erectile tissue of the clitoris and perivaginal plexus and carry sensory fibers for the perception of pain and distention from the bladder and rectum. The sympathetic fibers distributed through the superior and inferior hypogastric plexuses and pudendal nerves as well as those coming directly from the sympathetic ganglia provide motor innervation to the involuntary sphincters of the rectum and bladder and mediate detumescence.

Sensory nerves from the perineum and distal end of the vagina travel with the pudendal (somatic) nerves to S-2, S-3, and S-4. Those from the remainder of the vagina and cervix of the uterus travel with the pelvic splanchnic (parasympathetic) nerves to S-2, S-3, and S-4. The nerves from the body and fundus of the uterus go through the hypogastric plexus and enter the spinal cord at the level of T-11 and T-12. The sensory nerves from the ovaries follow the ovarian arteries, which arise from the aorta just inferior to the renal vessels and enter the spinal cord at the level of T-10.

The lymphatics of the pelvis and perineum are clinically important but difficult to visualize (Fig. I-18). The lymphatic vessels from these areas drain into pelvic, abdominal, and inguinal lymph nodes. The pelvic lymph nodes are located either inside the pelvic cavity itself or along the pelvic brim. Those in the pelvic cavity include nodes associated with the vessels supplying the area, such as the internal iliac, vesical, rectal, lateral sacral, and medial sacral; those in the broad ligament near the cervix; perirectal nodes posterior to the rectum; and others along the course of the superior rectal artery. Along the pelvic brim are found external iliac and common iliac nodes, as well as some that are just superior to the promontory of the sacrum. Many nodes are associated with the abdominal aorta; those receiving drainage from pelvic structures include the inferior mesenteric and the lateral and preaortic nodes that lie between the renal and the common iliac arteries. The inguinal lymph nodes include the superficial nodes that lie just inferior and parallel to the inguinal ligament, and the deep inguinal nodes that lie along the femoral vessels and in the femoral canal.

Lymphatics from the ovary follow the ovarian vessels to the lateral aortic and preaortic nodes in the abdomen. Lymph from the uterus drains into abdominal, pelvic, and inguinal nodes. From the fundus and uterine tubes, lymphatics course laterally and follow the ovarian vessels to the lateral aortic and preaortic nodes. From the body of the uterus, they pass via the broad ligament to the external and common iliac nodes, but the areas near the attachments of the round ligaments of the uterus drain to the superficial inguinal nodes. Thus, it is possible for disease in the uterus to manifest itself first in nodes that can be easily palpated just inferior to the inguinal ligament. The vessels from the cervix and superior part of the vagina pass laterally to the external and internal iliac nodes along the course of the uterine and vaginal arteries and posteriorly in the uterosacral folds to the lateral sacral nodes and those near the promontory.

In general, lymph from the vulva drains to the superficial inguinal nodes, but like that of the anus and anal canal, some of it follows the course of the internal pudendal vessels to the internal iliac nodes. The entire female urethra is drained by the internal iliac nodes. Lymphatics from the glans of the clitoris follow its deep dorsal vein and pass to the deep inguinal nodes.

Lymph from the urinary bladder drains mainly to the pelvic nodes, both the external iliac and internal iliac. Lymphatics from the superior and inferolateral surfaces of the bladder follow the superior vesical vessels to the side wall and up to nodes along the external iliac artery. Some of the

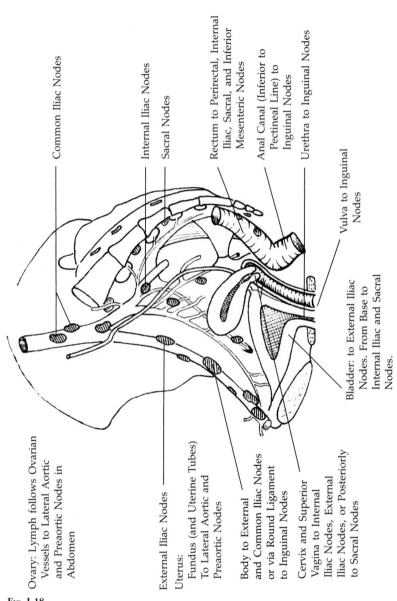

Common Iliac Nodes

Internal Iliac Nodes

Sacral Nodes

Rectum to Perirectal, Internal Iliac, Sacral, and Inferior Mesenteric Nodes

Anal Canal (Inferior to Pectineal Line) to Inguinal Nodes

Urethra to Inguinal Nodes

Vulva to Inguinal Nodes

Ovary: Lymph follows Ovarian Vessels to Lateral Aortic and Preaortic Nodes in Abdomen

External Iliac Nodes

Uterus:
Fundus (and Uterine Tubes) To Lateral Aortic and Preaortic Nodes

Body to External and Common Iliac Nodes or via Round Ligament to Inguinal Nodes

Cervix and Superior Vagina to Internal Iliac Nodes, External Iliac Nodes, or Posteriorly to Sacral Nodes

Bladder: to External Iliac Nodes. From Base to Internal Iliac and Sacral Nodes.

Fɪɢ. I-18.

lymphatic vessels from the base of the bladder also pass to the external iliac nodes, whereas others drain into the internal iliac nodes or follow the superior surface of the levator ani to the sacral nodes posteriorly.

The rectum drains primarily to the perirectal nodes posteriorly and in turn to the superior rectal and inferior mesenteric nodes. Lymph from the rectum also drains to the lateral and median sacral nodes. The distal portion of the rectum and the part of the anal canal proximal to the pectinate line drain along the middle rectal vessels to the internal iliac nodes. Most of the lymphatics from the anus and the anal canal distal to the pectinate line drain to the superficial inguinal nodes, but some of them follow the inferior rectal vessels to the internal iliac nodes.

Peritoneum covers all of the pelvic structures on their superior surfaces to a greater or lesser extent. Peritoneum coats the inside of the abdominal wall inferiorly to the symphysis pubis, from which it is reflected posteriorly over the superior surface of the urinary bladder to a point about 2 cm short of the anterior fornix of the vagina. From there the peritoneum is reflected over the anterior surface of the uterus, creating the vesicouterine pouch. The peritoneum continues over the fundus and posterior surface of the uterus across the posterior fornix of the vagina for about 1 cm before being reflected posteriorly and superiorly to the anterior and lateral surfaces of the rectum. Just as the peritoneal reflection from the superior surface of the urinary bladder to the anterior surface of the uterus creates the vesicouterine pouch, the reflection from the posterior surface of the uterus and posterior fornix onto the rectum forms the rectouterine pouch. When the bladder is empty, the vesicouterine pouch is nothing more than a transverse slit, but the rectouterine pouch is a sizeable excavation in which loops of bowel may lie. The rectouterine pouch is the most dependent part of the peritoneal cavity. It is possible to drain pus and other fluids from this pouch through the posterior fornix of the vagina.

Lateral to the uterus, the peritoneum is draped over the oviducts to form the broad ligaments. The broad ligament comprises the mesovarium, mesosalpinx, and mesometrium. The mesovarium suspends the ovaries from the posterior leaf of the broad ligament. The mesosalpinx is the part superior to the mesovarium that encloses the uterine tubes. The mesometrium is inferior to the mesovarium; its two layers separate to enclose the uterus. A continuation of the broad ligament from the superior pole of the ovary to the side wall of the pelvis is called the suspensory ligament of the ovary. It contains the ovarian vessels, nerves, and lymphatics. Peritoneum from the broad ligaments and lateral walls of the pelvis drapes over the uterosacral ligaments to form the rectouterine folds. The peritoneum then extends into the rectouterine pouch between the uterus and rectum and the pararectal fossae on the sides of the rectum. Between the anterior and posterior folds of the broad ligament along the sides of the uterus is the parametrium.

The development, anatomy, and physiology of the breast are discussed on p. 295.

The Gynecologic Examination

Every gynecologic and obstetric examination should be preceded by a review of systems and a general physical with particular attention to blood pressure, heart, lungs, and eyegrounds. Whenever a patient is examined by a male gynecologist a female assistant should remain in attendance. The patient should void before pelvic examination except when stress incontinence of urine is to be demonstrated. It is easier to palpate the pelvic organs if the patient's rectum is empty. An outline of the examination of breasts and pelvic organs is given in Table 2.

Table 2. Gynecologic Examination

```
  I. Breasts
     A. Inflammatory lesions
     B. Symmetry
     C. Masses
        1. Cystic or solid
        2. Fixation to overlying skin
        3. Retraction of skin
     D. Discharge from nipple
     E. Tenderness
     F. Lymphadenopathy
        1. Axillary
        2. Supraclavicular
 II. Abdomen
     A. Masses and organomegaly
     B. Tenderness
     C. Rigidity
     D. Bowel sounds
     E. Ascites or encapsulated fluid
     F. Scars
III. Pelvic Examination
     A. External genitalia
        1. Congenital anomalies
        2. Hair distribution
        3. Size of clitoris
```

Table 2. Continued

---

     4. Inflammation, masses, or lesions of Bartholin's glands, ure-
       thra, and Skene's glands
     5. Masses, lesions, and ulcerations of the labia majora, labia
       minora, perineum, and anus
  B. Vagina
     1. Partial or complete atresia
     2. Transverse or longitudinal septa
     3. Relaxation of walls
     4. Inflammation and atrophy of the mucosa
     5. Masses or nodularity of the vaginal wall
     6. Discharge
  C. Cytologic examination of cervix and vagina (Papanicolaou smear)
  D. Cervix*
     1. Size and shape
     2. Configuration of external os
     3. Pain on motion
     4. Ulcers or masses
     5. Color and consistency
     6. Contact bleeding
  E. Corpus
     1. Size and configuration
     2. Mobility and position
     3. Pain on motion
  F. Adnexa
     1. Masses (size and consistency)
     2. Pain on motion
  G. Rectovaginal
     1. Nodularity of cul-de-sac
     2. Consistency of parametria
     3. Rectal or rectovaginal masses
     4. Rectal bleeding

---

*Colposcopy is frequently included as part of the routine examination of the cervix. Its use in the diagnosis of cervical abnormalities is described on pages 185 and 250.

Careful examination of the breasts should routinely precede gynecologic examination. Inspection and palpation may be supplemented by transillumination. In cases of doubtful findings, mammography (roentgenographic examination to detect cancer or fibrocystic disease) may be employed (p. 303). Inspection and palpation are performed with the patient in several positions in order to examine each quadrant of the breast with maximal efficiency. First, the patient sits at the edge of the table with her arms extended upward to optimize examination of the upper quadrants. She then bends forward with her arms extended outward so that the breasts are dependent. Asymmetry of the breasts is noted in these positions. Each portion of the breast is palpated to detect size, consistency, tenderness, and fixation of any masses. Bloody discharge from the nipple should be investigated by a cytologic smear as an initial study. Any retraction of the skin or nipple and any discrete firm mass require further investigation, usually including biopsy. The patient then assumes a recumbent position. She first turns on her right side for examination of the inner quadrants of her right breast and the outer quadrants of her left breast. She then turns on her left side for examination of the inner quadrants of the left breast and the outer quadrants of the right breast. The axilla is best examined with the tips of the fingers, which should be inserted while the patient's arms are raised. The palpation is carried out after the patient's arm is brought down against the chest wall. After examination of the axilla, an attempt should be made to palpate supraclavicular nodes. As the doctor inspects and palpates the patient's breasts he should teach her systematic self-examination. Additional information concerning the history and physical findings of diseases of the breast is found on p. 297.

The abdomen is next examined by inspection, palpation, percussion, and auscultation with the patient in the recumbent position. Scars, striations, diastasis of the recti, and hernias of the abdominal wall should be noted. Asymmetry of the abdominal contour suggests an abnormal mass. Large myomas are likely to be irregular, whereas a pregnant uterus is normally symmetric. An ovarian cyst may closely resemble a symmetric myoma. On inspection alone, cystic tumors may be indistinguishable from ascites.

Percussion may aid in delimiting the edges of tumors, the height of the urinary bladder, and loops of distended bowel. It may also differentiate the free fluid of ascites from the encapsulated fluid within an ovarian cyst. Paracentesis should not be performed diagnostically because of the risk of rupturing an ovarian cyst that may be malignant or contain irritating contents that could initiate a chemical peritonitis.

In the case of ascites, the abdomen is symmetric and there is shifting dullness, dullness in the flanks, and tympany in the anterior abdomen. With an ovarian cyst the upper abdomen is flat, and there is seldom shifting dullness, but there is tympany in the flanks and dullness in the anterior abdomen.

Palpation of the upper abdomen should precede that of the lower abdomen and pelvis. In thin women the lower pole of the kidney may normally be palpated. An attempt should be made to feel the lower edges of the liver and spleen. Tenderness in the costovertebral angles should be noted. The inguinal region should be palpated to detect hernias and lymphadenopathy. Palpation should begin as far away as possible from areas of tenderness. Persistence of spasm after a few moments of gentle depression of the anterior abdominal wall suggests peritoneal irritation. The other major sign of peritonitis is rebound tenderness.

For the pelvic examination proper, the patient's feet are placed in stirrups and her buttocks are brought well over the edge of the table. Her knees should be separated as widely as possible and the examiner positioned comfortably with a well-focused bright light. The external genitalia are examined in the following sequence: clitoris, urethral meatus, Skene's ducts, labia minora and majora including Bartholin's ducts, the perineal body, and the perianal region. Skene's ducts, the urethra, and Bartholin's ducts may be inflamed. In the case of acute gonorrhea they may produce a purulent discharge. Bartholin's gland is not normally palpable unless involved in a cyst or abscess and its opening onto the labia is not visible except in the presence of inflammation. The size of the clitoris should be noted and inflammation, atrophy, ulcer, or discharge involving the labia, mons, and perineum recorded. After the labia are separated, the fourchette and hymen should be examined for evidence of tears or scarring. In the virgin the labia majora are apposed. In the nonvirginal nulliparous woman various degrees of gaping and scarring are normal. In parous women these changes are exaggerated. In older women some degree of labial atrophy is normal. At this point in the examination the patient is asked to bear down to see whether she loses urine on coughing (stress incontinence). Descent of the anterior vaginal wall, posterior vaginal wall, or cervix represents cystocele, rectocele, and uterine prolapse, respectively.

The Papanicolaou Smear

The systematic examination of the genitalia is now interrupted to obtain a Papanicolaou smear of the vagina and cervix. Because lubricants interfere with preparation of the cytologic smear, the speculum should be inserted without lubrication but moistened with warm water. To minimize discomfort during introduction of the speculum, the perineum should be depressed, avoiding contact with the anterior portion of the vagina and the clitoris. For best results in cytologic diagnosis, bleeding should be minimal and the patient should be instructed to avoid douching for the 24 hours preceding examination.

Because the Papanicolaou smear is an integral part of the gynecologic examination, it is described in detail here. Its interpretation in connection with other diagnostic procedures is described on pages 184 and 251.

The most important specimens are obtained from the portio by scraping the squamocolumnar junction with a specially designed spatula and from the endocervical canal by scraping with a spatula or rubbing with a cotton-tipped applicator. Cells may be obtained by aspiration from the vaginal vault or scraping the side walls of the vagina. The smear should be fixed immediately in equal parts of 95% alcohol and ether or dry-fixed with a commercially available spray. The smear must be labeled carefully, preferably by marking the slide itself with a diamond pencil. The smears are generally stained by the Papanicolaou method and examined with the light microscope. Cytologic screening is a most important procedure that should be performed as part of the physical examination of any woman over the age of 25 and in even younger patients who are sexually active. No treatment of a cervical lesion should be attempted before the results of the cytologic screening are available. Electrocauterization, cryosurgical procedures, and use of the laser must be deferred until a diagnosis is obtained by colposcopic examination and appropriate biopsy.

A smear of material pipetted from the posterior fornix includes squamous cells from the vagina and cervix and glandular cells from the endocervix and endometrium. Carcinoma of the cervix is best detected in a smear obtained from around the external os, whereas a scraping from the lateral vaginal wall is best for hormonal cytodiagnosis. Several "do-it-yourself" kits are available for home use in cancer detection, but there are inherent errors in collection of the specimen. Furthermore, the patient is denied the benefit of a simultaneous pelvic examination. The Papanicolaou smear prepared from a single cervical swab is highly accurate in detecting carcinoma of the cervix, but a single vaginal aspiration is not sufficiently accurate for detection of endometrial carcinoma. Aspiration of cells from the endometrial cavity improves the rate of detection of carcinoma of the corpus, but definitive diagnosis of this lesion requires adequate histologic sampling of the endometrium.

The Papanicolaou smear may be used to assess the woman's hormonal status as part of the investigation of an endocrine disorder or infertility. The maturation index is the ratio of parabasal to intermediate to superficial cells. For example, a maturation index of 0/20/80 indicates a fair estrogenic effect. The maturation index is normally maximal at the time of ovulation. A maturation index (MI) of 20/75/5, for example, represents a poor estrogenic effect. The karyopyknotic index (KI) is the percentage of superficial cells with deeply pigmented (pyknotic) nuclei. A high karyopyknotic index (greater than 30) is considered to reflect a marked estrogenic effect.

Any suspicious lesion of the cervix should be subjected to biopsy when first detected (p. 184). The biopsy specimen may be obtained through a single punch of a localized lesion or a large mass. Selection of a site for biopsy is made during colposcopic examination (p. 185). Schiller staining (p. 184) may reveal areas of epithelium that fail to take up iodine and thus may be abnormal. Cone biopsy (p. 185) is never performed as an office procedure. Since the Papanicolaou smear is only a screening procedure, histologic confirmation is required before any treatment is initiated. The management of the abnormal Papanicolaou smear is diagrammed on page 251.

Before removal of the speculum, the color of the cervix is noted. A bluish discoloration may be an indication of pregnancy or a large tumor. The condition of the external os may indicate parity. The nulliparous cervix has a small circular external os, whereas in the parous woman the os is irregular or transversely lacerated.

The vagina itself is often inadequately inspected because the speculum covers a large part of its surface. Nevertheless, the entire surface of the vagina should be carefully inspected under bright light. The color of the mucosa and the condition of the rugae should be noted. Nodularities and ulcers should be described. Any suspicious lesion should be subjected to biopsy.

An attempt should be made to identify the etiologic agent in any profuse vaginal discharge. Organisms that may be identified on initial examination are Gonococcus, Candida (Monilia), and Trichomonas. Discharge from the urethral meatus, Skene's ducts, Bartholin's ducts, the external cervical os, the anal crypts, and the pharynx may be gram-stained and inoculated on a Thayer-Martin agar plate or another suitable culture medium, to identify gonococci. Culture is often performed without charge by local health departments.

Hanging-drop smears for trichomonads may be obtained from the urethra, external os, or posterior fornix. The material is suspended in normal saline and examined on a glass slide. The yeast-like organisms that cause candidiasis may be recognized if some of the cheesy exudate is suspended in 10% potassium hydroxide or cultured on a medium such as Nickerson's, where they will appear as brown or black colonies within 24 hours.

The remainder of the internal examination is completed with the patient in the lithotomy position. The patient may help to relax her abdominal wall by taking fast shallow breaths. The uterus and adnexa are palpated between the internal (vaginal) hand and the external (abdominal) hand during the bimanual examination. By depressing the patient's perineum and by resting his elbow on his thigh, the examiner may be able to reach further into the vagina.

The examiner may find it helpful to rest one foot on a low stool. At the beginning of the internal examination, the cervix is located and its size, mobility, and consistency noted. Pain on motion of the cervix should be recorded. The corpus should then be palpated between the abdominal hand, which makes downward pressure on the uterus, and the vaginal hand, which pushes it upward. The size, mobility, consistency, position, and shape of the uterus should be recorded.

Physical diagnosis is rendered difficult when the patient fails to relax, when the examination causes pain, when the patient is obese, and when the bladder or rectum is filled. The normal fallopian tube is rarely palpable even under ideal conditions of examination. Before an attempt is made to ascertain the size and consistency of the ovary, the position and size of the uterus must be known. If an ovarian enlargement is felt, it is most important to describe whether it is cystic or solid, and unilateral or bilateral. Because any solid ovarian mass may represent a malignant tumor, the description of any adnexal lesion must be accurately recorded. The size of a pelvic mass should be noted in centimeters rather than in terms of fruits, vegetables, or eggs of various birds. It is valuable to accompany the description of abnormal findings by a drawing because subsequent management may depend on whether a lesion has regressed, remained the same size, or grown since the last examination.

A normal ovary may be felt in a thin cooperative patient by even a relatively inexperienced examiner, but even a distinctly enlarged ovary may not be palpable by an expert in an obese or uncooperative patient. If there is any doubt about the presence of an adnexal mass, consultation should be obtained, because any ovarian enlargement is a potentially serious lesion. The average dimensions of the normal adult ovary are $3 \times 2 \times 1.5$ cm, although ovarian size varies considerably during the reproductive period. Any adnexal mass greater in size than the normal ovary should be carefully investigated. The average dimensions of the postmenopausal ovary are $2.0 \times 0.5 \times 0.5$ cm. Any palpable ovary in the postmenopausal woman must be considered abnormal. For accurate diagnosis of an adnexal mass, the pelvic examination must occasionally be performed under anesthesia, especially in children.

The rectovaginal examination should be performed last because it is usually the most uncomfortable, but it should never be omitted from the gynecologic examination. The middle finger is inserted into the rectum and the index finger into the vagina. The tissues of the rectovaginal septum are felt between the two fingers. Moving the fingers laterally from the cervix to the right and left permits systematic palpation of the parametria. The parametria and uterosacral ligaments, which may be involved in inflammatory or neoplastic diseases, are palpable only on rectovaginal examination. Lesions detected on rectovaginal palpation include a high rectocele, an enterocele (p. 221), endometriosis (p. 224), and masses on the posterior uterine wall and in the cul-de-sac and rectovaginal septum. Palpation of the parametria is requisite to clinical staging of carcinoma of the cervix (p. 252).

Occasionally in children and older virgins, the rectal examination is substituted for the vaginal. If the findings are suspicious or inconclusive, examination under anesthesia may be required. During rectal examination attention is directed to hemorrhoids, fistulas, fissures, anorectal polyps and tumors, and condylomas.

Women who have been raped or claim to have been raped may come, often with police escort, for examination and possible treatment. The physician's duty at such time is to record the history as accurately as possible, preferably in the patient's own words, and to record objectively the physical findings, as described on page 214.

Obstetric Examination

An outline of the physical examination of the obstetric patient is presented in Table 3, and further details are supplied on pages 59-61.

Table 3. Obstetric Examination

I. Uterine Size
II. Consistency and Shape of the Uterus (early in pregnancy)
III. Presentation and Position of the Fetus
IV. Size and Movements of the Fetus
V. Mobility of the Fetal Head
VI. Consistency, Size, and Engagement of the Head
VII. Presence of Fetal Heart Tones (by stethoscope or Doptone)
VIII. Vaginal Examination to Detect Position, Length, Consistency, and Dilatation of the Cervix
IX. Manual Pelvimetry
X. Papanicolaou Smear on the First Antepartum Visit If the Patient Has Not Had a Cytologic Examination Within the Last 12 Months
XI. Sonographic Examination During the First Trimester to Ascertain Developmental Age of the Fetus.[*]
XII. Cervical Culture for Gonorrhea

[*]Sonography may be repeated later in gestation to assess fetal growth and to detect abnormalities of the fetus or placenta.

II

Normal Obstetrics

Diagnosis of Pregnancy

Diagnosis of pregnancy is made on the basis of history, physical signs, and laboratory tests. The history must include an accurate account of the menses, the last normal menstrual period, exposure to pregnancy, and contraception. The signs of pregnancy have traditionally been classified as positive, probable, or presumptive.

The use of serum beta subunit human chorionic gonadotropin (β-hCG) titers and ultrasound has greatly diminished the importance of most of these signs and symptoms as definitive diagnostic indications of pregnancy. Definitive diagnosis of intrauterine pregnancy is now made by a β-hCG concentration greater than 6,500 m.i.u./ml and an intrauterine gestational sac identified by ultrasound. Both are usually present by the sixth week after the last menstrual period. Normal values for concentrations of β-hCG in the serum during the various stages of pregnancy are shown in Figure II-1. The times of appearance of the various indicators of pregnancy are shown in Table 4. Figure II-1 also shows the corresponding values for the other important trophoblastic polypeptide hormone, human placental lactogen (hPL), or human chorionic somatomammotropin, which is described on p. 78.

Table 4. Times of Appearance of Important Indicators of Pregnancy

POSITIVE TEST OR OBSERVATION	INTERVAL AFTER ONSET OF LAST NORMAL MENSTRUAL PERIOD
Serum β-hCG (RIA)	24 Days
Serum β-hCG (ELISA, "Icon")	26 Days
Urine β-hCG (ELISA, "Icon")	28 Days
Softening of the cervix	4–5 Weeks
Intrauterine gestational sac (Ultrasound)	5–6 Weeks
Other urinary pregnancy tests	5–8 Weeks
Softening of the lower uterine segment (Hegar's Sign)	6 Weeks
Fetal cardiac activity (Ultrasound)	7–8 Weeks
Fetal cardiac activity (Doppler)	10–12 Weeks
Perception of fetal movement	16–20 Weeks
Auscultation of fetal cardiac sounds	18 Weeks

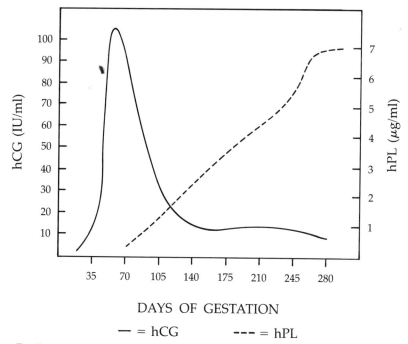

DAYS OF GESTATION

— = hCG   - - - = hPL

Fɪɢ. II-1. Concentrations of chorionic gonadotropin and placental lactogen in serum during various stages of pregnancy.

The traditional positive signs of pregnancy are not elicited before the second trimester by conventional clinical techniques. They include seeing or feeling fetal movements by the examining physician, hearing and counting the fetal heart rate separately from the maternal pulse, and radiologically delineating the fetus. Fetal movements can normally be felt by the fifth month. The fetal heart beat can be detected by stethoscope by the eighteenth week and by Doppler ultrasound by the twelfth week. The fetus can be visualized radiologically by the sixteenth week and a gestational sac may be detected sonographically as early as the fifth week (p. 83).

Probable signs of pregnancy include enlargement of the abdomen, enlargement of the uterus, a globular change in shape of the uterus, softening of the cervix and the lower uterine segment (the area between cervix and corpus), irregular painless contractions of the uterus (Braxton Hicks contractions), ballottement of the uterus (repercussion of the fetus after tapping the lower uterine segment), and positive urinary hormonal tests for pregnancy. The hormonal tests, which may be immunologic or biologic, depend essentially on the detection of human chorionic gonadotropin, the level of which is normally highest between the fiftieth and ninetieth days of gestation. Progestin-induced withdrawal bleeding is no longer an acceptable technique to rule out pregnancy. Examination of the cervical mucus in pregnancy will reveal either a beaded (cellular) or an intact fernlike pattern. An intact fern is not compatible with normal early pregnancy.

Presumptive signs and symptoms of pregnancy include amenorrhea, fullness and tenderness of the breasts, enlargement and darkening of the areola, prominence of sebaceous glands of the areola (Montgomery's tubercles), and secretion of thick yellow fluid (colostrum) from the nipple after the first few months. Additional presumptive symptoms include lassitude, nausea and vomiting (morning sickness), frequency of urination, and quickening (appreciation by the patient of fetal movements after the fourth month). Presumptive physical signs include bluish discoloration of the vagina and cervix, increased pigmentation of the skin , and abdominal striae.

The average duration of human pregnancy is 40 weeks (p. 61). To calculate the estimated date of confinement (EDC), count back three months from the last menstrual period (LMP) and add seven days. For example, if the LMP was March 18, 1988, the EDC is December 25, 1988.

About 40% of women will deliver within 5 days of the EDC and about two thirds within 10 days of the EDC. Because women experience vaginal bleeding during the first 2 months of pregnancy (p. 122), erroneous calculation of EDC is not uncommon.

Urinary immunologic pregnancy tests have replaced the biologic tests. All are semiquantitative, utilizing an immunologic reaction to human chorionic gonadotropin; the preferable tests are specific for β-hCG. Accuracy and sensitivity vary among the individual tests. The "Icon" test is specific, with a sensitivity of 50 m.i.u./ml. It gives a positive reaction as early as 10 days after ovulation and in normal pregnancy is consistently positive by the time of the expected menses. Use of the first voided morning urine increases the concentration of hCG and therefore the effective sensitivity of the test. Other tests available for home use are less specific and less sensitive, but all should give a positive reaction in normal pregnancy within 6 weeks after the last normal menstrual period (4 weeks after ovulation). False-positive reactions are rare, particularly if the test has been repeatedly positive, but a negative reaction does not necessarily indicate the absence of pregnancy. The urinary concentration of hCG may simply be too low to elicit a positive response. Because concentrations of hCG rise rapidly in early normal pregnancy, a negative test in the presence of a high clinical suspicion of pregnancy should be repeated after 1 week and, if still negative, after a second week. Persistently negative tests, including at least one performed more than 3 weeks after the "missed" period, provide a fairly reliable indication of the absence of normal pregnancy.

Newer tests to detect urinary chorionic gonadotropin use an enzyme-linked immunoassay involving monoclonal antihuman chorionic gonadotropin antibody.

The differential diagnosis of pregnancy includes myomas, ovarian cysts, pseudocyesis (false, or spurious, pregnancy), and hematometra (collection of blood within the uterus). None of these conditions is accompanied by a positive test for pregnancy or a gestational sac on sonographic examination. With myomas there is usually no amenorrhea and the uterus is firmer. With ovarian cysts the mass may be felt separate from the uterus. Both myomas and ovarian cysts, however, may coexist with pregnancy. With pseudocyesis, a normal-sized uterus may be palpated under anesthesia. The signs of false pregnancy may occasionally be reversed under hypnosis.

The definitive sign of fetal death is absence of a fetal heart beat in real-time sonographic examination. Suggestive signs of fetal death include failure of growth or regression in size of the uterus, regression of mammary changes, and disappearance of fetal heart tones and fetal movements. Radiologic examination is much less commonly performed today. Radiologic signs include collapsed cranial bones, exaggerated curvature of the spine, gas in the heart and great vessels, and failure to demonstrate swallowing of amnionic (amniotic) fluid into which a contrast medium has been injected (amniography).

Some of the physical signs in a first pregnancy are different from those in later pregnancies. In a woman pregnant for the first time, the abdominal wall is tenser, the uterus and breasts are firmer, the labia may be apposed, and tags of hymen and vaginal rugae are more obvious. The primigravid cervix is more likely to be conical and closed with a regular circular external os. The vagina of the multipara is wider, the vulva gapes, and the external os is irregular.

Maternal Physiology

The average duration of human pregnancy is 40 weeks (280 days) from the first day of the LMP, or 38 weeks (266 days) after ovulation. The growth of the uterus is a response to hormones in the first few months of pregnancy. Thereafter the growth is related to the mechanical effects of the enlarging products of conception. The uterus changes in shape from pyriform in the nonpregnant state to globular in early pregnancy and to ovoid in later pregnancy. It is frequently rotated laterally, more often to the right (dextrorotated). The uterus increases in length from 7 cm in the nonpregnant state to 35 cm at term and from 500 to 1000 times in volume. By the third lunar month of gestation, the top of the uterus reaches the pelvic brim. By the fourth month it is four fingerbreadths above the symphysis. By the fifth month the top of the uterus is almost at the level of the umbilicus. By the sixth month it is slightly above the umbilicus. By the seventh month it is three fingerbreadths above the umbilicus. By the eighth month it is three fingerbreadths above the level reached in the seventh month. By the ninth month it is just below the xiphoid, and by the tenth month it has fallen back to its position in the eighth month. An estimate of fundal height can be made by measuring from pubic symphysis to top of fundus with a tape measure.

The descent of the fetal head into the true pelvis, particularly in the primigravida, often occurs about 2 weeks before term. This phenomenon, which suggests that the fetal head is not too large for the pelvis, is called lightening.

The uterus increases in weight from 60 g in the nonpregnant state to 1000 g at term. Myometrial fibers stretch and hypertrophy but undergo little if any hyperplasia. The myometrial fibers are disposed in figure-of-eight arrangements, which serve as living ligatures to effect hemostasis. Uterine blood flow increases to 600 ml/min at term with a parallel increase in oxygen consumption. Myometrial contractions progress from an irregular and painless (Braxton Hicks) pattern to regular and painful contractions at term. The decidual reaction of the endometrium involves hypertrophy of the endometrial glands and formation of large polygonal stromal cells filled with glycogen and lipid (decidual cells). The basal cells of the cervical epithelium undergo hyperplasia. The cervix increases in vascularity and softens as its glands hypertrophy. It remains occluded by a mucous plug until near the onset of labor. This mucus forms a beaded (cellular) rather than a fernlike pattern when allowed to dry on a glass slide.

A fernlike pattern is a manifestation of estrogenic dominance, which does not obtain in normal pregnancy. The estrogen is associated with a high content of electrolytes in the mucus, particularly sodium, which is responsible for the fern. As labor approaches, the cervix effaces, thins, and becomes increasingly dilatable as term approaches, probably because estrogens depolymerize the acid mucopolysaccharides that form the ground substance.

The uteroplacental circulation develops as a low-resistance system. Uterine blood flow is only 1 to 2% of cardiac output in the nonpregnant state, whereas at the end of pregnancy it accounts for over 10% of the cardiac output, which itself may be increased almost 50%. Uterine blood flow remains fairly constant, however, throughout the course of gestation when calculated in terms of flow to uterus and products of conception. The figure remains close to 10 to 15 ml/100 g of tissue/min. Oxygen consumption is fairly constant at 1 cc/100 g tissue/min. The weight of evidence suggests that the uterine blood flow is not autoregulated. Lack of autoregulation of uterine blood flow is relevant to the use of antihypertensive drugs in pregnant women. The reduction in blood pressure probably decreases uterine blood flow, which is already half or less than half of normal in hypertensive gravidas.

The vagina undergoes an increase in vascularity early in pregnancy, developing a bluish discoloration that may aid in the diagnosis of pregnancy (p. 60). The increased production of lactic acid from glycogen by lactobacilli maintains the acidic pH of the vagina.

The primary change in the ovary is the formation of the corpus luteum of pregnancy, with accompanying cessation of ovulation and menstruation. The ovarian vessels undergo a huge increase in caliber.

The breasts undergo an increased growth of ductal and alveolar tissue. Development of the ducts is under the control of estrogen and that of the alveoli under the control of progesterone. Additional hormones involved in mammary development include prolactin, growth hormone, insulin, cortisone, and thyroxine. In addition to the general increase in size of breasts, areolae, and sebaceous glands (p. 60), the nipples enlarge and become more deeply pigmented and erectile.

The normal average weight gain in pregnancy is about 20 to 25 pounds. Two pounds are normally gained in the first trimester and about 11 pounds in each of the last two trimesters. The average weight gain in pounds at term is distributed roughly as follows: fetus, 7.5; placenta, 1.0; amniotic fluid, 2.0; uterus, 2.5; breasts, 2.0; blood, 2.5; and interstitial fluid, 5.5.

Many of the physiologic changes in pregnancy are maximal, or nearly so, by the sixth week of gestation, including increase in concentration of renin in plasma and decrease in plasma oncotic pressure. The net gain in protein amounts to about 1 kg, about half of which is in the products of conception and half in the uterus, breasts, and blood. About 7 liters of water are retained until delivery; about half of this volume is lost at the time of delivery of the fetus, placenta, and amniotic fluid. Additional important metabolic changes include a lowering of glucose tolerance (p. 158), a positive nitrogen balance, and an increase in free fatty acids, phospholipids, and total lipids. The mother ordinarily needs about 800 mg of iron during the course of gestation (500 mg for increased mass of maternal erythrocytes and 300 mg for the fetus and placenta).

Hypochlorhydria and vomiting in pregnancy may interfere with absorption of iron by the mother. The mother stores more calcium than the fetus requires until the last month of pregnancy, when the fetus needs about twice as much as the mother can ordinarily assimilate. The maternal reserves are then taxed and the mother may require additional calcium during lactation.

The increase in blood volume in pregnancy amounts to about 30 to 40% above nonpregnant levels. The maximum is achieved at about 34 weeks of gestation and is maintained throughout pregnancy without a terminal decrease. The elevation of the diaphragm with displacement of the heart to the left creates the false impression of cardiomegaly in normal pregnancy. Increases occur in cardiac rate, stroke volume, and cardiac output. The circulation time is somewhat decreased in the upper portion of the body and increased below the pelvis. Soft systolic apical and pulmonic murmurs are common, but diastolic murmurs indicate disease (p. 161).

The rise in femoral venous pressure is a result of compression of the vena cava by the enlarging uterus. Arterial blood pressure, however, is normally somewhat decreased in the second trimester.

Edema is common in normal pregnancy. About three quarters of all pregnant women have pedal edema that increases while they are erect and regresses while they are recumbent. Many women also have edema, which is normally slight, of the hands and face. The pedal edema, caused mechanically, is attributable to the increase in femoral venous pressure that occurs when the woman in late pregnancy sits, stands, or lies supine. The bulky uterus occludes the vena cava while she is supine and blocks the common iliac veins while she is erect. The generalized nondependent edema is an effect of estrogens; the depolymerization of the ground substance permits increased binding of sodium and water. In the absence of preeclampsia, women with such edema have larger babies, as do those with larger plasma volumes, more total body water, and greater gains in weight.

The arterial blood pressure, especially the diastolic, decreases some time during the first trimester and begins to rise again late in the second. Inasmuch as the cardiac output has increased by 30 to 40% by the end of the first trimester, there must be a remarkable decrease in total peripheral vascular resistance. Suggested explanations for the decrease have invoked progesterone, prostaglandin E_2, and prostacyclin, but they all increase while the blood pressure is rising late in pregnancy.

The extent of the hemodynamic increases is as follows; erythrocyte mass, 25 to 30%; plasma volume, 40 to 50%; cardiac output, 30 to 40%; uterine blood flow, 1000%; and cardiac rate, 10 to 15 beats/min.

Hematocrit and hemoglobin concentration normally decrease as a result of the hemodilution of pregnancy, reaching their lowest values at about 26 to 28 weeks of gestation. The leukocyte count may normally increase to 15,000 in pregnancy and to 25,000 in labor and the puerperium. There is no morphologic or numeric change in platelets, but increases in fibrinogen, and in Factors VII, VIII, IX, and X are found. Fibrinolytic activity, however, is depressed. An increased erythrocyte sedimentation rate and tendency to thrombosis may result from these changes.

Fibrinogen normally increases about 50% over nonpregnant levels from an average of 300 mg% to about 450 mg%. The decrease in concentration of plasma proteins amounts to about 1 g%. Most of the decrease is in the albumin fraction, with perhaps a slight increase in globulins. As a result, the A/G ratio falls. Among the numerous changes in serum enzymes, the increases in alkaline phosphatase and cystine aminopeptidase are consistent.

Glomerular filtration rate (GFR) and renal plasma flow (RPF) both increase about 30 to 50% in normal pregnancy. Glucosuria, sometimes heavy, and aminoaciduria are common in pregnancy; their occurrence and intensity vary sporadically. Proteinuria, however, is abnormal. Increased renal excretion results in decrease in blood urea nitrogen and creatinine. Urinary stasis results from hypomotility and dilation of the ureters and renal pelves, a consequence primarily of the relaxation of smooth muscle by progesterone.

Dilatation of the ureter in pregnancy begins before the mechanical effect of the enlarging uterus is brought into play. The ureter in pregnancy is dilated, angulated, and elongated. The trigone of the bladder is elevated and edema of the base of the bladder predisposes to trauma. The combination of trauma, stasis, and increased urinary dextrose and amino acids leads to ascending infection of the urinary tract.

Because the average increase of 50% in the filtered load of glucose is presumed to be constant, tubular function must vary for unknown reasons. Experimental expansion of the blood volume is known to inhibit the renal tubular reabsorption of dextrose, sodium, and urate, and probably of other substances, but the hypervolemia of pregnancy does not fluctuate significantly.

The increased GFR and progesterone and the expanded plasma volume tend to increase the excretion of sodium. Estrogen and corticosteroids tend to retain sodium. For accurate results in pregnancy, the GFR and RPF must be measured in the lateral recumbent rather than the supine position.

Since tidal volume and respiratory rate increase in pregnancy, minute volume is increased. This hyperventilation may be a result of an increased sensitivity of the maternal respiratory center to carbon dioxide, perhaps as an effect of progesterone. Respiratory alkalosis may occur, but is compensated by a decrease in serum bicarbonate with resulting stability of pH of the blood.

Elevation of the diaphragm lowers the functional residual capacity, but vital capacity and maximum breathing capacity are not altered significantly.

Progesterone causes decreased motility of the gastrointestinal tract and, by inference, delayed absorption and constipation.

Additional changes in the digestive tract include reduction in free HCl, reflux esophagitis (the probable cause of "heartburn"), increased stasis in the gallbladder (possibly leading to formation of stones), and upward displacement of the appendix (possibly interfering with the diagnosis of acute appendicitis in pregnancy). Ptyalism (excessive salivation) and hyperemia of the gums, alterations in appetite, increased size of hemorrhoids, and constipation are commonly encountered in pregnancy.

The hypochlorhydria is especially marked in the first half of pregnancy. For that reason, even severe vomiting seldom results in hypochloremic alkalosis, as it would in nonpregnant women.

General endocrine changes in pregnancy include alterations in secretory and excretory rates, in binding by globulins, and in metabolic interactions, and increase in size and vascularity of the endocrine organs. The most pronounced changes affect the ovary, with persistence of the corpus luteum, cessation of ovulation, and increased and prolonged elaboration of progesterone.

Moderate enlargement of the thyroid gland is accompanied by increases in basal metabolic rate (up to 25%), thyroid-binding globulin (TBG), and thyroxine (T_4). Triiodothyronine (T_3) uptake is decreased and serum cholesterol increased. Free thyroxine levels are essentially unchanged.

Pregnancy and hyperthyroidism share the following: increase in BMR, total T_4, and RAI uptake (which should not be performed during pregnancy); palpitation; tachycardia; perspiration; and emotional lability. Pregnancy and hyperthyroidism differ in the following respects: cholesterol is increased in pregnancy but decreased in hyperthyroidism; TBG is increased in pregnancy but is normal in hyperthyroidism; unbound thyroxine is not increased in pregnancy but is increased in hyperthyroidism; absolute iodine uptake is not increased in pregnancy but is increased in hyperthyroidism; and resin T_3 uptake is decreased in pregnancy but increased in hyperthyroidism.

The pancreas in pregnancy is subjected to a diabetogenic stress. Since islet cell function and secretion of insulin are increased while the antagonism of insulin by placental lactogen (chorionic somatomammotropin) and, much less important, its destruction by placental insulinase increase, the pancreas in taxed in order to produce enough insulin to maintain the hyperinsulinemia of pregnancy (p. 158).

Production of cortisol increases although much of the steroid is bound by corticosteroid-binding globulin, or transcortin, which is increased in pregnancy. Some increase in free cortisol can be measured, however.

Concentrations of aldosterone, renin substrate, and angiotensin, and both concentration and activity of renin in plasma increase from twofold to tenfold. The change in plasma renin activity is attributable chiefly to changes in plasma renin substrate, the hepatic synthesis of which is influenced by estrogens. The increase in aldosterone protects against the natriuretic and antikaliuretic effects of progesterone. Enlargement of the adrenal cortex involves primarily the zona fasciculata, with the result that glucocorticoids but not 17-ketosteroids are considerably increased. The pituitary gland enlarges and, rarely, may compress the optic chiasma and reduce the visual fields. Parathormone levels are regulated by calcium levels in the blood, which ordinarily do not undergo great change. The concentration of ionized calcium remains almost unchanged but that of total calcium decreases somewhat because of the decrease in the fraction bound to albumin.

Hyperpigmentation in pregnancy involves the areola, vulva, and linea nigra. Facial hyperpigmentation may result in chloasma, or the mask of pregnancy, which generally regresses post partum. These changes may be the result of an increase in melanocyte-stimulating hormone. Striae on the abdominal wall and breasts are pink during pregnancy, but may later become silvery, providing evidence of prior pregnancy. Vascular spiders and palmar erythema develop as effects of estrogen. Cutaneous blood flow increases about sevenfold; this effect serves to dissipate the extra heat associated with the changes in basal metabolic rate. Changes in the musculoskeletal system include progressive lumbar lordosis, with increased mobility of the pelvic joints and an anterior displacement of the center of gravity.

The commonly encountered increase in emotional lability is manifested by anxiety, apprehension, identity crises, and changes in libido. Alterations in appetite may include craving for unusual substances not normally considered as food (pica), such as starch and clay. Mild postpartum depression is common, although frank psychotic reactions reflect a preexisting tendency.

Gametogenesis and Fertilization

Somatic cells divide by mitosis, which results in two daughter cells with the same diploid number of chromosomes as the parent cell. Gametogenesis (ovogenesis, or oogenesis, and spermatogenesis) requires meiosis, or reduction division, during which the chromosomal number is halved to produce haploid gametes. The diploid number is restored during fertilization.

Ovogenesis begins around the middle of the third month of gestation, when primary ovocytes (oocytes) can first be defined. All ovogonia (oogonia) have become primary ovocytes by the seventh month. Ovogenesis begins with the entrance of ovogonia into prophase of the first meiotic division. The lengthy prophase in the female is divided into five phases: leptotene, zygotene, pachytene, diplotene, and diakinesis. During pachytene, the longest phase, pairing of homologous chromosomes and exchange of genetic material occur. At the end of the pachytene phase, ovocytes enter the diplotene phase, in which they remain until they resume maturation or become atretic.

As many as 7 million ovocytes are present in the ovary during the fifth month of fetal development. At birth only two million remain. By the age of 7 years the number is reduced to between 200,000 and 400,000. The decline continues throughout life, few ovocytes surviving beyond menopause.

Primordial germ cells migrate from the endoderm of the yolk sac to the gonadal ridge, where they increase in number by mitotic division in the gonadal anlage. Ovogonia are primordial germ cells that have ceased mitosis but have not yet begun to enlarge or entered the meiotic prophase. Upon entering prophase I, ovogonia become primary ovocytes, which when surrounded by a single layer of flattened follicular cells form primary follicles.

In each menstrual cycle between 5 and 20 follicles begin to develop but normally only one will ovulate. As many layers of follicular, or granulosa, cells are formed, spaces appear between the individual cells. As these spaces coalesce to form an antrum, the antral, or secondary, follicle develops. As the follicle enlarges and ovulation approaches, the mature, or graafian, follicle is formed. During folliculogenesis an acellular layer, the zona pellucida, is deposited around the ovocyte by the granulosa cells.

During the follicular (proliferative) phase of the menstrual cycle, increasing titers of estradiol produced by the developing follicle eventually result in a surge of both FSH and LH from the pituitary. This release of pituitary hormones occurs on about day 14 of the normal cycle. The surge of LH is responsible for ovulation.

Follicle-stimulating hormone is a glycoprotein with a large sialic acid moiety and a half-life of about two hours. It is secreted by the basophilic cells of the anterior pituitary and is released by gonadotropin releasing hormone (GnRH). Negative feedback to estradiol occurs in both the pituitary and the hypothalamus. FSH effects follicular growth to the antral stage by promoting uptake of amino acids by the follicle. LH, probably through its steroidogenic action, is required for complete follicular maturation.

Luteinizing hormone is a glycoprotein with a small sialic acid moiety and a short half-life of about 30 minutes. It too is secreted by the basophilic cells of the anterior pituitary and is released by GnRH. Negative feedback to progesterone and low levels of estradiol, and positive feedback to high levels of progesterone, as found in the mature graafian follicle, occur. The action of LH is to stimulate steroidogenesis in the ovary.

The portion of the brain with the greatest concentration of GnRH is the hypothalamus, from the septal-preoptic region anteriorly to the premamillary nucleus posteriorly. GnRH fibers originating from the arcuate nucleus and from cell bodies in the anterior hypothalamic region terminate in the median eminence of the hypothalamus near the long portal vessels. Originating in the hypothalamus, these vessels descend along the pituitary stalk to the anterior pituitary gland. GnRH is secreted directly into this specialized vasculature and thus reaches the pituitary gland undiluted by passage through the peripheral circulation. Biologic activity of GnRH requires interaction with a specific membrane receptor on the gonadotrope.

Follicular development requires both FSH and LH. The surge of LH triggers resumption of meiotic activity within the ovocyte. After the LH surge, the ovocyte rapidly completes the first meiotic division, with production of a large secondary ovocyte and a small first polar body. No synthesis of DNA occurs at this point and the secondary ovocyte proceeds immediately to the metaphase of the second meiotic division, which is completed only after fertilization.

After ovulation the corpus luteum is formed, but luteinization may sometimes occur without ovulation. Luteinization results in two changes in the ovary: an alteration in the biosynthesis of steroids and a proliferation of granulosa cells. In the follicular phase of the menstrual cycle, the follicle synthesizes estrogens from progesterone and androgenic precursors as well as de novo from cholesterol. In the luteal phase, the granulosa cells lose the capacity to convert progesterone into androgens. As a result, a large amount of progesterone is released from the ovary. The theca interna, which secretes estrogen during the follicular phase, continues to produce estradiol during the luteal phase. The concentration of progesterone rises from the time of the midcyclic surge of gonadotropin to a peak that occurs about 7 days later. The variability in the length of the normal ovulatory cycle is a function primarily of the length of the follicular phase, for the corpus luteum has a finite life span of about 14 days.

Development of spermatozoa begins with spermatogonia, which comprise Type A and Type B elements. Spermatogonia of Type B grow and divide mitotically to produce primary spermatocytes, which give rise through meiotic division to haploid secondary spermatocytes and then spermatids, half of which carry an X chromosome and half a Y. The process by which spermatids are transformed into spermatozoa is called spermiogenesis. When the spermatozoon achieves its definitive shape, it is released into the seminiferous tubule. Ability of the spermatozoon to fertilize is not achieved until its passage through the epididymis. The biochemical changes that render the spermatozoon capable of fertilization are known as capacitation, which occurs in the uterus, oviduct, or both. Capacitation is stimulated by estrogen and inhibited by progesterone.

Fertilization requires a capacitated spermatozoon, a mature secondary ovocyte, and a milieu in which union of sperm and egg can occur. Fertilization generally occurs in the ampulla of the oviduct.

The secondary ovocyte presents three barriers to spermatozoa: the mass of cumulus cells, the zona pellucida, and the vitelline membrane. In the process of penetration, spermatozoa undergo the acrosome reaction. This reaction involves fusion of the plasma membrane of the spermatozoon with the outer acrosomal membrane, vesiculation of both membranes, and finally their disappearance. The result is the release of several enzymes. The two most important are hyaluronidase, which disperses the cells of the cumulus and allows spermatozoa to reach the zona pellucida; and acrosin, a proteinase that lyses a path for the spermatozoon through the zona pellucida. In addition, acid phosphatase and neuraminidase are released. After penetration by a spermatozoon, the Golgi apparatus of the ovocyte disintegrates into small membrane-bound cortical granules, which migrate to a position immediately beneath the vitelline membrane. Release of material from the granules into the perivitelline space effects a block to polyspermy.

After fusion of the membranes of spermatozoon and ovum to form the zygote, meiosis resumes and the second polar body is extruded. The haploid sets of chromosomes from spermatozoon and ovum are quickly surrounded by pronuclear membranes to form the male and female pronuclei. Fertilization is completed when the pronuclei move to the center of the zygote, the pronuclear membranes disintegrate, and the maternal and paternal chromosomes are aligned on the metaphase plate of the first cleavage division. In the human being, the two-cell stage is not attained until 24 to 36 hours after fertilization.

After ovulation the ovocyte normally remains capable of being fertilized for not longer than 12 hours. Although it may be penetrated at a later stage, it will probably degenerate before implantation. Breakdown of the metaphase II spindle may result in trisomy (a condition of three homologous chromosomes resulting from nondisjunction) or failure of extrusion of the second polar body (triploidy). During aging of the ovocyte, cortical granules move toward the center of the ovocyte, where they are no longer in a position to block polyspermy.

Early Development of the Fetus

For the first 24 hours after fertilization the zygote remains in the one-cell stage. The two-cell stage begins 24 hours after fertilization and ends 12 hours later. The four-cell stage lasts from hour 36 to hour 48; the eight-cell stage lasts from hour 48 to hour 72; and the 16-cell stage lasts from hour 72 to hour 96. The zygote enters the uterine cavity as a solid ball of cells, the morula, between three and five days after fertilization. In the uterus the morula is transformed into a fluid-filled blastocyst, which consists of an outer covering of trophoblast and a small inner cell mass (embryo-forming cells). The zona pellucida is lost at this stage and the blastocyst then implants on approximately day 6 with the embryonic pole in contact with the endometrium. During the second week the bilaminar embryo is formed and during the third week the trilaminar embryo develops. The embryonic period comprises the second through the eighth weeks and the fetal period the remainder of gestation (third through tenth lunar months). Organogenesis is completed by 16 weeks or earlier.

By day 16 the trilaminar embryonic disc comprises ectoderm, endoderm, and mesoderm. At about day 20 the paraxial mesoderm begins to divide into paired cuboidal bodies called somites, the primordia of the axial skeleton and associated musculature. Each column of paraxial mesoderm is continuous laterally with the intermediate mesoderm, the primordia of the urogenital system (p. 317). Laterally, the intermediate mesoderm thins and becomes continuous with the lateral mesoderm, the primordia of the body wall and the wall of the primitive gut.

The most significant event in the establishment of general form of the developing body occurs during the embryonic period, namely, the process of folding, which transforms the flat, ovoid trilaminar disc into a cylindrical embryo. This folding in both longitudinal and transverse planes is caused by rapid growth in the region of the neural tube, a slower rate of growth at the periphery of the embryonic disc, and a slight constriction in the region of the future umbilical cord.

Development of the Placenta and Fetal Membranes

The human placenta is basically a chorioallantoic structure, for although a vesicular allantois is lacking, the precociously developed allantoic mesenchyme, which later forms the umbilical cord, gives rise in situ to the allantoic vessels that vascularize the chorion. Because maternal blood is in direct contact with trophoblast-covered villi, the human placenta is classified as hemochorial. Because only one layer of trophoblast (the syncytium) is continuous throughout pregnancy, the human placenta is considered hemomonochorial.

The yolk sac, or umbilical vesicle into which it develops, is prominent at the beginning of pregnancy. The embryo is at first a flattened disc, situated between the cavities of amnion and yolk sac. As the embryo grows, it bulges into the amnionic cavity, and the dorsal part of the yolk sac is incorporated into the body of the embryo to form the gut. The yolk sac may occasionally be recognized even in the mature placenta as a crumpled vascular sac between amnion and chorion.

The allantois may project into the base of the body stalk. Its mesoderm normally contains two arteries and one vein. The right umbilical vein disappears early, leaving only the original left vein.

The amnion forms around the eighth day of development by cavitation. Distention of its sac brings the amnion into contact with the internal surface of the chorion. Apposition of the mesoblasts of chorion and amnion occurs between the fourth and fifth months of gestation with the result that the extraembryonic celom is obliterated.

The changes that culminate in the transformation of the endometrium to decidua are not complete until several days after implantation (nidation). Directly beneath the site of implantation is the decidua basalis. Surrounding the ovum and separating it from the rest of the uterine cavity, in the early months of gestation, is the decidua capsularis, which forms as a result of deep, or interstitial, implantation, with the endometrium relining the uterus over the site of the implanted blastocyst. The remainder of the pregnant uterus is lined by decidua parietalis.

The human blastocyst is completely embedded in the endometrium by day 11 or 12 after fertilization. The greater part of the chorion, in contact with the decidua capsularis, loses its villi between the third and fourth months of gestation and forms the smooth chorion, or chorion laeve. The villi on the side of the chorion toward the decidua basalis enlarge and become elaborately branched to form the chorion frondosum. By the third month the decidua capsularis degenerates and the chorion laeve comes into contact with the parietal decidua of the opposite wall of the uterus. The human placenta is thus of dual origin, comprising fetal (chorion frondosum) and maternal (decidua basalis) elements.

Once the cytotrophoblast has penetrated the deepest layer of decidua, continued growth of normal placenta cannot be accomplished by further trophoblastic invasion. Increased thickness of the placenta must therefore be the result of growth in length and size of the villi of the chorion frondosum, with accompaning expansion of the intervillous space. Until the end of the fourth month, the placenta grows in thickness and circumference; thereafter, there is no appreciable increase in thickness, but growth in circumference continues almost throughout pregnancy.

The earliest form of nutrition is derived from endometrial secretion; later, maternal blood is the source. During and after implantation there appear within the syncytiotrophoblast numerous vacuoles, the coalescence of which creates lacunae, which merge to form the intervillous space. Maternal venous sinuses are tapped early, but until day 14 or 15 no arterial blood enters the intervillous space. By day 17 the chorionic villi are vascularized, but until villous and fetal vessels are connected and the fetal cardiac pulsations are initiated (in the second month), no true circulation can be described.

Villi may first be distinguished on or about day 12. The period between days 9 and 20 is characterized by intense growth and differentiation of the chorion. The trophoblastic trabeculae develop a cellular core as a result of multiplication of cytotrophoblastic elements. These highly modified trabeculae may then be designated primary villi. The villous stems later develop mesodermal cores, which convert primary into secondary villi. Vascularization of the secondary villi transforms them into tertiary villi, the principal organs of exchange in the human placenta. Proliferation of cellular trophoblast at the tips of the villi forms the cytotrophoblastic cell columns, which are not invaded by mesenchyme but are anchored to the decidua at the basal plate.

As the placental villi mature, several morphologic changes render them more efficient in maternofetal transfer. The early villi are less finely branched (Fig. II-2), have a smaller surface-to-volume ratio, and are less well vascularized than are the terminal villi of the mature placenta (Fig. II-3). In the early villi a prominent layer of cytotrophoblast (Langhans cells) is evident (Fig. II-4), whereas in the mature villi the trophoblastic covering is thinner, with capillaries more numerous and closer to the surface (Fig. II-5). Although the Langhans layer thins and becomes discontinuous as pregnancy advances, it never disappears completely from the normal human placenta. Electron microscopy shows that the syncytium is the differentiated form of trophoblast whereas the Langhans layer, to which mitotic activity is confined (Fig. II-6), comprises the less well differentiated cells that are the source of syncytiotrophoblast.

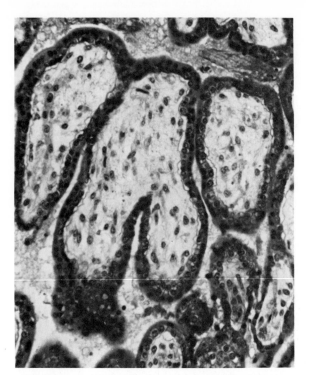

Fig. II-2. First-trimester placenta, showing villi with well defined syncytial and cytotrophoblastic layers.

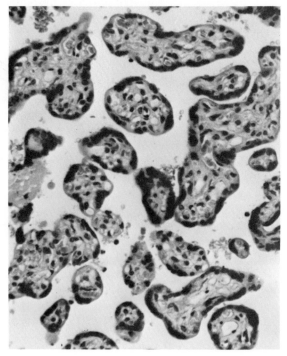

Fig. II-3. Term placenta, showing mature, well vascularized villi.

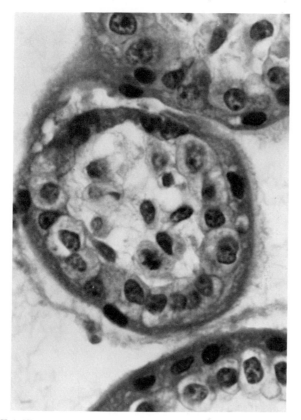

FIG. II-4. High-power view of first-trimester placenta, showing details of trophoblast.

Some changes that accompany maturation of the placenta cannot be interpreted as indications of increased efficiency of placental transfer. They include thickening of basement membranes of endothelium and trophoblast, obliteration of villous capillaries, fibrosis of placental connective tissue, and deposition of calcium. A knot of syncytium in one part of the villus may accompany intimate approximation of endothelial and trophoblastic membranes to form a very thin vasculosyncytial membrane in another part.

Fetoplacental Physiology

The fetus derives all its nutrition from the mother through the placenta, which serves as a fetal kidney, liver, lung, and endocrine organ. The unusual dual circulation of the placenta allows for effective fetomaternal exchange. Maternal blood enters the basal plate of the placenta, whence it is driven by the maternal systolic blood pressure toward the chorionic plate. As the blood falls back toward the basal plate, exchange takes place. The deoxygenated blood then returns to the uterine veins through the basal plate.

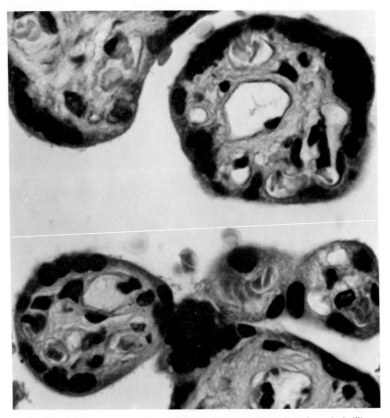

FIG. II-5. High-power view of term placenta, showing well vascularized terminal villi.

The unique features of the placenta include its extracorporeal location, its limited life span, its multiplicity of functions, and its apparent escape from immunologic rejection. The retention of fetal (placental) tissue within the mother for a period of time far exceeding that of allograft rejection depends primarily on the special properties of the trophoblast. An absence or a deficiency of trophoblastic histocompatibility antigens, presence of extracellular sialomucin coatings of the trophoblast, and perhaps effects of progesterone and immunologic enhancement have been considered principal factors in retention of the foreign tissue.

Two maternal proteins, uteroglobin and transglutaminase, have recently been shown to protect the mammalian embryo from immunologic rejection during early pregnancy. Additional factors that have been invoked to explain retention of allogeneic fetoplacental tissue include: anatomic separation of maternal and fetal circulations; afferent blockade of the immunologic reflex arc by decidua; inactivation of maternal immunologic

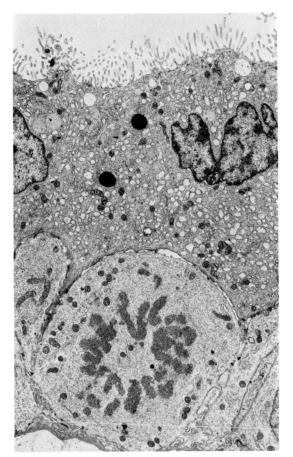

FIG. II-6. Electron micrograph of placenta from six weeks' gestation, showing well differentiated syncytium with microvillous border and Langhans cells (cytotrophoblast), one of which displays a prominent mitotic figure.

effector agents by trophoblast; production by the fetus of immunosuppressive agents such as alpha-fetoprotein; and production by the mother of immunoregulatory agents that confer protection upon the fetoplacental unit.

Placental Hormones

The trophoblast produces both protein and steroid hormones. The proteins are synthesized by the trophoblastic syncytium; synthesis of the steroids involves participation by the mother and fetus as well as the syncytium. The level of human chorionic gonadotropin (hCG) is elevated abruptly in early pregnancy, reaching a peak at about 80 days and gradually declining to a level that remains low throughout pregnancy. The production of hCG by the trophoblast is the basis for hormonal pregnancy tests (p. 60).

Chorionic gonadotropin is a glycoprotein with a large sialic acid moiety, which gives it a long half-life of 6 to 24 hours. This hormone has primarily LH-like properties on bioassay, with a very small amount of FSH-like activity. It substitutes for pituitary gonadotropins in maintaining steroidogenesis in the corpus luteum of pregnancy. Cellular gonadotropin is produced by a variety of human tissues but is glycosylated to its physiologic form only by placenta.

Chorionic gonadotropin reaches a peak of 100,000 to 300,000 IU/liter of maternal urine by the end of the second month of pregnancy. By the fourth month the level is down to 25,000 to 50,000 IU/liter. A low level is maintained to term. Between 45 minutes and 6 days after expulsion of the placenta, hCG normally disappears from the urine.

The other important protein hormone is human placental lactogen (hPL), also named human chorionic somatomammotropin (hCS), which undergoes a gradual increase from 6 weeks' gestation to term. It is diabetogenic and shares certain physiologic and chemical properties with human growth hormone.

Placental lactogen is a polypeptide with both prolactin-like and growth-hormone-like activities. It may substitute for prolactin in supporting ovarian function in early pregnancy and may promote development of the breast, inasmuch as growth hormone is necessary for expression of the effects of estrogen and progesterone on mammary tissue.

The plasma level of hPL reaches a maximum of between 20 and 25 μg/ml near term. The level of this hormone may be an index of placental function (Fig. II-1). Levels below 4 μg/ml after the thirtieth week of gestation have been associated in some but not all studies with poor perinatal outcome.

The placenta has recently been shown to produce a luteinizing hormone releasing hormone that is immunologically identical with that of the hypothalamus.

Progesterone is synthesized by the placenta from maternal precursors. The concentration of this steroid, which is essential for the maintenance of pregnancy, gradually increases in the plasma to term. The main estrogen excreted in pregnancy is estriol. Its production requires a supply of androgens by the fetal adrenal cortex and metabolic participation by the fetal liver and placenta. Its production rises throughout pregnancy with a sharp increase at 28 weeks. Defective function of the fetal adrenal or liver or of the placenta may lead to low levels of estriol in the maternal urine or plasma. A decrease in the level of maternal estriol may result from administration of steroids and certain antibiotics. Measurement of estriol was formerly thought to be an indicator of fetal well-being. Because of high variability and low sensitivity, however, estriol is not frequently measured today.

The principal metabolite of progesterone in pregnancy is pregnanediol, which reaches a maximum at about 32 weeks' gestation. It is not a reliable index of placental function. At the fourteenth week of pregnancy the maternal excretion of urinary estrogen is 1 mg/day. At term the level is normally 30 mg/day, about 90% of which is estriol (E_3).

Maternal cholesterol is converted to pregnenolone by the placenta. This compound is then converted to dehydroisoandrosterone sulfate (DHAS) by the fetal adrenal. DHAS is then hydroxylated at the 16-position in the fetal liver. This is the rate-limiting reaction. The 16-alpha-OH-DHA is converted to estriol in the placenta. It is conjugated to a glucosiduronate or a sulfate and is excreted as E_3G or E_3S in the maternal urine. The placenta does not synthesize corticosteroids. TSH-like activity has also been identified in the placenta. The placenta is somewhat permeable to thyroxine but not to TSH, parathormone, posterior pituitary extract, or insulin.

Placental Transfer

Placental transfer in either direction may be active or passive. The rate of transfer depends principally on the following factors: the rates of maternal and fetal blood flows, the respective concentrations of substances in the maternal and fetal plasmas (concentration gradients), the area and thickness of the placental membrane, the molecular weight and electrical charge of the compound, the physical properties of the barrier, the biochemical mechanisms for active transfer, and the metabolism by the placenta itself.

Since most drugs administered to the mother—including antibiotics and anesthetics, as well as gases, nutrients, many hormones, and some immunoglobulins—cross the placenta, everything prescribed for the mother during pregnancy must be considered in terms of effects on the fetus as well. A few agents, such as succinylcholine, d-tubocurarine, and heparin, however, cross very slightly or not at all. Other substances are concentrated preferentially in the fetal circulation.

The fetus meets its requirements for iron even in the presence of maternal anemia. It maintains oxygenation of its blood by several mechanisms. First, fetal erythrocytes have a higher affinity for oxygen than do maternal erythrocytes. The higher hemoglobin level of the newborn resembles that seen in the adult at high altitude. Fetal blood has a greater oxygen capacity, but has a lower saturation and a higher hematocrit than does adult blood. Accumulation of iron in the fetal liver occurs mainly in the third trimester.

Placental transfer occurs as a result of several mechanisms. Respiratory gases and some electrolytes are transferred by simple diffusion. Sodium is probably transferred actively, with chloride then diffusing to maintain electrostatic balance. Carbohydrates are transferred by facilitated diffusion, and amino acids and some vitamins by active transport. Ascorbic acid, for example, is concentrated on the fetal side. Differential rates of transfer of stereoisomers, such as D- and L-histidine, are evidence of enzyme-mediated carrier mechanisms. In general, the greater the degree of lipid solubility and the smaller the molecular weight, the greater is the rate of transfer. Certain molecules of high molecular weight, however, such as some of the immunoglobulins, cross the placenta, whereas other of equal molecular weight do not. In general, uncharged particles are transferred more readily. Macromolecules may be transported across the placenta by pinocytosis. Water is transferred by bulk flow in response to small hydrostatic or osmotic pressure gradients. Breaks in placental villi lead to leakage of fetal erythrocytes into the maternal circulation and possible Rh-isoimmunization in certain circumstances (p. 155). Some viruses such as rubella may cross the placenta and produce fetal disease (p. 164).

IgG passes the placenta, whereas IgM and IgA do not. Passive immunity to some diseases may be conferred on the fetus as a result of the transfer of these antibodies. In addition, the fetus may produce some of its own antibodies after midpregnancy.

The fetus receives most of its nitrogen as amino acids and synthesizes its own protein. Although the placenta transfers phospholipids, which are subsequently degraded, most of the fetal lipid is synthesized by the fetus itself. Similarly, the fetus synthesizes its own nucleic acids. Glucose is readily transferred in both directions, but the maternal level is usually higher than the fetal. The levels of calcium and phosphorus, however, are higher on the fetal side.

Fetal Development

A fetus reaches term at 40 weeks. It is considered mature at 2500 g, which corresponds to about 36 weeks' gestation. It is sometimes considered viable at 500 g, which corresponds to about midpregnancy.

The fetal hypogastric arteries continue extraabdominally as umbilical arteries, which carry deoxygenated blood to the placenta. The umbilical vein carries relatively well-oxygenated blood from the placenta back to the fetus. Various shunts of oxygenated blood characterize the fetal circulation. Some blood from the umbilical vein is shunted through the ductus venosus to avoid the liver, the only organ to receive undiluted freshly oxygenated blood. The upper half of the fetal body receives more oxygen than does the lower half. The foramen ovale shunts blood to the left side of the heart to supply the head. The ductus arteriosus shunts much of the pulmonary arterial flow to the aorta, thus bypassing the lungs.

At birth, the lungs expand as the infant draws it first breath. As blood begins to flow through the pulmonary vessels, the ductus venosus, foramen ovale, and ductus arteriosus undergo functional closure (Fig. II-7).

The high cardiac output of the fetus and the high hemoglobin content and better oxygen dissociation of fetal hemoglobin compensate for the relatively poor oxygen content of fetal blood. The fetal heart rate of 135/min drops to about 110/min in the newborn.

By the third month of fetal life, the genitalia are sufficiently differentiated to allow diagnosis of sex. By the second trimester the liver has replaced the placenta as the principal organ for storage of carbohydrate.

The growth of the fetus by weight and length is as follows:

Gestational Week	Length (cm) (Crown-heel)	Weight (g)
8	3	1
12	10	18
16	18	100
20	25	300
24	32	600
28	37	1,000
32	42	1,700
36	47	2,500
40	50	3,200 or more

The composition of the amniotic (amnionic) fluid is determined in part by metabolic products of the fetus. The fluid is at first isotonic with maternal serum and is later diluted by hypotonic fetal urine. The volume of fluid increases to a maximum of slightly over 1000 ml at about 35 weeks and gradually decreases to between 500 and 800 ml at term. Examination of the amniotic fluid can be used to assess fetal well-being and maturity. The cells and fluid are examined to detect sex of the fetus and many metabolic and chromosomal abnormalities.

Severe diminution in the volume of amniotic fluid (oligohydramnios) is associated with a poor prognosis if it occurs during the second trimester. If oligohydramnios does not occur until the third trimester, however, it may respond to therapy. Causes of severe oligohydramnios include chromosomal anomalies such as triploidy and genitourinary disorders such as bilateral obstruction of the urethrovesical junctions, posterior urethral valves, and renal agenesis. A marked decrease in amniotic fluid also may occur with retardation of intrauterine growth.

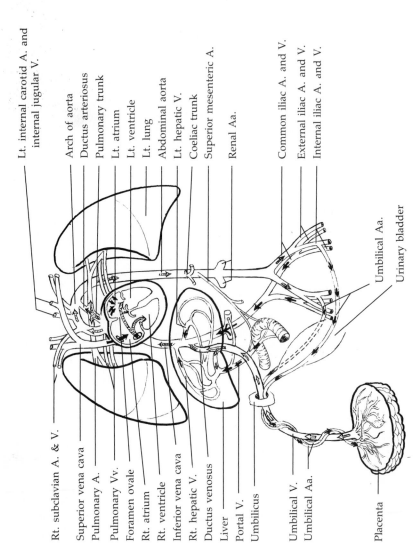

Lt. internal carotid A. and internal jugular V.

Arch of aorta

Ductus arteriosus

Pulmonary trunk

Lt. atrium

Lt. ventricle

Lt. lung

Abdominal aorta

Lt. hepatic V.

Coeliac trunk

Superior mesenteric A.

Renal Aa.

Common iliac A. and V.

External iliac A. and V.

Internal iliac A. and V.

Umbilical Aa.

Urinary bladder

Rt. subclavian A. & V.

Superior vena cava

Pulmonary A.

Pulmonary Vv.

Foramen ovale

Rt. atrium

Rt. ventricle

Inferior vena cava

Rt. hepatic V.

Ductus venosus

Liver

Portal V.

Umbilicus

Umbilical V.

Umbilical Aa.

Placenta

Fig. II-7. The fetal circulation.

Fetal maturity may be assessed by a variety of clinical and laboratory methods. An accurate knowledge of the last menstrual period, auscultation of the fetal heart by standard fetoscope by 20 weeks, and several early measurements of the size of the uterus (before 16 weeks) are the best means of assessing gestational age and fetal maturity by history and physical examination. Ultrasonic detection of the onset of fetal cardiac activity at 5 to 7 weeks and measurements of crown-rump length between 7 and 14 weeks and of biparietal diameter and femoral length between 16 and 30 weeks also provide accurate assessments of gestational age. Ultrasonic measurements of crown-rump length have proved most accurate. In each case, serial measurements are always more accurate than a single measurement. Assessment of gestational age during the third trimester is considerably less accurate than during the first or second trimester. A biparietal diameter of 9.0 cm or more or a femoral length of 7.1 cm or more usually indicates a fetus that weighs at least 2500 grams. Serial measurements of fundal height in centimeters above the symphysis (with a tape measure) provide another simple means of assessing fetal growth. Radiologic examination of the fetus for assessment of gestational age is contraindicated. Illustrations of the sonographic assessment of gestational age are presented in Figures II-8 through II-10.

Placentas may be graded from 0 (least mature) through I and II to III (most mature). A grade III placenta has a chorionic plate with indentations extending to the basal layer, a placental mass divided into compartments with echo-free areas, and a basal layer with dense, almost confluent echogenic areas.

Several chemical studies of the amniotic fluid have proved fairly reliable in ascertaining fetal age. The most important chemical indices of fetal maturity are the phospholipids in the amniotic fluid. The lecithin/sphingomyelin ratio is approximately 1.0 at the thirty-fifth week. An L/S ratio of about 2.0 indicates pulmonary maturity and little likelihood of respiratory distress syndrome (Fig. II-11). A lower ratio, however, does not necessarily indicate the likely development of respiratory distress syndrome. Measurement of phosphatidyl glycerol (PG) is also a very useful means of assessing pulmonary maturity, especially in diabetic pregnancies. In mature fetuses the ratio of PG to the other phospholipids in the amniotic fluid is increased. A "shake test" (foam stability test) is a rough guide to the presence of surface-active substances.

Several additional chemical tests are less commonly employed today. The concentration of creatinine, for example, should be 2 mg% or more

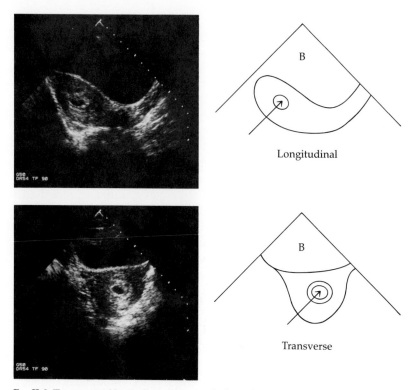

FIG. II-8. Transverse and longitudinal sonograms of a five to six weeks' intrauterine gestation. A 1 cm sac with an echogenic rim is seen within the uterus but no fetus is yet visible. Sac (arrow) and bladder (B) are shown. The early sac of an intrauterine gestation may be confused with a decidual reaction or "pseudosac" that is associated with ectopic pregnancy.

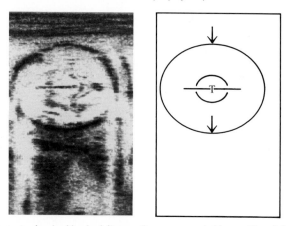

FIG. II-9. Sonogram showing biparietal diameter (between arrows) of fetus at 22 weeks' gestation. The image was obtained at the level of the thalamus (T). This method, although frequently used, is somewhat less accurate than the crown-rump length. Accuracy of both methods, however, varies with gestational age. For the biparietal diameter (BPD), accuracy at 16 weeks is ± 1 week; near term it is ± 3 weeks.

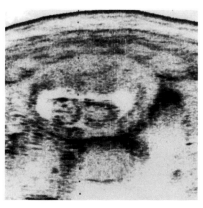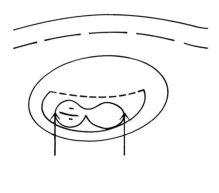

Fig. II-10. Transverse sonogram showing crown-rump measurement of a fetus judged to be of 12 weeks' gestational age. The bilobed structure demarcated by the arrows is the fetus. The head is identified by the intracerebral echoes. Crown-rump measurements are the most accurate sonographic means of assessing gestational age and are most useful from 7 to 13 weeks of gestation.

after the thirty-seventh week of gestation. In the normal term fetus the bilirubin concentration should be negligible. In the mature fetus the osmolality, which is measured by depression of the freezing point and reflects predominantly the concentration of sodium, should be less than 250 milliosmoles.

Measurement of the optical density of the amniotic fluid at 650 nm is another rapid, inexpensive test of fetal pulmonary maturity.

Genetic Disorders

Examination of the amniotic fluid and cells can be used for the following additional purposes: detection of biochemical disorders (enzymatic defects) such as Tay-Sachs disease; ascertaining fetal blood type; detection of the sex of the fetus (by Barr body analysis or karyotype) in cases of sex-linked disorders; and detection of chromosomal disorders (by karyotype), such as Down's syndrome in fetuses of elderly mothers (those over the age of 35).

In a description of the karyotype the first item to be recorded is the total number of chromosomes (including sex chromosomes) followed by a comma (,). The sex chromosomal constitution is recorded after the comma:

46,XX	Normal female
46,XY	Normal male
45,X	Turner's syndrome
47,XXY	Klinefelter's syndrome

Numerical aberrations of the autosomes are indicated by the group letter or individual chromosomal number followed by a plus (+) or minus (−) sign after the sex chromosomal designation:

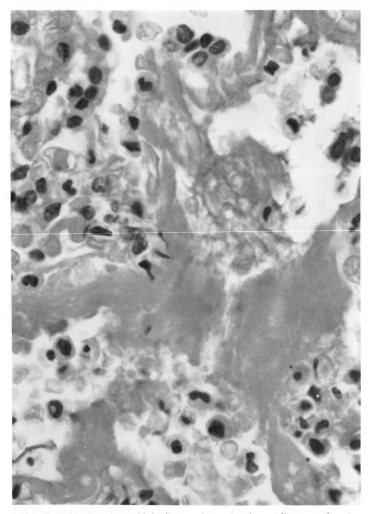

FIG. II-11. Newborn lung with hyaline membranes (respiratory distress syndrome).

45,XX,C−   45 chromosomes, XX sex chromosomes,
                and a missing C-group chromosome
46,XY,18+21−   46 chromosomes, XY sex chromosomes, an
                extra chromosome 18, and a missing chro-
                mosome 21

Chromosomal mosaicism is indicated by two karyotypic designations separated by a diagonal (/):

45,X/46,XY   A chromosomal mosaic with two cell
                  types—one with 45 chromosomes and a
                  single X and the other with 46 chromo-
                  somes and XY sex chromosomes

46,XY/47,XY,G+   A chromosomal mosaic with a normal
                  male cell line and cell line with an extra
                  G-group chromosome

The short arm of a chromosome is designated by the lowercase letter "p" and the long arm by the letter "q". Increase in the length of an arm of a chromosome is indicated by placing a plus (+) sign and decrease in length by placing a minus (−) sign after the designation of the arm:

46,XX,2p+   46 chromosomes with an increase in length of
             the short arm of chromosome 2

A translocation is indicated by the letter "t" followed by parentheses, which include the chromosomes involved:

46,XY,t(Bp−;Dq+)   A balanced reciprocal translocation be-
       or   tween the short arm of a B-group chro-
                    mosome and the long arm of a D-group
46,XX,t(Bp+;Dq−)   chromosome

In a centric fusion translocation in which only one translocation chromosome is present, the semicolon is omitted:

45,XX,D−,G−,t(DqGq)+   45 chromosomes, XX sex chro-
                       mosomes, one chromosome
                       missing from the D-group and
                       one from the G-group, their long
                       arms having united to form a DG
                       translocation chromosome

Trisomy 21 (47,XX,+21, or 47,XY,+21) is the most common trisomy compatible with life. It accounts for 95% of all cases of Down's syndrome. Virtually all affected persons are mentally retarded and 30% have congenital cardiac disease. Less common forms of Down's syndrome involve translocations and mosaicism.

The risks of having a child with Down's syndrome at various maternal ages are as follows:

Maternal Age	Risk of Down's Syndrome
20	1/1,923
25	1/1,205
30	1/885
35	1/365
40	1/109
45	1/32
49	1/12

The risk of having an aneuploidy of any sort at maternal age 44 or above is of the order of 1 in 10. The empirically calculated risks for several common congenital defects in the general population are as follows: anencephaly and meningomyelocele, 1—2/1000; cleft lip with or without cleft palate, 1/1000; and cleft palate, 0.4—1/1000. The frequencies of the more common chromosomal anomalies found in the newborn are as follows: Trisomy 21, 1/800-1/1000 births; Trisomy 18; 1/8000 births; Trisomy 13, 1/20,000 births; XXY, 1/1000 male births; XYY, 1/1000 male births; XXX, 1/950 female births; and X (XO), 1/10,000 female births.

Because congenital malformations account for about 20% of infant deaths in the United States today, the question of amniocentesis to detect these defects assumes great importance. The risk of abortion of about 0.5% after amniocentesis precludes its routine use, but certain conditions are clear indications for the procedure including: advanced maternal age, a prior child with a chromosomal anomaly, a parent with a translocation or other chromosomal anomaly, carriers of inborn errors of metabolism (mendelian disorders), and a prior child with a neural tube defect.

Alpha-fetoprotein (AFP) is produced by the fetus and passes into the amniotic fluid. It is not normally found in the adult, but small amounts diffuse into the pregnant woman's blood. At the site of a neural tube defect that is open (not covered by skin), additional AFP escapes, elevating the level of this protein in the amniotic fluid and usually in the maternal plasma as well. The major open neural tube defects that can be detected by an elevated AFP are anencephaly and open spina bifida. Multiple fetuses and fetal death may also elevate the AFP in amniotic fluid and maternal plasma. Additional causes of elevated AFP include omphalocele, congenital nephrosis, and atresias of duodenum and esophagus.

Approximately one to two neural tube defects occur in every 1000 live births in the United States. Ninety to 95% of these disabling and often fatal defects appear in infants with no family history of such disorders. If a couple have had a child with a neural tube defect in a prior pregnancy, there is a 2% chance of having another affected child. The initial screening test, performed at 16 to 18 weeks' gestation, detects elevated values of AFP in maternal blood. Further testing is accomplished with sonography and amniocentesis.

Indications for amniocentesis and measurement of AFP in the fluid include: a prior pregnancy that resulted in an infant with a neural tube defect, a mother or father who has had a neural tube defect, and probably pregnancy in the siblings of the parents of an affected child. Elevation of acetylcholinesterase in the amniotic fluid is another indication of an open neural tube defect.

Fetal surgery has made possible the correction of certain neural tube defects. Other conditions amenable to this approach include congenital hydronephrosis, congenital diaphragmatic hernia, and obstructive hydrocephalus. The ethical as well as the scientific implications of fetal surgery remain to be elucidated.

More recently, clinical significance has been attached to the finding of a low value of AFP in maternal plasma. Genetic amniocentesis in such patients has led to the detection of fetal aneuploidy in women under the age of 30 years.

Several classes of inherited biochemical disorders are detectable in the middle trimester through analysis of fluid obtained by amniocentesis. Among the disorders of lipid metabolism are Gaucher's disease, GM_2 gangliosidosis type I (Tay-Sachs disease), and the varieties of Niemann-Pick's disease. The disorders of carbohydrate metabolism include galactosemia, glucose-6-phosphate dehydrogenase deficiency, and the glycogen storage diseases. Disorders resulting from disturbances in mucopolysaccharide metabolism are Hurler's, Hunter's, Sanfilippo's, and Morquio's syndromes. Inborn errors of amino acid and organic acid metabolism include homocystinuria, maple syrup urine disease, methylmalonic acidemia, and phenylketonuria. The Lesch-Nyhan syndrome is listed among the miscellaneous disorders.

Cystic fibrosis is the most common autosomal recessive disorder in western Europe and in white Americans. The incidence is about one in 2000 births. An immunoassay based on monoclonal antibodies specific to each of the three major isoenzymes of alkaline phosphatase has been used in diagnosis of cystic fibrosis in the second trimester. The immunoassay, which employs amniotic fluid, is highly sensitive when used in high-risk mothers.

An alternative to amniocentesis for diagnosis of fetal sex and fetal chromosomal disorders is chorionic biopsy. This technique may be performed earlier in gestation than can amniocentesis. Because villi are obtained transcervically, the risks attendant upon invasion of the amniotic sac are avoided. A small risk of abortion, nevertheless, complicates this procedure.

Fetoscopy allows direct visualization of the fetus and sampling of fetal tissues, including blood and skin, for the antenatal detection of fetal defects. Diagnosis of α-thalassemia, sickle cell anemia, and some cases of β-thalassemia are possible through analysis of patterns of DNA from cells in the amniotic fluid without fetoscopy. Genetic disorders that require analysis of fetal serum are hemophilia-A (Factor VIII deficiency), Christmas Disease (Factor IX deficiency), and chronic granulomatous disease. Biopsies of fetal skin have led to the prenatal diagnosis of harlequin ichthyosis, epidermolysis bullosa lethalis, and epidermolytic hyperkeratosis. Biopsy of fetal muscle may soon become a reliable method for detection of Duchenne muscular dystrophy.

Prior to fetoscopy, ultrasonographic examination is required to confirm fetal viability, diagnose placental location and plural gestation, verify gestational age, and ascertain fetal position. Diagnosis of disorders of fetal hemoglobin is also possible during the first trimester by means of trophoblastic biopsy in conjunction with restriction endonuclease analysis of fetal DNA.

Dysmaturity is a discrepancy between birth weight and gestational age. It is associated with increased perinatal mortality and morbidity. The obstetrician must identify predisposing factors and affected fetuses. Dysmaturity may be of the small-for-gestational-age (SGA) or the large-for-gestational-age (LGA) varieties. In SGA the fetal weight is at or below the tenth percentile of the weight appropriate for that gestational age; in LGA the fetal weight is greater than the 90th percentile. The former is often called intrauterine growth retardation (IUGR) and the latter, fetal macrosomia. Both are disorders of the third trimester. Serial measurements of fundal height in centimeters above the symphysis (obtained by tape measure at each antepartum visit) provide clinical assessment of fetal growth. If these clinical measurements suggest an abnormality, ultrasonic assessment of the fetal biparietal diameter, abdominal circumference, and femoral length, as well as the ratios of these measurements, provides accurate information. All diagnoses of abnormalities of growth depend on accurate knowledge of the gestational age.

Fetuses with IUGR are at increased risk for the adverse effects of hypoxia. As neonates they have deficient subcutaneous fat and are at increased risk for hypoglycemia, hypocalcemia, aspiration of meconium, hypothermia, and polycythemia. LGA fetuses are at increased risk for shoulder dystocia.

One third of all cases of IUGR are of the symmetrical type and two thirds are of the asymmetrical type. Symmetrical IUGR is caused by a fetal insult early in gestation, such as infection, a chromosomal anomaly, or radiation. The ratio of circumference of the head to that of the abdomen is below the 95th percentile and both number of cells and content of DNA in the brain are reduced. Such a fetus has a guarded prognosis. Asymmetrical IUGR is caused by an insult later in gestation, such as preeclampsia, chronic hypertension, or diabetes. The ratio of circumference of the head to that of the abdomen is above the 95th percentile and the number of cells is decreased but the DNA content of the brain is normal. "Catch-up" growth is possible in these infants and although intrapartum distress may occur, the prognosis is usually good.

Many maternal, placental, and fetal factors are associated with intrauterine growth retardation. The more important include: hypoperfusion of the placenta; maternal undernutrition and hypoxia; low maternal socioeconomic status; small placenta; maternal smoking, strenuous exercise, and consumption of alcohol during pregnancy; high altitude; maternal disorders, including cardiac disease, anemia, pulmonary insufficiency, essential hypertension, preeclampsia, chronic renal disease, and some hemoglobinopathies; transplacental viral infection, for example rubella or cytomegalovirus; infection with mycoplasmas or *Chlamydia trachomatis;* chromosomal abnormalities in the fetus, including trisomies and deletion syndromes; and pregnancy prolonged beyond 42 weeks. Women who have had a baby with IUGR in a prior pregnancy are at risk for repetition of that complication.

Two important metabolic disorders, phenylketonuria and hypothyroidism, can be detected soon after birth and both are amenable to treatment. The incidence of phenylketonuria (PKU) is approximately 1/20,000 live births. If not diagnosed and treated early in the neonatal period, it causes severe mental retardation. Hypothyroidism, which occurs more commonly, with an incidence of approximately 1/4000 live births, is also associated with mental retardation if the disorder is not detected and treated soon after birth. Phenylketonuria is identified by a simple test of the urine, and hypothyroidism by measurement of TSH in serum. Many states require that both tests be performed routinely.

Infants may be large for gestational age for the following reasons: constitutionally large by heredity, transposition of the great vessels, recipient twin in the transfusion syndrome, and overproduction of insulin. Infants who produce an excess of insulin include those born to diabetic mothers and those with certain cases of erythroblastosis fetalis. Fetal macrosomia secondary to maternal diabetes can be greatly diminished, if not eliminated, by strict control of the diabetes during the antepartum period.

Antepartum Care

A major purpose of antepartum care is education of the patient about pregnancy, labor, and delivery. Pregnancy should be explained as a physiologic process rather than an illness. The antepartum period is a good time to practice preventive medicine, since ideally the patient is under a physician's supervision for at least half a year. During this time dental care may be obtained, an adequate diet planned, and advice about sexual activity and contraception given.

Diet should be well-balanced to include meat, eggs, fresh fruits and vegetables, and a total intake of 2500 calories. Iron should be prescribed with meals (p.168). Prenatal vitamins may be given routinely, although a well-balanced diet with iron supplementation is usually adequate for a healthy woman. The pregnant patient must be urged to discontinue smoking cigarettes and drinking alcoholic beverages for at least the duration of the gestation.

The patient should be told that bathing is permissible, especially since bath water does not enter the vagina, and that coitus may be continued, if desired, so long as there are no abnormalities of pregnancy and it causes no discomfort. Normal physical activity should be permitted to the point of fatigue. The patient should be encouraged to walk about a half mile a day and to continue work as long as she is physically and emotionally comfortable. Short-distance travel is associated with no increased risk, but long trips may be hazardous during the third trimester, especially if opportunities for ambulation and recumbency are limited.

Vigorous exercise during pregnancy is contraindicated in the following circumstances: history of three or more spontaneous abortions, ruptured membranes, premature labor, plural gestation, incompetent cervix, bleeding and cardiac disease.

Classes for both parents are valuable to allay fear of labor and delivery. The patient should be informed that any drug taken during pregnancy may affect the fetus (Table 5) and that maternal infectious diseases may affect the fetus and neonate (Table 6). The obstetrician must therefore be consulted before the patient undergoes any diagnostic investigation or treatment. In general, no drug or treatment, including over-the-counter preparations, should be given to the pregnant woman unless the benefits clearly outweigh the risks to mother and fetus. The mother should receive no immunizations with live virus during pregnancy. Vaccines with killed organisms and tetanus toxoid may be administered during pregnancy.

Table 5. Effects of Maternal Drugs on the Fetus and Newborn

Maternal Drug	Effect
Alcohol	Deficiencies in growth; mental retardation; facial anomalies
Amethopterin	Anomalies; abortion
Ammonium chloride	Acidosis
Androgens	Masculinization
Cephalothin	Positive direct Coombs' test
Chlorambucil	Anomalies; abortion
Chloramphenicol	"Gray baby syndrome"
Coumadin	Fetal death; hemorrhage; osseous deformities
Diethylstilbestrol	Vaginal adenosis; uterine anomalies
Diphenylhydantoin (Phenytoin)	Dysmorphic facies; cardiac defects; abnormal genitalia
Diuretics	Imbalance of electrolytes
Heroin	Neonatal death or convulsions
Hexamethonium	Neonatal ileus
Iodine-containing preparations	Abnormal development of thyroid

Table 5. Continued

Isoretinoin	Abortion; multiple fetal defects
Lead	Abortion; stillbirth
Methimazole	Goiter; mental retardation
Morphine	Neonatal death or convulsions
Novobiocin	Hyperbilirubinemia
Phenobarbital	Neonatal bleeding
Potassium iodide	Goiter; mental retardation
Progestins	Masculinization; possible cardiovascular anomalies
Propylthiouracil	Goiter; mental retardation
Reserpine	Nasal congestion and drowsiness
Salicylates (excess)	Neonatal bleeding
Smoking (cigarettes)	Low-birth-weight babies
Streptomycin	Damage to acoustic nerve
Sulfonamides	Kernicterus
Tetracyclines	Discoloration of teeth; inhibition of osseous growth
Thalidomide	Phocomelia
Thiazides	Thrombocytopenia
Trimethadione	Craniofacial and cardiac anomalies
Valproic acid	Neural tube defects
Vitamin K analogues (excess)	Hyperbilirubinemia

During the antepartum visits the various methods of analgesia and anesthesia should be discussed and the patient informed about the available forms of contraception. She should be given the opportunity to decide whether she prefers breast feeding or a bottle. She should also be encouraged to select possible names for the baby. The patient must be taught to recognize uterine contractions, or "hardening" of the uterus, and the feeling of pelvic pressure that is associated with premature labor. She should also be taught to recognize the onset of labor, that is, the regular, painful, progressive contractions, and to report any "bloody show" (blood-tinged mucous discharge from the vagina that accompanies dilatation of the cervix during the first stage of labor) or rupture of the membranes (definite or suspected). The patient should be instructed to take no food after the onset of labor. It is important that the patient be taught to report any of the danger signs of pregnancy, including vaginal bleeding, abdominal pain, edema, blurred vision, headache, or any significant change in well-being.

Table 6. Effects of Maternal Infections and Radiation on the Fetus and Newborn

Maternal Insult	Effect
Cytomegalovirus	Microcephaly; retardation of somatic growth; cerebral damage; hearing loss
Rubella	Cataracts; deafness; cardiac lesions; expanded syndrome including effects on all organs
Syphilis	Fetal death with hydrops (severe); abnormalities of skin, teeth, and bones (mild form)
Toxoplasmosis	Chorioretinitis; hydrocephalus; calcification in CNS; and possible effects on all organs
Varicella-zoster	Intrauterine and persistent postnatal disease; possible effects on all organs, including scarring of skin and muscular atrophy
X-Radiation	Microcephaly; mental retardation

The daily diet should contain 150 g of carbohydrate, 100 g of fat, and 85 g of protein. Six to 8 glasses of fluid including a quart of milk a day are desirable. The diet should specifically contain adequate amounts of calcium, iron, vitamin A, thiamine, riboflavin, niacin, folic acid, and vitamins C and D. The sodium content of carbonated beverages and beer and the caloric content of alcohol must be considered in planning the diet. Consumption of alcohol should be discontinued during pregnancy to minimize the likelihood of "the fetal alcohol syndrome," which includes dysfunction of the central nervous system, deficiency of linear growth before and after birth, and underdevelopment of the midface, especially the eyes. If specific dietary problems arise, a professional dietician should be consulted.

A maternity girdle and low-heeled walking shoes may add to the patient's comfort. No hand-bulb syringes must be used for douching because of the danger of air embolism, and the douche bag should be held not more than two feet above the level of the hips to avoid undue pressure. Coitus may be continued unless premature labor, rupture of the membranes, vaginal bleeding, or infection supervenes. Cunnilingus during pregnancy may introduce air into the vagina and cause fatal air embolism.

High-Risk Pregnancy

An important aspect of antepartum care is identification of the high-risk pregnancy. First, a history of medical, surgical, or obstetric complications in prior pregnancies must be elicited. Risk is increased in patients of low socioeconomic status and possibly unwed mothers, in whom the effects of environment and heredity are often difficult to separate. Extremes of age (under 15 and over 40) are associated with more obstetric complications. Obesity, addiction or habituation to drugs, and heavy intake of ethanol are all associated with an increased rate of complications. Heavy smoking by the mother leads to lighter but not necessarily premature infants. High parity itself, moreover, is associated with a significantly increased rate of obstetric complications.

In obtaining the obstetric history the doctor should inquire specifically about diabetes mellitus, preeclampsia-eclampsia, tuberculosis, rheumatic fever, cardiac disease, renal disease, syphilis, rubella, pelvic operations, hereditary diseases, and a familial history of twins. History of the menses and prior pregnancies should be recorded in detail. The most common complication leading to serious perinatal morbidity and mortality in the United States today is preterm labor. A major factor associated with preterm labor is a prior preterm birth (p. 133).

Many findings obtained on examination of the mother give clues to high-risk pregnancy. The more important include: abnormal growth of the uterus (suggesting plural gestation, hydramnios, and hydatidiform mole), dead fetus, contracted pelvis, abnormal presentation, and large or abnormal fetuses. Fetal indications of a high-risk pregnancy include retardation of growth and abnormal cardiac sounds.

Laboratory tests used to detect possible complications of pregnancy include: serologic test for syphilis; examination of urine for glucose and protein; urine culture (particularly with a history of urologic infection); hemoglobin and hematocrit; Papanicolaou smear; glucose tolerance test in the presence of glycosuria, a history suggestive of diabetes, or a history of prior newborns weighing greater than 9 pounds. It is advisable to perform a single measurement of plasma glucose after an oral glucose load at about the twenty-sixth week of gestation. If this value is elevated, a full 3-hour glucose tolerance test is performed. Cultures for gonorrhea should be obtained from urethra, cervix, and anus. Fetal disease may be anticipated by identifying the mother's blood group (ABO) and Rh-type. In cases of Rh-negative mothers, antibody titers are indicated (p. 155).

Antepartum visits should be made monthly during the first six months, every two weeks from the twenty-eighth to the thirty-sixth week of gestation, and weekly during the last month. The patient should consult the obstetrician as early in pregnancy as possible. Advantages include early assessment of gestational age and careful surveillance during the period of early fetal growth. In the first few months of pregnancy the fetus is most susceptible to the effects of ingested drugs and environmental factors such as radiation.

Accurate records must be kept in an effort to optimize maternal and fetal well-being. The patient must be encouraged to ask questions during her visits and the obstetrician must answer them factually and completely. Several suitable books are readily available to provide further information to the patient.

At each antepartum visit the blood pressure, weight, and urinary protein should be checked, primarily to detect preeclampsia (p. 150). The normal midtrimester drop in blood pressure should be recognized. Weight gain is normally kept to 20 to 25 pounds, but in the absence of fluid retention a greater weight gain in itself may not be harmful to the outcome of the pregnancy. In no case should the patient be placed on a program of weight reduction, and "diet pills" of all varieties are contraindicated in pregnancy. In cases of suspected recent exposure to rubella, antibody titers should be obtained. (p. 164).

The height of the fundus should be measured at each visit and the fetal heart tones recorded (by stethoscope or Doptone). The presence of plural gestation or abnormalities of presentation should be noted as soon as they are suspected. In the third trimester it is appropriate to repeat the hemoglobin, the serologic test for syphilis, and the gonococcal cultures. A pelvic examination including Papanicolaou smear is performed at the initial visit, but it may be easier to perform manual pelvimetry later in pregnancy when the pelvic tissues are more relaxed. Frequent vaginal examinations are helpful in identifying early cervical dilatation in patients who are at risk for preterm delivery.

Manual pelvimetry should include an estimate of the diagonal conjugate (the distance from the promontory of the sacrum to the inferior border of the pubic symphysis), which is normally about 12.5 cm. The true conjugate is the distance from the promontory of the sacrum to the superior border of the symphysis. It cannot be measured manually, but is estimated by subtracting between 1 and 2 cm from the diagonal conjugate, depending on the height and inclination of the symphysis, to give a figure of about 11 cm. The intertuberous diameter (the distance between the inner aspects of the ischial tuberosities) is the transverse diameter of the outlet and is generally about 11 cm. If the diagonal conjugate is below 11.5 cm, further study is often indicated (p. 146).

Other pelvic features of obstetric importance are the shape of the pubic arch, the width of the sacrosciatic notch, the prominence of the ischial spines, the shape of the forepelvis, the convergence of the side walls, and the thickness of the bones. Because X-ray pelvimetry exposes mother and fetus to ionizing radiation and because appropriate clinical management is usually possible without it, the technique is rarely used today.

In discussing common complaints with the patient it is important to distinguish physiologic alterations of pregnancy from disease and to discourage the use of drugs whenever possible. Lassitude, urinary frequency without dysuria, ptyalism, tingling of the breasts, palpitation, tachypnea, and occasional syncope ordinarily require no special therapy. Backache may be relieved by supportive garments and a firm mattress. Constipation may be treated with mild laxatives, a high intake of fluids, and a diet high in bulk. Varicosities may require supportive stockings and elevation of the legs. Leukorrhea, hemorrhoids, and heartburn occasionally require symptomatic therapy. Painful uterine contractions must be distinguished by continued observation from true progressive labor (p. 140). Any severe abdominal pain requires ruling out appendicitis, cholecystitis, partial abruption of the placenta, and urinary tract infection.

Pica, which may interfere with a regular diet, should be recognized and discouraged. Emotional liability, as opposed to a true psychiatric disturbance, usually responds well to simple support and reassurance.

Hyperemesis gravidarum is an exaggeration of nausea and vomiting of pregnancy, with systemic effects such as acetonuria and substantial weight loss. It is best treated with multiple small feedings high in carbohydrates and sometimes antiemetics.

Hyperemesis gravidarum appears to be less common than formerly and is no longer considered a form of preeclampsia. Etiologic factors may include elevated levels of gonadotropins and steroids, delayed gastric emptying, and emotional predisposition. It is most common between the second and fourth months of pregnancy. The important components of therapy include maintenance of fluid and electrolyte balance, correction of other diseases, and avoidance of obnoxious odors. Other causes of nausea and vomiting must be ruled out, including viral hepatitis and ulcers. Hyperemesis gravidarum is often associated with immature personalities but is not apparently increased in unwed mothers. Psychologic support is important and antiemetic agents such as cyclizine, meclizine, and dicyclomine have been useful and have not proved to be teratogenic. Despite its value the drug Bendectin was taken off the market by its manufacturer in 1983. Drastic and punitive measures have no place in the management of hyperemesis, and abortion is rarely indicated.

Labor and Delivery

Labor is divided into three stages. The first stage begins with the onset of true labor and ends with full dilatation of the cervix (10 cm). The second stage begins with full dilatation of the cervix and ends with birth of the fetus. The third stage begins with birth of the fetus and ends with the expulsion or extraction of the placenta and membranes.

Labor is characterized by progressive dilatation and effacement of the cervix, which accompany regular painful uterine contractions normally associated with descent of the presenting part (that part of the fetus that is lowest in the pelvis). The presenting part is the part of the fetus that is palpated by the examining finger on vaginal examination, for example, occiput, sacrum, or acromion. Dilatation of the cervix is the enlargement of the external cervical os caused by the upward retraction of the myometrial fibers during labor. Effacement of the cervix is accomplished when the cervix is completely retracted, the cervicovaginal angle has disappeared, and only the external os remains to be dilated.

During the course of pregnancy painless irregular uterine contractions (Braxton Hicks contractions) increase in intensity and regularity and eventually become true labor pains. The contractions of true labor begin in the lumbar region at intervals of 20 to 30 minutes. At the onset of labor the mucous plug is expelled from the cervical canal.

Normal uterine contractions are characterized by fundal dominance (contractions that are strongest in the top of the uterus and weakest in the bottom) and symmetry (contractions that arise simultaneously from both cornual areas). The intensity of normal uterine contractions increases progressively so that at the height of a contraction the intrauterine pressure rises to between 40 and 60 mm Hg and the myometrium can be indented only with strong digital pressure. Uterine contractions with an intensity of less than 15 mm Hg are ineffective. The tonus of the uterus is the pressure between contractions, when the myometrium can be indented with only moderate digital pressure. Tonus is normally less than 25 mm Hg. The frequency of uterine contractions gradually increases to about one every 2 to 3 minutes and the duration to between 45 and 60 seconds at the end of labor.

The upper segment of the uterus is the thick contractile portion; the lower segment is thin and passive. A retraction ring may divide the two.

The first stage of labor is concerned with overcoming cervical resistance and the second stage with the passage of the fetus through the birth canal. Although the lengths of the stages of labor may normally vary within fairly wide limits, the first stage lasts about 6 to 8 hours in the multipara and 10 to 14 hours in the primigravida. The second stage usually does not last longer than 2 hours. The third stage usually lasts about 15 to 30 minutes and should be terminated after 1 hour at the latest.

The three main factors determining the course of labor are the powers (uterine contractions), the passages (bony pelvis and maternal soft tissues), and the passenger (size and position of the fetus). Progress in labor is determined by the gradual descent of the presenting part, or change in station (the location of the presenting part in the birth canal). Designation of station as "+" or "−" refers to the level in cm below (+) or above (−) the ischial spines. Station 0 is attained when the presenting part has reached the level of the ischial spines. Station +2, for example, is attained when the presenting part is 2 cm below the spines. When the occiput is at station 0, the vertex is said to be engaged clinically. Engagement occurs when the fetal biparietal diameter has passed the plane of the pelvic inlet.

Presentation, or lie, is the relation of the long axis of the fetus to the long axis of the mother. It may be either longitudinal or transverse. With a longitudinal lie the presenting part is either the head (cephalic) or the breech. With a transverse lie the shoulder is the presenting part. Cephalic presentations are classified according to the relation of the head to the body of the fetus. When the head is fully flexed and the chin contacts the thorax, the occiput, or vertex, presents. When the neck is fully extended and the occiput contacts the back, a face presentation results, with the chin, or mentum, the presenting part. Intermediate conditions include the sinciput, in which the large fontanelle presents, and the partially extended head, in which the brow presents. Sinciput and brow presentations usually convert spontaneously to vertex or face presentations by flexion or extension, respectively, during the course of labor.

Position is the relation of a designated point on the presenting part of the fetus to a designated point in the maternal pelvis. For example, if the occiput occupies the right anterior portion of the maternal pelvis, the position is designated ROA or ORA. In the case of a breech the designated point is the sacrum (as in LST) and in the case of a face it is the chin, or mentum (as in RMA).

Labor is divided into latent and active phases. The latent phase is the time between the onset of regular contractions and appreciable cervical dilatation. During this phase the cervix effaces but dilates only slightly. The active phase extends from the end of the latent phase to the end of the first stage of labor. The events of labor normally occur in an orderly sequence at accelerating rates. Variations from this pattern may indicate impending abnormalities (p. 140).

The latent phase in a primigravida lasts about 8.5 hours and ends when the cervical dilatation is about 2.5 cm. The accelerated phase lasts about two hours and occurs while the cervix dilates from 2.5 to 4 cm. The phase of maximal slope lasts about two hours and occurs while the cervix is dilating from 4 to 9 cm. The phase of deceleration lasts about two hours and occurs during the last centimeter of dilatation of the cervix. In the second stage intrauterine pressures in excess of 100 mg Hg may result from bearing down. The total length of labor in the multigravida is normally several hours shorter than in the primigravida.

During labor the fetal head may be in various degrees of flexion or extension (habitus or attitude). A fully flexed vertex occurs in about 95% of all deliveries. The fetal head may undergo certain changes in shape to accommodate to the configuration of the maternal pelvis. Molding is a change in shape of the fetal head in labor that is brought about by the forces of labor, the resistance of the bony pelvis, and the loose connections between the bones of the fetal skull. The head may also undergo lateral flexion (asynclitism). Synclitism exists when the fetal head presents with the sagittal suture midway between the maternal symphysis pubis and the sacral promontory. In anterior asynclitism, the sagittal suture approaches the sacral promontory and the anterior parietal bone of the fetus is the most dependent portion of the head in the birth canal. In posterior asynclitism the sagittal suture approaches the symphysis pubis and the posterior parietal bone is most dependent.

During long labor a caput succedaneum may be formed. In the process, the portion of the fetal scalp immediately over the cervical os becomes edematous and may prevent the differentiation of sutures and fontanelles by the examiner. Molding, asynclitism, deflexion, and caput may all lead to an erroneous diagnosis of station, since the head feels lower than it actually is.

Throughout labor the fetal status must be monitored by the recording of heart rate by stethoscopic auscultation or electronic methods. The maternal status must be monitored by the recording of vital signs every 30 to 60 minutes, urinary output, and the quality and frequency of uterine contractions. Fetal position should be ascertained by abdominal and vaginal examination. When the fetal position or presentation is in doubt, consultation is mandatory. Failure of progress of labor for 2 hours and detection of a small pelvis or a fetal abnormality also require consultation. The method of pain control, analgesia and anesthesia, may affect the progress of labor and the status of the fetus (p. 110)

If no vaginal bleeding is detected, vaginal examination should be performed to ascertain station, cervical dilatation, and effacement. The vaginal examinations must be repeated under aseptic conditions at appropriate intervals. During the first stage the patient may have an enema, but the perineal preparation need not include shaving of all pubic hair. A large-bore intravenous needle should be inserted, especially if there is increased likelihood of blood transfusion. The patient should take nothing by mouth after the onset of labor. The bladder should not be catheterized unless the patient cannot void or a difficult delivery or cesarean section is anticipated. During the second stage, as the patient begins to bear down, maternal vital signs and fetal heart rate are monitored more frequently. The multipara is often transported to the delivery room when the cervix is 7 to 8 cm dilated, and the primigravida at full dilatation, depending on the rapidity of labor.

The normal mechanism of labor in a vertex involves: engagement, descent, flexion, internal rotation, extension, external rotation, and expulsion. When the fetal head has negotiated the pelvic outlet and its largest diameter is encircled by the vulvar ring, crowning is said to take place. After the head is born the shoulders are delivered, followed more or less rapidly by the remainder of the body.

The cause of the onset of labor is basically unknown, but important factors may include: release of the progesterone block of myometrial activity, changing relations or oxytocin and oxytocinase, and fetal endocrine activity. The enzymatic release of arachidonic acid, a precursor of prostaglandins, may be important in the initiation of parturition. The increased synthesis of prostaglandin E_2 in the amnion may be stimulated by a substance in fetal urine. Thus, the fetus may play a major role in determining the onset of labor. Oxytocin may stimulate uterine contractions by acting both directly on the myometrium and indirectly on the production of decidual prostaglandin. The principal problem in diagnosis of labor is its differentiation from false labor, which unlike true labor is unaccompanied by progressive dilatation of the cervix or increasingly forceful contractions. It can be differentiated from the latent phase of labor with certainty only on retrospective evaluation. The hazards of false labor include maternal exhaustion, apprehension, and premature intervention by the obstetrician.

Diagnosis of presentation and position is made by abdominal palpation, vaginal examination, auscultation of the location of the fetal heart, and sonography. The breech feels softer than the head, and the back feels larger, smoother, and firmer than the small parts, which are nodular and irregular. If the cephalic prominence is felt on the same side as the small parts, the head is flexed. If the cephalic prominence is on the same side as the back, the head is extended.

The typical obstetric inlet has an anteroposterior diameter of 11.5 cm and a transverse diameter of 13 cm. The plane of least pelvic dimensions in the midpelvis has an anteroposterior diameter of 12 cm and a transverse diameter of 10.5 cm. If the inlet and midpelvis are adequate, it is unlikely that the outlet will cause difficulty in delivery. The normal biparietal diameter of the term fetus is about 9.25 cm and the bitemporal about 8.0 cm. When there is difficulty in engagement in the transverse diameter, the bitemporal diameter is often substituted for the biparietal diameter and extension is the result. In normal circumstances, flexion results in making the suboccipitobregmatic (9.5 cm) rather than the occipitofrontal (11.5 cm) the engaging diameter.

The anterior fontanelle (bregma) is the diamond-shaped junction of the parietal and frontal bones. The posterior fontanelle is the triangular junction of the two parietal bones and the occipital bone.

X-ray pelvimetry, though used frequently before the advent of obstetric sonography, has been virtually replaced by a trial of labor with electronic fetal monitoring.

If the membranes rupture during the first stage of labor, the size of the uterine cavity decreases and the pressure of the head directly on the lower uterine segment may improve the efficiency of labor. Immediately after rupture of the membranes the fetal heart should be auscultated and a vaginal examination should be done to detect prolapse of the umbilical cord. If the origin of the fluid is in doubt, nitrazine paper may be used to detect the alkaline pH that is characteristic of amniotic fluid but not urine. Microscopic examination may be employed to detect fetal epithelial cells, globules of fat, and hair, which are normally released into the amniotic fluid. Ferning is also characteristic of amniotic fluid but not urine.

Fetal monitoring during labor is greatly improved by adding electronic surveillance to clinical methods. In the first stage of labor the fetal heart rate may drop during contractions but rises again to between 120 and 160/min between contractions. Occasionally detection of tachycardia, bradycardia, or irregularity of the fetal heart rate by stethoscope calls attention to the need for more precise electronic monitoring. The combination of abnormalities of the fetal heart rate and passage of meconium is serious. Auscultation of the fetal heart should be even more frequent during the second stage.

Several patterns emerge when simultaneous electronic monitoring of the fetal heart rate and uterine contractions is carried out. In normal tracings beat-to-beat variability is found. When deceleration of the fetal heart rate occurs immediately after the onset of uterine contractions, the pattern known as early deceleration results (Fig. II-12). This pattern should suggest compression of the fetal head and is not an ominous sign. Bradycardia occurring late after the onset of uterine contractions is called late deceleration (Fig. II-13). This pattern usually indicates uteroplacental insufficiency. A variable onset of deceleration with respect to the uterine contraction often indicates compression of the umbilical cord (Fig. II-14).

Late decelerations may be caused by placental insufficiency, maternal hypotension, or excessive uterine activity resulting from administration of oxytocin. If correction of maternal hypotension and discontinuation of the oxytocin do not correct the pattern, prompt delivery may be indicated. Variable deceleration is often corrected by repositioning of the mother and administration of oxygen. If these factors do not reverse the pattern, operative delivery may be required to avoid the hazards of prolonged compression of the cord. Analysis of the pH of blood from the fetal scalp is helpful in deciding the management. Acidosis (pH of less than 7.20) suggests a more serious degree of fetal compromise necessitating delivery (Table 7).

Whether to use electronic fetal monitoring in all labors is still controversial. The technique is clearly indicated, however, in all high-risk pregnancies including, but not limited to: meconium-stained amnionic fluid, retardation in intrauterine growth, oligohydramnios, preterm or postterm gestation, antepartum medical complications, the use of oxytocin in labor, and abnormalities of the fetal cardiac rate identified by other methods. Inasmuch as a low-risk pregnancy may become high-risk intrapartum, electronic monitoring should always be available. If intermittent cardiac auscultation is used instead of electronic monitoring, it must be done at least every 30 minutes during the first stage of labor and at least every 15 minutes during the second stage; in both stages it should be performed for a period of 30 seconds after the uterine contraction.

The oxytocin challenge test, or contraction stress test, indicates the response of the fetal heart rate to transient reduction in uteroplacental blood flow, and thus fetal oxygenation. A positive test is the occurrence of late deceleration with uterine activity below the level of three to four contractions in 10 minutes. The test is considered negative, or normal, when late decelerations are absent at this level of stress. The test usually requires 1 to 2 hours.

Self-stimulation of the nipple is a simple way to assess fetal well-being. The patient rubs one nipple to stimulate the release of endogenous oxytocin. If sufficient uterine activity is thus produced, infusion of intravenous oxytocin is avoided.

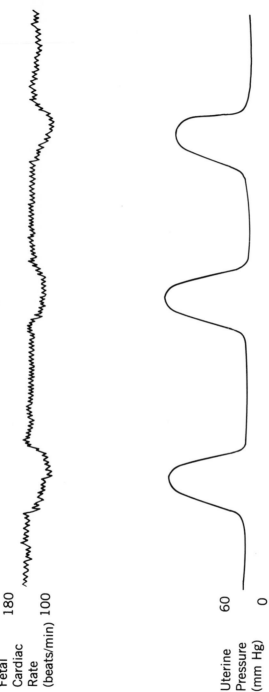

Fetal
Cardiac
Rate
(beats/min)

180

100

Uterine
Pressure
(mm Hg)

60

0

Early Deceleration (Compression of Fetal Head)

Fɪɢ. II-12. Early deceleration, showing uniform pattern with onset and end of deceleration synchronous with onset and end of uterine contraction. Pattern is related to pressure on fetal head.

104

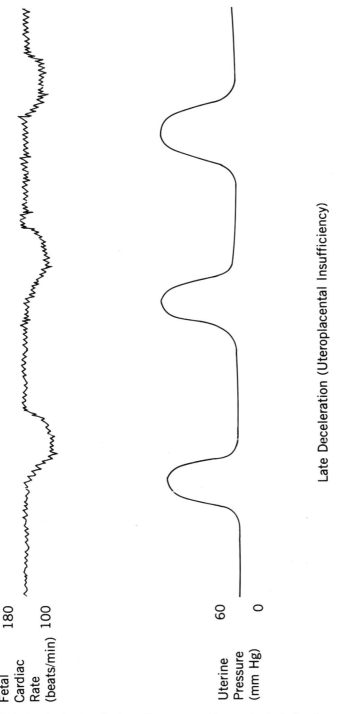

Fig. II-13. Late deceleration, showing uniform pattern with onset after beginning of uterine contraction and recovery after end of uterine contraction. Pattern is related to uteroplacental ischemia.

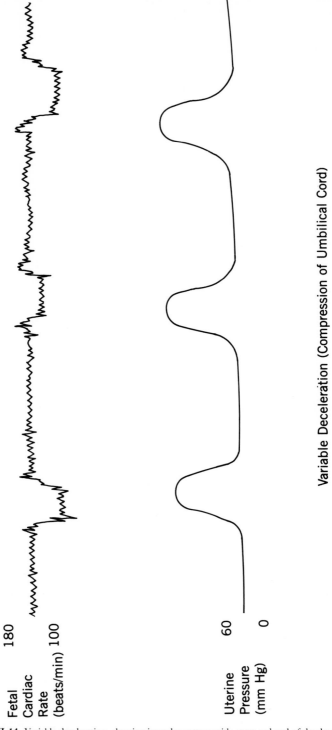

Fig. II-14. Variable deceleration, showing irregular pattern with onset and end of deceleration bearing no consistent relation to onset and end of contraction. Pattern may be related to compression of cord.

Table 7. Management of Fetal Distress

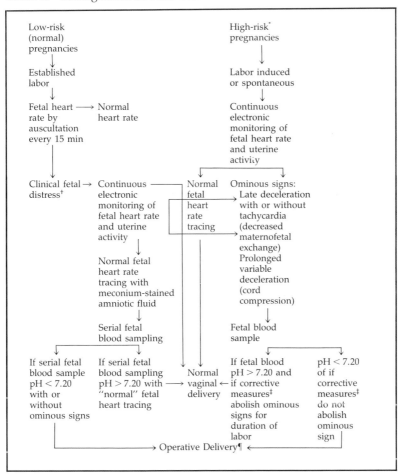

*For example: diabetes, chronic hypertension, preeclampsia, premature labor, and third-trimester bleeding.

†Auscultated fetal hear rate >160 of <120/min or meconium staining of amniotic fluid.

‡Change in maternal position to alleviate maternal hypotension or compression of the umbilical cord. Decrease or discontinuation of intravenous oxytocin to alleviate uterine hyperactivity.

¶Anticipate birth of depressed newborn and have available obstetric or pediatric personnel skilled in direct resuscitation.

The nonstress test is another valuable means of assessing fetal well-being. The baseline and variability of the fetal heart rate and the occurrence of accelerations of the rate with fetal movement are taken as indications of the integrity of the reflexes controlling cardiac rate. The pattern is considered reactive if the baseline rate is between 120 and 150 beats per minute, the baseline variability is 10 beats per minute or more, and two or more fetal movements accompanied by accelerations of 15 beats per minute or more occur during a period of 20 minutes. The advantages of nonstress monitoring include the virtual absence of contraindications, the avoidance of drugs, and the short period of only 30 minutes required for its completion.

The test is not useful before the thirtieth week because the fetal response is not present until then.

In both stressed and nonstressed monitoring the prediction of fetal compromise is less certain than the confirmation of fetal well-being. These tests must be used in conjunction with indices of fetal maturity and other relevant clinical data in deciding the need for delivery.

Fetal well-being may be assessed by the so-called biophysical profile, which includes the nonstress test and measurements of fetal breathing movements, gross fetal movements, fetal tone, and volume of amniotic fluid. A normal fetus will have, in addition to a reactive nonstress test, the following responses: at least one episode of fetal breathing of at least 60 seconds' duration within a period of 30 minutes; at least three discrete fetal movements within the 30-minute period; upper and lower extremities in full flexion, trunk in flexion and head flexed on chest, and extension of extremities or spine with return to flexion; and amniotic fluid throughout the uterine cavity with the largest pocket of fluid greater than 1 cm in vertical diameter.

Amnioscopy is a technique for evaluation of the color and turbidity of the amniotic fluid by means of transcervical examination through an endoscope. Meconium staining is associated with a lower Apgar score and a higher perinatal mortality. It is used more often in countries other than the United States and is valuable principally in conjunction with other tests of fetal well-being.

Most fetuses engage in the occiput transverse position and deliver as occipitoanteriors. In a typical labor the head is born by extension over the perineum, followed by external rotation back to the transverse or anterior position. The patient should be instructed not to bear down before the second stage.

Delivery is most safely accomplished spontaneously or by low forceps extraction. Excessive or premature administration of anesthesia results in the need for more difficult forceps deliveries.

The head should be delivered between contractions. During spontaneous delivery the obstetrician should cover the patient's anus with a towel and apply upward pressure on the chin through the perineum. The obstetrician's other hand should be used to control the egress of the head by gentle pressure on the occiput. As soon as the head is delivered, loops of cord should be removed from the infant's neck. Delivery of the shoulders should be delayed until they are in the anteroposterior diameter of the outlet. One shoulder should be delivered at a time. The rest of the body ordinarily follows with ease. In normal circumstances, the newborn should be suspended by its feet below the level of the placenta to allow transfusion of placental blood.

The third stage of labor comprises separation and expulsion of the placenta. Its successful spontaneous termination depends primarily on uterine activity. After the placenta separates, the shape of the uterus changes from discoid to globular and the top of the uterus is felt at a somewhat higher level. At the same time there is a gush of blood and a lengthening of the cord, which yields when slight traction is applied. Uterine bleeding after expulsion is controlled by occlusion of blood vessels by sustained uterine contraction.

The placenta should be routinely inspected for completeness and the birth canal should be examined for injuries. A missing placental cotyledon or a torn vessel on the chorionic surface indicates retention of a placental fragment within the uterus.

The vital signs of the mother and the uterine tone should be monitored for at least one hour post partum. The patient should remain in the recovery room for two to three hours before being returned to her room.

The average blood loss during normal vaginal delivery without episiotomy is about 300 ml. The blood loss is often greater than it appears without accurate measurement. Loss of blood of 500 ml or more is considered postpartum hemorrhage (p. 148).

The placenta is best delivered as soon as possible after it has separated, with care taken to remove all the membranes as well. In the presence of excessive bleeding or after 30 minutes in the third stage, it is wisest to remove the placenta manually under appropriate anesthesia. No traction should be applied to the cord until the placenta has separated. Premature or forceful traction may result in inversion of the uterus, a serious accident that may lead to shock and may require hysterectomy.

Many regimens for the administration of oxytocic agents after delivery of the fetus are employed. One satisfactory method is the addition of 10 units of oxytocin to the intravenous infusion. The oxytocin should not be given in a single intravenous push. To avoid trapping of the placenta, it is wisest to defer the administration of oxytocin until after the completion of the third stage, although some obstetricians use it at the time of delivery of the shoulders. Derivatives of ergot are used less often now immediately post partum and should be avoided in the presence of hypertension or preeclampsia.

When uterine atony is anticipated, as in cases of overdistension of the uterus or prolonged labor, it is best to keep the oxytocin infusion running for several hours after the third stage.

Obstetric Anesthesia

The problems of obstetric anesthesia differ from those of anesthesia in general because of the altered maternal physiologic functions in pregnancy, the presence of the fetus (which is particularly sensitive to anesthetic agents), alterations in maternal homeostasis resulting from anesthesia, and often the emergency during which obstetric anesthesia must be administered. In particular, the changes in maternal respiratory and cardiovascular function tend to alter the speed of induction of inhalation anesthesia; the diminished volumes of spinal canal and epidural spaces necessitate smaller amounts of local anesthetic agents to achieve a similar level of anesthesia; furthermore, there is the effect of the diminished venous return, which results from the compression of the inferior vena cava by the gravid uterus (supine hypotensive syndrome). The drop in peripheral resistance and the venous dilatation secondary to sympathetic blockade resulting from major regional anesthesia, in combination with compression of the inferior vena cava, may cause life-threatening hypotension. Finally, all general and local anesthetic agents, barbiturates,tranquilizers, and narcotics cross the placenta. Most relaxants of skeletal muscle (curare, pancuronium, and succinylcholine), however, cross the placenta poorly or not at all. Analgesia may be achieved during labor and delivery by means of narcotics and other types of analgesic agents, regional blocks, or general anesthetics.

General anesthesia must be avoided when the patient's stomach is full, unless intubation can be promptly carried out. Analgesia (such as 100 mg of meperidine) should be withheld until labor is clearly established, and regional blocks should not be performed until the cervix is at least 4 to 5 cm dilated. The choice of anesthetic agent depends on the availability of the technique and the skills of the personnel. It should be tailored to the type of delivery and the desires of the patient whenever possible. For example, a low forceps or a normal spontaneous delivery of a multipara can often be effected by analgesia and a pudendal block. A forceps delivery of a primigravida, however, may often be managed best by lumbar epidural, caudal, or low subarachnoid (saddle) block. Deliveries that require extensive intrauterine manipulations should be conducted with maximal uterine relaxation, such as is provided by halothane.

Analgesia during labor is most often accomplished by means of narcotic agents. These drugs rapidly cross the placental barrier and may depress the fetus' respiratory center. The intravenous and intramuscular routes of administration are both acceptable. Narcotics are often used in combination with tranquilizers because of a possible synergistic effect. Barbiturates, unless used in anesthetic amounts, are not analgesic but reduce anxiety. Tranquilizers alone are often helpful during early first stage of labor when anxiety rather than pain is the principal problem. Use of these drugs, particularly diazepam, may, however, result in depressed newborns. Scopolamine in large doses and in combination with narcotics causes amnesia, but also excitation, which may be difficult to control. Inhalation anesthetic agents such as nitrous oxide and methoxyflurane may be used in subanesthetic concentrations to obtund painful sensations during labor and delivery. Inhalation analgesia may be used in conjunction with narcotics. The patient must be carefully watched and protected from unnecessarily deep anesthetic levels.

Anesthesia remains a major cause of maternal mortality in the United States (p. 173), where general anesthesia is still widely used to achieve relief of pain during delivery. General anesthesia, however, is responsible for most of the deaths attributable to anesthesia; 50% are attributed to aspiration of gastric contents. This form of anesthesia must be approached with the greatest care if the patient has eaten within 6 hours of the onset of labor. Even if 6 hours have elapsed, however, the stomach is not necessarily empty. All patients in labor must therefore be considered to have full stomachs. Aspiration of gastric contents is often fatal. All inhalation anesthetic agents, with the exception of nitrous oxide, depress the myometrium and can abolish uterine contractions. Halothane is most effective for inducing uterine relaxation.

The purpose of regional anesthesia is to block sensations arising from the cervix, uterus, and perineum. The pain pathways during the first stage of labor involve visceral afferent nerve fibers that arise from the uterus and cervix. The pains of the second stage of labor arise from somatic afferent receptors and fibers in the vulva and perineum and travel by way of the inferior hemorrhoidal nerve, the labial nerve, and the dorsal nerve of the clitoris. These nerves join to form the pudendal nerves.

Paracervical blocks administered in the vaginal fornices block pain impulses at the level of the uterine plexus. Lumbar epidural and caudal blocks interrupt pain sensations in the epidural space before the nerve's entrance into the spinal canal. Subarachnoid anesthesia blocks the nerves in the spinal canal where they bathe directly in the cerebrospinal fluid. Pudendal blocks interrupt only pain sensations arising from the perineum and vulva and are useful only in the second stage of labor. Paracervical anesthesia does not block the sacral segments and therefore does not relieve pain arising from the perineum. Spinal, lumbar epidural, and caudal blocks may be used to interrupt painful sensations from the uterus, cervix, and perineum. Because paracervical anesthesia is frequently associated with fetal bradycardia, it is not popular in modern obstetrics.

Toxic reactions to local anesthetics are most often related to overdosage. This result can occur after careless use of any of the aforementioned techniques, although least frequently with spinal anesthesia. Hypotension can occur after any major block that results in sympathetic blockade. Therapeutic measures must be taken immediately if hypotension develops. The steps include lifting the uterus off the inferior vena cava or placing the patient on her left side; rapidly hydrating the patient with 1 liter of a balanced salt solution; and administering vasopressors intravenously if the prior measures do not return the pressure to normal levels. Since the drop in blood pressure must be quickly noted and treated, major regional blocks must be preceded by: the application of a blood pressure cuff that is to be left in place, constant monitoring of vital signs, and the establishment of a dependable means of intravenous medication (intravenous cannulas or catheters).

Less local anesthetic is required to achieve a given level of anesthesia in late pregnancy than in the nonpregnant state. Hypotension resulting from regional blocks must be treated to maintain a maternal systolic pressure of at least 100 mm Hg. Lower pressures may impair perfusion of the intervillous space and result in fetal hypoxia, hypercarbia, and acidosis.

Complications resulting from major regional blocks such as spinals and epidurals include overdosage, with respiratory depression or arrest and convulsions; chemical and septic meningitis; constrictive arachnoiditis; and postpuncture headaches. The complications are generally preventable.

Regional anesthesia is preferred over other forms of anesthesia because the complications arising from these methods are preventable or treatable, and they appear to be less dangerous to the fetus. Spinal, caudal, and lumbar epidural anesthesia are contraindicated, however, if: the patient is hypovolemic or suffers from a complication that is accompanied by blood loss; the patient is hypotensive; the skin is infected at the site of puncture; there is an active neurologic disorder; the patient is receiving anticoagulants; the patient refuses the procedure; and the physician lacks the experience or adequate equipment for administration, monitoring, and resuscitation.

The need for highly skilled physicians to administer major regional blocks or general anesthesia has not been met. The safest, easiest way of achieving pain relief during parturition thus appears to be the careful administration of small doses of narcotics and tranquilizers during labor, followed by a pudendal block and subanesthetic concentrations of general anesthetic agents for delivery.

General anesthetic agents in obstetrics may be employed for three purposes: in subanesthetic concentrations for analgesia; general anesthesia of a degree sufficient for delivery or cesarean section; and as myometrial relaxants for intrauterine manipulations such as breech extraction or version and extraction, replacement of an inverted uterus, relaxation of tetanic contractions, and removal of a retained placenta. Because of the danger of aspiration of gastric contents, endotracheal intubation is always indicated when general anesthesia is administered. Endotracheal intubation can be performed with the patient awake after topical anesthesia of the pharynx and larynx or with the patient asleep after the rapid administration of a fast-acting barbiturate, followed immediately by a muscle relaxant. Cricoid pressure should be maintained to compress the esophagus and prevent regurgitation. Pressure should be maintained until the endotracheal tube cuff has been inflated and the airway protected.

Aspiration of gastric contents can cause death by two different mechanisms. First, obstruction of the airway renders the capillary-alveolar gas exchange impossible. Second, if the pH of the gastric juice is below 2.5, contact with the respiratory tree often results in bronchospasm, pulmonary edema, and death. If the patient survives the immediate injury, severe atelectasis and chemical pneumonitis may ensue. The treatment consists in quickly clearing the airway by suction, administering 100% oxygen by means of an endotracheal tube, treating the bronchospasm with isoproterenol, and using mechanical ventilation with positive end expiratory pressure (PEEP) and high doses of steroids and broad-spectrum antibiotics.

The first and most important factor in the prevention of aspiration pneumonitis is the awareness that every parturient is at high risk. It has been recommended that patients receive nonparticulate oral antacids throughout labor. Although these drugs do not protect against aspiration of solid material, they probably lower the risk of damage to the lung by acidic fluids.

The use of vasopressors for the treatment of hypotension secondary to major regional blocks is based on their ability to increase venous return by activating adrenergic receptors and therefore causing a rise in peripheral resistance and venous constriction. Furthermore, they can increase venous return by activating beta-adrenergic receptors and cause an increase in cardiac inotropism and chronotropism. Some vasopressors do both. In obstetrics the use of alpha-adrenergic stimulants such as methoxamine or phenylephrine is contraindicated because the rise in maternal blood pressure is accompanied by uterine arterial vasoconstriction, diminished perfusion of the intervillous space, and resulting aggravation of fetal distress. Agents that have mainly beta-adrenergic receptor-activating effects are preferred. The principal agent is ephedrine. In preeclampsia-eclampsia, vasopressors must be used in smaller doses because of the increased adrenergic receptor sensitivity. Derivatives of ergot must not be used after vasopressors have been administered. There is a synergistic effect between these two types of medications that may lead to lethal hypertension.

The rate at which an inhalation agent will affect a fetus is difficult to predict because it is dependent upon many variables involving the mother, placenta, and fetus. An intravenous anesthetic agent such as thiopental, however, rapidly reaches the fetus. After an injection of thiopental, equilibrium between mother and fetus is reached in less than two minutes. Thereafter the fetus continues to accumulate thiopental. As the concentration of thiopental in the mother diminishes, however, as a result of redistribution to various spaces, so does that in the fetus. The concentration in the umbilical vein is always higher than in the umbilical artery. It is therefore impossible to deliver the baby before equilibrium is reached. The anesthesiologist should not hurry the obstetrician, but the obstetrician should work with careful speed. Despite the rapid placental transfer of thiopental, this agent in conjunction with nitrous oxide, oxygen, and succinylcholine is preferred when general anesthesia is chosen.

When spinal anesthesia is to be administered it is important to be proficient in the use of 25-gauge or 26-gauge spinal needles. The incidence of postpuncture headaches is directly related to the size of the rent made in the dura in the course of the administration of a spinal block. During administration of an epidural block, a small test dose must be given to ascertain whether the subarachnoid space has been inadvertently entered. The accidental subarachnoid injection of the usual doses of local anesthetics used for epidural anesthesia may result in a very high or total spinal block, which may cause respiratory arrest. Resuscitation equipment and drugs must be on hand at all times.

Popular local anesthetics for use in obstetrics include esters such as procaine, chloroprocaine, and tetracaine, and amides such as lidocaine, mepivacaine, and bupivacaine. The amides generally diffuse and penetrate better and have a longer duration of action. The esters are metabolized in the plasma by pseudocholinesterase. Tetracaine is used almost exclusively for spinal anesthesia. For local infiltration and pudendal or epidural blocks the maximal recommended doses for procaine and chloroprocaine are 1000 mg; for lidocaine and mepivacaine the maximal dose is 500 mg. The doses for spinal anesthesia are, of course, much smaller.

Toxic reactions are usually caused by high levels of the local anesthetic agent in the blood, as a consequence of exceeding the maximal recommended dose or inadvertent intravascular administration. The toxic effects include stimulation of the central nervous system (confusion, vertigo, tinnitus, twitching, or convulsions), cardiovascular collapse, or both. Allergic reactions are uncommon. The treatment is as follows: maintenance of the airway, oxygen, intravenous anticonvulsants such as diazepam to counter stimulation of the central nervous system, intravenous fluids, and cardiac massage or defibrillation for cardiovascular collapse. Chloroprocaine and bupivacaine are popular agents for epidural anesthesia. Bupivacaine in a concentration of 0.75% is no longer recommended for obstetric anesthesia because of reports of cardiac arrest. Only concentrations of 0.25% and 0.5% should be used in obstetrics.

Normal Puerperium

The puerperium is the period of time, usually about six weeks, from delivery until the genital tract returns to the normal nonpregnant condition. After an uncomplicated spontaneous delivery the multiparous patient may often be discharged as early as 24 hours post partum. Primigravidas and many patients with episiotomies usually remain for a few days in the hospital post partum. In all cases the patient should be allowed to ambulate and to use the bathroom as soon after delivery as she can comfortably do so. She should be encouraged to empty her bladder at least every 8 hours to avoid overdistension, which may predispose to infection. A mild cathartic may be prescribed after 48 hours if the patient has not moved her bowels. Codeine (0.06 g) and aspirin (0.6 g) may be prescribed for afterpains. These pains are more common in the multipara but usually subside by 48 hours post partum. The perineum should be kept clean during the puerperium. Painful sites of episiotomy or lacerations may be treated symptomatically with sitz baths and a heat lamp. If the lochia (vaginal discharge during the puerperium) are particularly bloody, methergine (methylergonovine maleate) may be prescribed in 6 doses of 0.2 mg at 4-hour intervals.

Postpartum chills are common but not necessarily indicative of infection. The temperature should be recorded every 6 hours for the first 24 hours at least. A slight elevation (rarely over 100.4° F) is common after a difficult labor or delivery, but it usually falls to normal within 24 hours. A sustained elevation or a rising temperature suggests infection (p. 171).

In certain situations in which Rh-isoimmunization is thought to have been initiated, anti-D globulin (RhoGAM) should be given shortly after delivery (p. 155). Since the patient may ovulate very soon after delivery, contraceptive advice should be given while she is still in the hospital and repeated at the time of the postpartum checkup. Coitus is best avoided until all discomfort has subsided and all wounds have healed.

The postpartum examination usually takes place between 4 and 6 weeks after delivery. At that time the physical examination should include measurement of the blood pressure and hematocrit; examination of the breasts, abdomen, and pelvis; and a Papanicolaou smear if it has not been done in the preceding 6 months.

Colostrum is secreted for about 2 days after delivery, at which time lactation begins. The mammary ducts usually fill with milk between the second and fifth days post partum. Suckling and the administration of oxytocin stimulate the let-down of milk. The milk attains a stable composition after the first month. If the mother does not intend to breast feed the baby, lactation may be suppressed by steroids early in the puerperium. One method is estradiol valerate and testosterone enanthate (Deladumone) in a single intramuscular injection of 4 ml. Treatment with steroids after lactogenesis is initiated will not suppress the process. A newer method of suppressing lactation is the use of bromocriptine. When no drugs are used, painful engorgement of the breasts normally disappears within 36 to 48 hours. Symptomatic relief of engorgement is provided by supportive binders, ice bags, fluids by mouth, and analgesics. The obstetrician must be aware that many drugs administered to the nursing mother may be transferred to the newborn in the milk.

Prolactin (LTH, lactogenic hormone, mammotropic hormone) is required for lactogenesis (initiation of the secretion of milk) and galactopoiesis (continuation of secretion of milk). The hormone also serves to maintain the cholesterol precursors in the ovary for the secretion of steroids.

Prolactin is a polypeptide similar in structure to growth hormone. It is secreted by acidophils of the hypophysis. Its release is promoted by thyrotropic releasing hormone (TRH) and inhibited by prolactin inhibiting factor (PIF) of the hypothalamus. PIF and GnRH are generally released and repressed together. Thus, when LH and FSH are secreted, prolactin is inhibited. An exception occurs during the midcycle gonadotropic surge, when there is also marked release of prolactin, presumably an action of TRH. During lactation and occasionally in women receiving phenothiazine tranquilizers, both PIF and GnRH are repressed, with resulting anovulation. Lactation may be induced via the central nervous system from stimulation of the breast or psychologic factors associated with nursing.

By the tenth postpartum day the uterus has descended into the pelvis, that is, has regressed to the size of a 3 months' gestation. During the puerperium the weight of the uterus decreases from 1000 to 100 g. In this process, known as involution, individual myometrial cells decrease in size. The endometrial lining is usually restored after several weeks as the placental site regresses. Involution of the placental site is normally complete by 6 weeks post partum. Interference with this process may result in late postpartum hemorrhage (p. 172). The lochia gradually change from red (lochia rubra) to pinkish or yellowish (lochia serosa) to whitish (lochia alba) as the proportions of erythrocytes, leukocytes, and decidual debris change. Lochial discharge normally continues for 4 to 8 weeks post partum.

The first normal menstrual period usually occurs between 4 and 8 weeks post partum and is often heavy. Although the first ovulation usually occurs about 4 to 6 weeks post partum, the patient may ovulate as early as the second or third day post partum. Lactation may delay or suppress menstruation, but does not in itself provide sufficient contraception.

During the puerperium a diuresis resulting in a loss of about five pounds takes place between the second and the fifth postpartum days. The loss of fluid may be even greater in preeclampsia (p. 150).

Leukocytosis immediately after labor may rise to as high as 30,000. The hemoglobin and hematocrit may vary somewhat during the postpartum period, but normally do not fall below the values before delivery unless the blood loss has been considerable. At 1 week post partum the blood volume is normally back to the level before pregnancy.

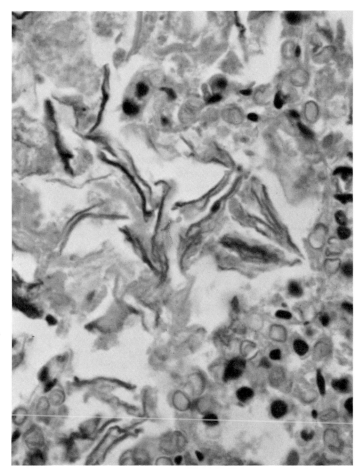

FIG. II-15. Newborn lung with aspirated amniotic fluid containing numerous squamous cells seen on end.

The Neonate

As soon as the head is delivered, the infant's nose and throat should be aspirated with a bulb syringe to clear the airway. Particularly when the fetus has been stressed it is necessary to take these measures to prevent aspiration of amnionic fluid (Fig. II-15). After delivery the infant should be held with the head dependent above the obstetrician's lap but below the level of the perineum to facilitate transfusion of placental blood. The cord of a normal infant should be allowed to stop pulsating before it is clamped. Double clamping is best performed about 4 cm from the umbilicus. The infant should be kept warm before transfer to the nursery. Handling of the newborn, particularly the premature, should be minimized. The newborn's eyes should be treated with penicillin or erythromycin ointment or silver nitrate (1% solution) to prevent gonorrheal ophthalmia.

The Apgar score should be recorded at 1 minute and 5 minutes after birth to permit objective transfer of information among obstetrician, anesthesiologist, and pediatrician (Table 8). Apgar scores of 0 to 3 denote a severely depressed infant; scores of 4 to 6 suggest a fair general condition; and scores of 7 or above indicate a baby in good condition. All newborns with scores of 0 to 3 and many with scores of 4 to 6 need resuscitation.

TABLE 8. Apgar Score

SIGN	0	1	2
Cardiac rate	Absent	Slow (Below 100)	Over 100
Respiratory effort	Absent	Weak cry; hypoventilation	Good effort; strong cry
Muscular tone	Limp	Some flexion of extremities	Active motion; extremities well flexed
Reflex irritability (Response to stimulation) of skin of feet	No response	Some motion (Grimace)	Crying and active
Color	Blue, pale	Body pink; extremities blue	Completely pink

The newborn's footprints should be obtained and identification bracelets applied as soon after delivery as possible.

The pediatrician should be forewarned of any complications during pregnancy, labor, or delivery and should be informed about any drugs that the mother may have taken. If the baby is jaundiced soon after birth, it may require an exchange transfusion. In such a case the umbilical cord should be left long and a pediatric consultation obtained immediately.

The placenta should be examined carefully to see whether it is intact and to detect gross lesions. A cross section of the cord should be inspected to detect the absence of one umbilical artery, an anomaly that is found in 1% of infants and is often associated with other congenital malformations.

Circumcision is performed in a sizable majority of newborn males in the United States. Although the American Academy of Pediatrics has stated that there are no strictly medical indications for routine neonatal circumcision, cultural and personal preferences have maintained the popularity of the procedure in the United States. Among the stated advantages are prevention of penile carcinoma and facilitation of penile hygiene. Alleged additional benefits include prevention of phimosis and paraphimosis, decrease in urinary tract infections, and avoidance of pain, risks, costs, and psychologic effects of late circumcision. Good technique and instruments minimize the risks, which, although uncommon, include hemorrhage and infection. The procedure should be deferred in premature or sick infants and those with a bleeding tendency or a penile anomaly such as hypospadias. The operation should not be performed immediately after delivery but at least 24 hours later, or until the infant has been observed to remain well. The American College of Obstetricians and Gynecologists refers to the decision about neonatal circumcision as a "personal choice." In this context, an informed written consent for the procedure must be obtained.

Resuscitation

The delivery room must have immediately available at all times equipment for resuscitation, including endotracheal tubes and laryngoscopes, umbilical vein catheters, oxygen, and suction devices.

A newborn may be incapable of maintaining normal respiration for several reasons including: intrauterine asphyxia or inadequate placental exchange, prematurity, congenital anomalies, drugs administered to the mother, trauma during labor or delivery, and anemia secondary to blood group incompatibility.

Intrauterine hypoxia or asphyxia may result from maternal disorders such as diabetes, hypertension, hypotension, preeclampsia, and renal disease. Additional factors include premature separation of the placenta, compression of the umbilical cord, and tetanic uterine contractions. Prematurity is associated with incomplete development of the lung and inadequate production of surfactant, leading to alveolar instability and predisposition to respiratory distress syndrome. Narcotics, barbiturates, and all anesthetic agents administered to the mother may depress the fetal central nervous and cardiovascular systems.

In resuscitating an infant the first step is rapid clearing of the airway. The second step is administration of oxygen by positive pressure ventilation. Resuscitation by bag and mask connected to a source of oxygen will permit the administration of 30 to 100% oxygen, depending on the type of equipment used. In performing positive pressure ventilation, the infant's head should be elevated and extended without exerting any pressure on soft tissues. When the babies are severely ill and when the results of the efforts at resuscitation are poor, oral endotracheal intubation under direct vision with a laryngoscope should be performed, but only by personnel trained in this technique. Improper or premature use of endotracheal intubation may result in further jeopardizing the baby by delaying the administration of oxygen and prolonging asphyxia. Careful external cardiac massage is mandatory if the baby suffers from severe bradycardia and appears pale.

Hypoxemia rapidly leads to anaerobic metabolism and acidosis, which should be counteracted by the administration of 4.5 to 9 mEq/kg of sodium bicarbonate. This drug should be administered into the fetal circulation by means of a catheter introduced into the umbilical vein or one of the umbilical arteries. Fetal blood pH and base excess should be checked repeatedly and, if necessary, compensated by further administration of sodium bicarbonate.

Narcotic antagonists should be administered only if respiratory depression can be clearly attributed to prior administration of narcotics to the mother. Asphyxia or hypoxia results in delayed closure or in reopening of the ductus arteriosus, pulmonary hypertension, and decreased pulmonary blood flow, which together form the syndrome of persistent fetal circulation. In addition, it leads to loss of alveolar surfactant, unstable alveoli, acidosis, and cardiovascular depression. All these factors, if untreated, increase hypoxia and create a vicious cycle.

III

Obstetric Complications

Spontaneous Abortion

The most common causes of vaginal bleeding in women in the reproductive age group are related to complications of pregnancy. Abortion is the termination of pregnancy before fetal viability, or when the fetus weighs less than 500 g. Abortion may be spontaneous (occurring through natural causes) or induced (by mechanical or medicinal means). Most spontaneous abortions occur in the second or third month of gestation. Induced abortion may be medically indicated or elective. Local laws rather than medical grounds determine whether an abortion is legal or criminal.

Spontaneous abortions occur in more than 10% of all pregnancies. The true rate is probably closer to 20%, for many of the earliest abortions are not recognized by the patient. The cause of spontaneous abortion is unknown in the majority of cases, although blighted ova and other less profound fetal genetic abnormalities (proved by chromosomal analysis) may be detected in a significant proportion of conceptuses. Local and systemic maternal disorders and environmental factors may all be operative. Maternal diseases include acute and chronic infections (such as those caused by Toxoplasma, *Listeria monocytogenes*, and T-mycoplasmas), chronic wasting diseases, and endocrinopathies (particularly thyroid dysfunction). Local factors include anomalies of the reproductive tract, myomas, or incompetence of the cervix. External environmental factors include trauma, radiation, and cytotoxic drugs.

Threatened abortion is diagnosed on the basis of any vaginal bleeding in the first 20 weeks of pregnancy. Only half of all cases of threatened abortion will progress to abortion regardless of treatment. Diagnosis requires a gynecologic examination to rule out other causes of vaginal bleeding, such as cervical polyps and neoplasms as well as injuries to the lower genital tract. With threatened abortion the uterine bleeding may be accompanied by cramps and backache, the uterine size is consistent with the menstrual history, and the cervix is not dilated. Especially if the pain accompanying uterine bleeding is severe, other complications of pregnancy must be ruled out, such as ectopic pregnancy and hemorrhagic corpus luteum.

Treatment of threatened abortion is conservative, namely, mild sedation and a few days of bedrest. Longer periods are not justified, for abortion cannot be forestalled by further bedrest. There is no drug therapy of proven effectiveness. When threatened abortion progresses to incomplete abortion, part of the product of conception is passed. Usually a portion of the placenta is retained and the incompletely emptied uterus continues to bleed. Hemorrhage may be slight or sufficient to produce shock. Abortion is usually preceded by fetal death and histologic examination generally reveals necrosis and hemorrhage in the decidua. The most effective treatment of incomplete abortion is curettage (suction or sharp), with oxytocin employed in the larger uteri (10 to 12 weeks' size or larger). An intravenous infusion should be started; in the presence of moderate or severe bleeding blood should be crossmatched and available. Complications (more common before the laws governing induced abortion were liberalized) include sepsis and shock. Septic abortion is a major cause of maternal mortality in the United States.

In cases of complete abortion, the entire product of conception is passed. Bleeding is usually minimal and no treatment is ordinarily required.

In cases of missed abortion, the fetus dies but is retained in utero for more than two months. Diagnosis is made on the basis of regression of the signs of pregnancy or absence of fetal heart beat on sonographic examination followed by lack of spontaneous abortion. The uterus should be evacuated as soon as the fetus is known to be dead. Early missed abortion may often be managed by intravenous oxytocin followed by curettage. Later abortions may require stimulation of uterine contractions by prostaglandin.

Habitual abortion is defined as three or more consecutive spontaneous abortions. Known causes include uterine anomalies, incompetence of the cervix, inadequate corpus luteum, hypothyroidism, vascular and renal maternal diseases, and immunologic incompatibilities (or perhaps excessive similarities) between the parents.

Since half of all threatened abortions fail to progress to frank abortion, any treatment will have a 50% chance of success. Progestin therapy has not been proved effective; it may, furthermore, cause retention of the products of conception and possible masculinization of the genitalia of the female fetus. One quarter to one half of all abortuses will have chromosomal anomalies such as autosomal trisomy (50%), monosomy X (25%), polyploidy (20%), and others (5%).

Threatened abortion becomes imminent when the cervix continues to dilate, usually in conjunction with an increase in abdominal pain. The abortion is considered inevitable when the membranes rupture through a dilated cervix. In patients with imminent and inevitable abortions the abortions should be completed.

An unusual complication of a missed abortion is hypofibrinogenemia, which ordinarily does not occur until 5 weeks or more after fetal death.
Late abortions occurring in the second trimester may be caused by

placental abnormalities and maternal diseases such as chronic hypertension. Syphilis may be a cause of late abortion (after the fourth month). Late abortions usually have no discernible cause; they resemble premature deliveries rather than early abortions in the relatively slight bleeding and the moderately severe pain.

The incompetent os is a cause of habitual midtrimester abortion that is not common but is amenable to surgical treatment. It is diagnosed by a history of signs and symptoms that appear in a sequence different from that of the usual incomplete abortion. In the case of incompetent os, the painless, bloodless dilatation of the cervix is followed by rupture of the membranes and then abortion. The pregnancy may be saved by the timely placement of a suture around the internal os. If the pregnancy is carried to term, a cesarean section may be performed or the suture may be cut.

Induced abortions, particularly those performed illegally, may be complicated by hemorrhage, sepsis, acute renal failure, and bacteremic shock. Treatment includes massive antibiotics, scrupulous regulation of fluids and electrolytes to tide the patient over the oliguric phase, and removal of necrotic foci that may be a source of toxins. Nephrotoxic antibiotics must be employed with great caution in patients with impaired renal function. Roentgenograms of the abdomen should be obtained to rule out a foreign body in the peritoneal cavity or free gas under the diaphragm, both of which indicate perforation of the uterus. Endotoxic shock complicating abortion leads to a high maternal mortality.

Abortion may be induced legally for medical (for example, cardiac, renal, and psychiatric) indications or electively, according to local statutes. Medical indications may be maternal (to preserve the life or health of the mother) or fetal (to prevent abnormalities, as with rubella, or genetic defects, as indicated by amniocentesis.) Techniques, with indications and contraindications for each, are discussed in Unit 7.

Very early abortions (before 6 weeks) and late abortions (after the sixteenth to twentieth weeks) may be complete. The common abortion (between the eighth and twelfth weeks), however, is usually incomplete, requiring a curettage. In spontaneous abortion many of the villi may show hydropic change.

Trauma is not a common etiologic factor in abortion. To prove a traumatic cause it must be shown that bleeding and abortion occur shortly after the trauma and that there is no abnormality of the conceptus. Habitual abortion requires careful investigation. In addition to a thorough history and physical examination, a minimal investigation includes a chest film, complete blood count, serologic test for syphilis, indices of thyroid function, glucose tolerance test, hysterogram, measurement of basal body temperature, endometrial biopsy, and progesterone assay.

Septic abortion usually results from instrumental or chemical interference. Uterine perforation, bacterial shock, and hemolysis may be associated. The prominent pathogens were formerly streptococci and staphylococci, which produced bacteremia. The principal offenders now are gram-negative bacilli (E. coli and related organisms), which may produce endotoxic shock, with hypotension, oliguria, and occasionally disseminated intravascular coagulation. Septic abortion caused by pathogenic clostridia may produce, in addition, hemolysis and jaundice. The treatment comprises massive antibiotics and attempts to maintain renal function and normal blood pressure. The patient may present with a foul purulent discharge, a boggy tender uterus, and temperature spikes. Prompt curettage to remove necrotic foci is indicated, except in the presence of extrauterine spread (parametritis).

Hypovolemia must be corrected and central venous pressure monitored to avoid overhydration. Metabolic acidosis must be corrected. Endotoxic shock should be suspected whenever hypotension and oliguria are not promptly reversed by intravenous fluids and blood transfusions. Corticosteroids are often given in the face of an inadequate response to fluids, blood, and antibiotics. The blood pressure must be maintained to assure renal perfusion, although the roles of vasoconstrictors and vasodilators are still somewhat controversial. Pressor amines are often given in the presence of warm, dry skin, and vasodilators in the presence of cold, clammy extremities. Mannitol may be used in an attempt to produce diuresis. The role of heparin in preventing or treating intravascular coagulation in cases of infected septic abortion is still controversial. If necrotic foci in the uterus are not accessible to curettage or if there is evidence of uterine perforation, laparotomy and possible hysterectomy may be required as lifesaving measures. The successful management of endotoxic shock depends upon early consultation with the dialysis team and prompt efforts to prevent permanent renal damage.

Ectopic Pregnancy

Pregnancy in any location other than the body of the uterus is considered ectopic. The vast majority of ectopic pregnancies occur in the oviduct (Fig. III-1). The diagnosis must be considered in any patient of reproductive age with menstrual irregularity, vaginal spotting, or abdominal pain. Diagnosis of ectopic pregnancy, ruptured or unruptured, is made by the finding of elevated concentrations of β-hCG in the serum (generally greater than 6,500 m.i.u./ml) and the absence of an intrauterine gestational sac on sonographic examination. The finding of a gestational sac in an extrauterine location is also indicative of ectopic pregnancy, but it is most often not recognized by ultrasound. If the β-hCG concentrations are lower than 6,500 m.i.u./ml, the measurement should be repeated in approximately 1 week. The levels of β-hCG in the serum should exceed 6,500 m.i.u./ml and a gestational sac should be visible by 6 weeks if the pregnancy is intrauterine and viable.

About 40,000 ectopic pregnancies occur per year in the United States, accounting for about 5.7% of all maternal deaths.

Ectopic pregnancy may be caused by any factor that retards passage of the fertilized egg from ovary to endometrium. The most

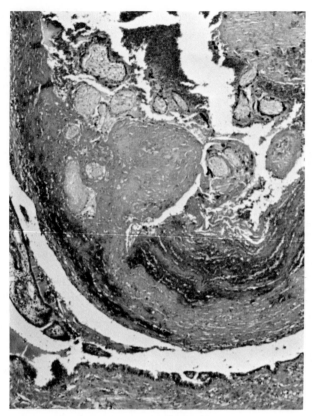

FIG. III-1. Ectopic pregnancy, showing chorionic villi involving wall of oviduct.

common cause is prior salpingitis. Rupture, which usually occurs at about 8 to 10 weeks' gestation, may be heralded by severe abdominal pain, clinical tenderness, syncope, a drop in hematocrit, and shock. Hemoperitoneum often causes pain referred to the shoulder and is frequently diagnosed by culdocentesis, although false-negative and false-positive taps may occur. Ultrasound is usually effective in identifying hemoperitoneum, but laparoscopy may be required for this purpose. Urinary pregnancy tests based on hCG are often misleading (false-positive and false-negative). If there is any doubt about the diagnosis, laparotomy is indicated.

The differential diagnosis, which is that of the acute abdomen in a woman of reproductive years, includes appendicitis, pelvic inflammatory disease, rupture of a follicle or corpus luteum cyst, and even threatened abortion. The primary treatment is surgical, with replacement of fluids and blood as soon as possible. If the patient desires future pregnancy, the tube is not severely damaged, and bleeding can be controlled, simple removal of the prod-

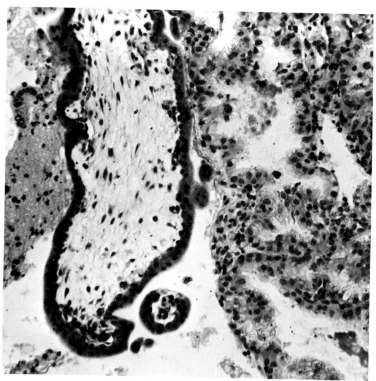

FIG. III-2. Tissue obtained by curettage from first-trimester pregnancy, showing early villus and Arias-Stella reaction in the adjacent endometrial epithelium.

ucts of conception through a linear salpingotomy may be performed. In all other situations, partial or total salpingectomy is the preferred procedure.

Tubal gestation appears to have tripled in frequency in the last 15 years, now occurring at the rate of about 14 per 1,000 reported pregnancies. Any factor that interferes with the function of the fimbriae or causes strictures or adhesions of the tubal wall may predispose to ectopic pregnancy. The intrauterine device and surgical procedures on the oviduct have been important factors in recent years, but prior tubal infection remains the most common cause. The uterus usually grows at a normal rate for about 6 to 8 weeks and a decidual reaction (without trophoblastic tissue) is commonly found in the endometrium. The Arias-Stella reaction, which comprises endometrial epithelial atypia and vacuolated cytoplasm, is not pathognomonic of oviductal pregnancy but may be found whenever there is functioning trophoblastic tissue anywhere in the body (Fig. III-2). The termination of the gestation depends largely on the location. Pregnancies in the ampulla, particularly the distal portion, frequently abort with minimal signs. Pregnancies in the isthmus usually rupture into the peritoneal cavity or between the leaves of the broad ligament. Rupture of a pregnancy in the interstitial portion of the tube may be rapidly followed by massive hemoperitoneum and severe shock. Such patients may die before reaching the hospital. Rupture is sometimes precipitated by a Valsalva maneuver, as with straining at stool.

The clinical picture of ectopic pregnancy usually includes a normal temperature and a normal or only moderately elevated white count. The classic triad of amenorrhea, vaginal bleeding, and pain occurs in only 25% of cases. An adnexal mass may be present or absent. None of the individual signs occurs in more than 75% of cases and the accuracy of diagnosis does not exceed 80%.

Conservative surgical treatment (expression of the pregnancy from the tube or removal of the products of conception through a linear salpingotomy) should be attempted in a woman who wishes to retain her potential for childbearing. Control of bleeding can often be achieved with pressure, cautery, or fine suture. If hemostasis is not complete, a partial salpingectomy must be performed. Total salpingectomy is performed only when the tube is severely damaged or the patient has no desire for further fertility. Oophorectomy should not be performed if the ovary is normal. Hysterectomy is indicated only for cornual pregnancy with severe damage to the uterus. If the uterus is not badly damaged and the patient desires further fertility, hysterectomy should not be performed because pregnancy is still possible after salpingectomy by means of embryo transfer. The use of intravenous methotrexate in conservative management of ectopic pregnancy is not yet standard practice.

Primary abdominal and ovarian pregnancies are rare. Most are secondary to tubal gestation. An abdominal pregnancy is characterized by easy palpation of the fetal parts, abnormal presentations (often transverse lie), and radiologic evidence of a fetus that appears to be overlying the maternal vertebral column. Although the fetus may be carried to term, it is usually removed abdominally as soon as it is diagnosed. The placenta should be left in place unless it can be easily removed without endangering the adjacent maternal structures. The fetus in cases of abdominal pregnancy may die and calcify to form a lithopedion. Ovarian pregnancy almost always requires oophorectomy. The rare cervical pregnancy usually requires hysterectomy to control hemorrhage, although gentle curettement and ligation of the internal iliac arteries occasionally have been successful.

Trophoblastic Growths

Gestational trophoblastic growths include hydatidiform mole, invasive mole (chorioadenoma destruens), and choriocarcinoma. Hydatidiform mole, a developmental anomaly that may have hy-

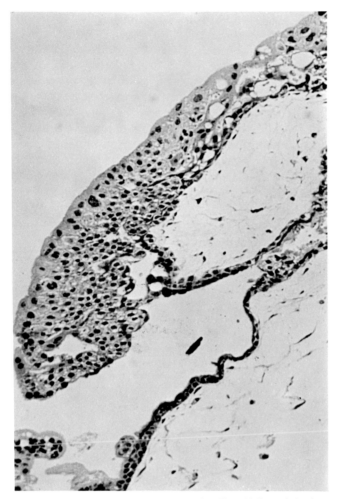

Fɪɢ. III-3. Benign hydatidiform mole, showing avascular villus with hyperplasia of syncytium and cytotrophoblast.

perplastic and dysplastic trophoblast, consists of grapelike vesicles without an embryo. Many moles may arise as blighted ova. The molar villi are edematous and avascular (Fig. III-3). The mole often presents with bleeding in the first half of pregnancy, occasionally with pain, particularly if the uterine growth is rapid. In about half the cases, the uterus is larger than the dates suggest. Abortion of the mole usually occurs at about 5 months' gestation or earlier, and the first indication of the disease is often the passage of vesicles. Severe hyperemesis, preeclampsia before the twenty-eighth week, and anemia are suggestive of the disorder. Since theca lutein cysts are present in about one third of the cases, the finding of adnexal masses may support the diagnosis. These tumors should not be excised because they regress after the trophoblastic tissue has been removed. An unusually high titer of chorionic gonadotropin, especially after the one-hundredth day of pregnancy, helps to confirm the diagnosis of mole. Twins and hydramnios must be excluded.

Diagnosis of mole can be made accurately by ultrasound. As soon as possible after diagnosis, the mole should be evacuated. Oxytocin is used to decrease the size of the uterus while the molar tissue is removed through a large-bore suction catheter. Sharp curettage is permissible only after the size of the uterus is sufficiently reduced to minimize the chance of perforation. Blood should be available during the procedure. In the rare event that the uterus does not respond to oxytocin, hysterotomy may be required. In older multiparas hysterectomy may be indicated. Because one in about five moles is followed by choriocarcinoma or invasive mole, follow-up by β-hCG titers to detect metastatic or persistent disease is mandatory. Invasive mole and choriocarcinoma are managed with great success by chemotherapy (methotrexate or actinomycin D).

Benign mole is followed by invasive mole in about 16% of cases (Fig. III-4) and by choriocarcinoma in about 2.5% of cases. Since hCG produced by persistent trophoblastic neoplastic tissue cannot be differentiated from that produced by a normal conceptus, pregnancy should be interdicted for a year to avoid confusion with persistent trophoblastic disease. Serum β-hCG should be measured weekly. The concentration is normally halved every 10 to 14 days. Patients in whom the serum β-hCG declines at a slower rate, remains at a plateau, or even increases should receive a thorough work-up and chemotherapy. Follow-up should be continued for 1 year. Curettage is repeated and the tissue submitted for histopathologic diagnosis, although the correlation between histologic appearance of the trophoblast and subsequent clinical behavior of the lesion is not good.

Choriocarcinoma comprises plexiform columns of trophoblast without a villous pattern (Fig. III-5). Whereas this disease was formerly almost 100% fatal, chemotherapy now effects cures of greater than 80%.

Moles occur only about once in 1200 to 2000 pregnancies in the United States, but the prevalence is greater in Indonesia, Hong Kong, and other parts of Asia. It is relatively more common at the extremes of reproductive life (particularly after age 30) and in women with a dietary deficiency of carotene, a precursor of vitamin A.

The classical, or complete, hydatidiform mole has a diploid chromo-

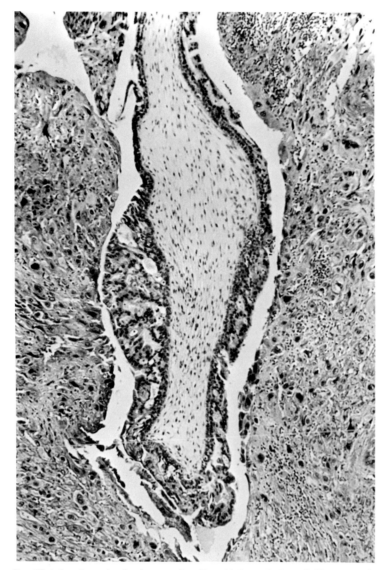

FIG. III-4. Invasive mole, showing avascular villus with hyperplastic trophoblast penetrating myometrium.

somal constitution. Cytogenetic studies have shown that all the chromo-somes in these moles are derived from the father. About 90% of complete moles have a 46, XX karyotype and about 10% have a 46, XY pattern. The evidence suggests that the female pronucleus is excluded at syngamy or earlier. The paternal chromosomes then undergo endoreduplication. In the complete mole, trophoblastic dysplasia and hyperplasia and general-ized hydatidiform swelling of the villi are conspicuous.

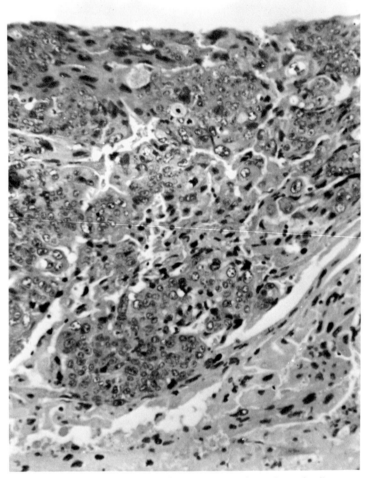

Fig. III-5. Choriocarcinoma, showing plexiform arrangement of syncytium and malignant cytotrophoblast.

In contrast to complete moles, partial moles are almost always triploid (either 69, XXY or 69, XYY with the extra set of chromosomes usually derived from the father. In addition, partial moles are associated with identifiable embryonic or fetal tissues (alive or dead), variably sized chorionic villi with focal hydatidiform swelling and cavitation, focal trophoblastic hyperplasia, marked scalloping of the chorionic villi, and prominent trophoblastic inclusions in the stroma. Partial moles are much less likely to be followed by metastatic trophoblastic gestational disease than are complete moles.

Pregnancy-specific β_1-glycoprotein (SP$_1$) and placental protein 5 (PP5) are found in higher concentrations in hydatidiform mole than in choriocarcinoma, although the β-hCG level is high in both forms of trophoblastic disease. Moles are said to occur less commonly in patients with group O blood.

Some authorities prefer to administer methotrexate or actinomycin before evacuation of a benign mole, but most reserve these drugs for proven or suspected metastatic or persistent disease.

An effective outpatient treatment for nonmetastatic gestational trophoblastic disease consists of methotrexate (1 mg/kg on days 1, 3, 5, and 7) and citrovorum (0.1 mg/kg on days 2, 4, 6, and 8). An alternative treatment is actinomycin D (10 to 13 μg/kg) intravenously daily for 5 days. Treatment must be stopped if leukopenia, a drop in platelets, or an elevation of SGPT or SGOT occurs. Chemotherapy must be continued until three consecutive negative hCG titers are obtained. Side effects of methotrexate may be reduced by citrovorum factor rescue.

Invasive mole, which at first spreads locally, may penetrate the myometrium deeply and cause serious hemorrhage. Unlike choriocarcinoma it maintains a villous pattern. Both hysterectomy and chemotherapy have been effective therapy for invasive mole. Choriocarcinoma metastasizes rapidly and widely. Its presenting sign may often be referable to a metastasis in the lung, vagina, liver, or brain. Although this lesion is preceded by mole in about half the cases, it may also be preceded by abortion, term intrauterine pregnancy, or ectopic pregnancy. Pregnancies have followed the successful treatment of choriocarcinoma.

Choriocarcinomas are placed in the category of high risk when any of the following pertains: duration of symptoms greater than 4 months, high initial titer of serum hCG (greater than 40,000 mlU/ml), metastases to brain or liver, failure of prior chemotherapy, or disease that follows term pregnancy. Such patients should receive triple therapy, which comprises methotrexate, actinomycin D, and chlorambucil, or an even more elaborate course of multiple agents that include hydroxyurea, actinomycin D, vincristine, methotrexate, cyclophosphamide (Cytoxan), folinic acid, and doxorubicin (Adriamycin). Radiotherapy and neurosurgical procedures have been employed successfully in the treatment of cerebral metastases.

Premature Labor

Prematurity is the leading cause of perinatal mortality and morbidity. The onset of labor is considered premature when it occurs before the 36th week, when the fetus normally weighs less than 2500 g (the lower limit of maturity). A fetus that weighs between 1000 and 2499 g is considered premature, and one between 500 and 999 g is immature. A fetus that is born weighing less than 500 g (the lower limit of viability) is an abortus.

The basic cause of premature labor is unknown although it is often associated with premature rupture of the membranes. Less commonly, premature labor may be ascribed to maternal systemic disorders including infections, second and third trimester uterine bleeding, and uterine anomalies.

Treatment of premature labor includes bedrest, hydration, mild sedation, and tocolysis. The most commonly used tocolytic agent is ritodrine, although considerable experience is available also with terbutaline and magnesium sulfate. Although attempts to stop premature labor are not always successful, they should always be made unless there are specific contraindications or the fetus is sufficiently mature. Narcotics that cross the placenta and depress the fetus should be avoided whenever possible. Delivery should be conducted under regional or local anesthesia, usually with episiotomy; it should be accomplished spontaneously or by elective outlet forceps. Fetal hypoxia and trauma must be avoided. The fetal prognosis depends on maturity and obstetric management. Expert neonatal care is a major factor in successful outcome. Preterm labor in a prior pregnancy is associated with repetition of the complication in subsequent pregnancy.

About 5 to 10% of all labors are premature. Prematurity is the cause of about two thirds of all cases of perinatal mortality and morbidity. In addition, it is a major etiologic factor in cerebral palsy and mental retardation. In only a minority of cases can a cause for prematurity be found. Conditions known to be associated with prematurity include prior preterm delivery, chronic vascular disease of the mother, preeclampsia-eclampsia, abruptio placentae, placenta previa, hydramnios, plural gestation, uterine malformations and tumors, and certain fetal anomalies.

Maternal genital infections are an important cause of potentially preventable prematurity. Increased rates of prematurity have been associated with maternal infection by Group B streptococci, *Neisseria gonorrhoeae*, *Chlamydia trachomatis*, and the virus of herpes simplex. Decreased birth weight, chorioamnionitis, and stillbirth have been associated with *Ureaplasma urealyticum*; febrile spontaneous abortion with *Mycoplasma hominis*; and prematurity and stillbirth with *Treponema pallidum*. Certain microorganisms, including *M. hominis*, *Gardnerella vaginalis*, and *Bacteroides* species, produce phospholipase A_2, an enzyme capable of cleaving arachidonic acid from the phospholipids of fetal membranes. The arachidonic acid thus released may result in the production of prostaglandins, which stimulate uterine contractions and premature labor.

Infants of mothers who smoke weigh less than those of mothers who do not, although the infants of smokers may not be premature by dates. Low socioeconomic status, poor nutrition, and stress appear to be conducive to prematurity.

Ritodrine hydrochloride is a betasympathomimetic drug that acts primarily on the β_2 receptors of the uterus. Other β_2-mimetics such as fenoterol, terbutaline, and salbutamol will probably receive FDA approval for use as tocolytic agents.

Patients who qualify for tocolytic treatment are those with uterine contractions leading to progressive effacement or dilatation of the cervix and whose fetuses are of 20 to 36 weeks' gestation or weigh less than 2500 g. Patients who do not qualify include those with amnionitis, vaginal bleeding, eclampsia or severe preeclampsia, a dead fetus or a major fetal malformation, maternal cardiac disease or hyperthyroidism, and any obstetric or medical complication that contraindicates prolongation of pregnancy. The chances of successful tocolytic therapy are limited by an incompetent cervix, ruptured membranes, advanced labor, and untreated infections.

When ritodrine is used intravenously, the maternal and fetal cardiac rates as well as maternal blood pressure and uterine activity must be monitored. The most common side effect is tachycardia. Additional effects include decrease in diastolic blood pressure, transient elevation of blood glucose and insulin, occasional elevations of free fatty acids and cAMP, and reduction of potassium. The initial dose is 0.1 mg/minute. The dose is then increased by 0.05 mg/minute every 10 minutes until contractions stop or unacceptable side effects occur. The dose should be reduced if side effects are poorly tolerated. The maximal dose is 0.35 mg/minute. Ritodrine should be discontinued if labor persists with the maximal dose, but if labor is successfully arrested the infusion should be continued for at least 12 hours.

When ritodrine is given orally, the initial dose should be 10 mg administered 30 minutes before the infusion is stopped. The drug is then given in doses of 10 mg every 2 hours for 24 hours. If contractions do not decrease, 10 to 20 mg are given every 4 to 6 hours until tocolysis is no longer indicated. The maximal oral dose should be 120 mg/day. If labor recurs during oral administration of ritodrine, an infusion may be repeated if it is clinically appropriate.

Premature Rupture of the Membranes

Rupture of the membranes is defined as premature when it occurs more than an hour before the onset of labor. The aggressive management of this condition includes delivery within 24 hours of rupture of the membranes. If the fetus is 1500 g or more in weight, prompt delivery is justified. The preferred method is induction with oxytocin if there are no contraindications to the drug. Otherwise, cesarean section is required, although this operation is rarely necessary on the basis solely of ruptured membranes. If the fetus is judged to weigh less than 1500 g, and the mother is afebrile, expectant management may be justified until the fetus reaches the desired weight. During this period, vaginal and rectal examinations should be avoided whenever possible. An initial vaginal examination is useful, however, to verify rupture of the membranes and to rule out prolapse of the umbilical cord. Digital examination of the endocervix provides no clinically valuable information but introduces indigenous pathogenic organisms into the uterine cavity. A daily leukocyte count and temperatures every 4 hours should be obtained to facilitate early detection of chorioamnionitis. Ultrasonic examination should be performed on all mothers with premature rupture of the membranes to ascertain whether the fetus has a serious congenital anomaly. Such a fetus is best delivered without prolonged hospitalization.

In many institutions aggressive management is carried out with fetuses estimated to weigh 1200 g or more. Still other centers with excellent facilities for intensive neonatal care prefer to deliver babies with even lower estimated weights, especially if the fetus is presenting by the breech.

If the patient is febrile and the cause is judged to be amnionitis, delivery is indicated regardless of the weight of the fetus. Antibiotics are usually given after the endometrial cavity is cultured. In all cases of premature rupture of the membranes, cultures should be obtained from the membranes and the infant's nasopharynx. The aggressive management is not universally practiced and many large centers have recently reverted to more conservative approaches to this complication.

Although premature rupture of the membranes may occur at any stage of pregnancy, its incidence increases as term is approached. The basic cause is unknown, but the condition is associated with premature delivery, maternal sepsis, and increased perinatal mortality and morbidity. Near term it is followed by the onset of labor within 24 hours in about 80% of cases, but the earlier in pregnancy premature rupture of the membranes occurs, the longer is the latent period (time between rupture and onset of labor). Diagnosis of rupture of the membranes may be difficult. Nitrazine (phenaphthazine) paper, which changes color in the range of pH from 4.5 to 7.5, is often used to detect alkaline fluid, which is presumably amniotic. A "fern" pattern, fetal epithelial cells, hair, or globules of fat suggest rupture of the membranes.

Placenta Previa

Placenta previa and abruptio placentae are the two most common causes of serious third-trimester bleeding. Placenta previa is characterized by painless vaginal bleeding in the third trimester. It is an important example of the principle that the incompletely separated placenta leads to maternal hemorrhage. If the fetus is judged to be under 2500 g (premature) and neither subsequent bleeding nor labor ensues, expectant management may be attempted; that is, no attempt at delivery is made until an estimated weight of 2500 g is attained. If severe or continuous bleeding occurs, if the patient goes into labor, or if the fetus is already mature, expectant management is inapplicable and the patient must be delivered promptly, usually by cesarean section.

In the most extensive variety of placenta previa (total), the entire internal os is covered by placenta. In the partial variety, only a portion of the internal os is covered. In the least extensive varieties (marginal placenta previa and low-lying placenta), the placenta barely encroaches upon the internal os.

Although the initial presumptive diagnosis is made most often by ultrasound (Fig. III-6), definitive diagnosis is made only by digital palpation of the placenta. This procedure must not be performed, however, except in the operating room, where immediate cesarean section may be accomplished if placenta previa is found. This is the double setup for examination and possible cesarean section. No vaginal or rectal examinations are permitted in a patient with suspected placenta previa except in the operating room.

Placenta previa occurs once in about 200 pregnancies. Its incidence increases with increasing maternal age and parity. It is associated with defective vascularization of the decidua and occasionally with partial placenta accreta. Abnormal presentations (transverse lie and breech) and twins are found more commonly with placenta previa. There is a tendency to repetition in subsequent pregnancies. Bleeding from placenta previa must be distinguished from heavy "show." In case of doubt the patient should be hospitalized for diagnosis.

With placenta previa the uterus is of normal consistency and is nontender, unlike that of typical abruptio placentae. Placenta previa rarely occurs before the seventh month, and the first hemorrhage is rarely, if ever, fatal. On initial examination a speculum should be gently inserted into the vagina to rule out nonobstetric causes of vaginal bleeding such as carcinoma of the cervix or lacerations. For all bleeding patients, blood should be typed and crossmatched and an intravenous infusion should be started through a large-bore needle. If the patient is anemic, blood should be transfused.

Most patients with placenta previa are delivered by cesarean section, including all primigravidas and all patients with total and partial varieties. Vaginal delivery by simple rupture of the membranes may occasionally be

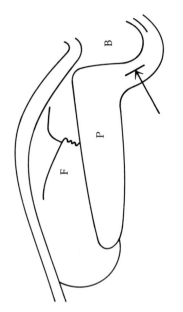

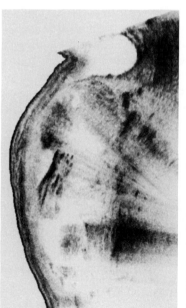

FIG. III-6. Longitudinal sonogram showing posterior placenta previa near term. The placenta (P) completely covers the cervix, which is identified by an echo from the endocervical canal (arrow). Bladder (B) and fetus (F) are also shown.

indicated in a case of low-lying placenta in a multipara with minimal bleeding. Cesarean section reduces both antepartum bleeding and traumatic bleeding at delivery and post partum from injury to the friable lower segment. Less than half of all cases of placenta previa may be managed expectantly. The maternal mortality of well-managed cases should approach zero, but the perinatal mortality remains high because of prematurity and fetal hypoxia.

Abruptio Placentae

Abruptio placentae, the premature separation of the normally situated placenta after the twentieth week of gestation, is the other major cause of third-trimester bleeding. Abruption is classified as either severe or mild, depending upon the degree of separation of the placenta from the uterine wall. The bleeding may be confined to the uterus, as in a retroplacental hematoma with no external bleeding (concealed hemorrhage), usually the more serious form of the disorder. If blood escapes into the vagina, external hemorrhage results.

Signs and symptoms depend on the degree and the duration of the separation. Maternal signs and symptoms may include vaginal bleeding, shock (if the bleeding is severe), and uterine tenderness and rigidity. With severe or rapid bleeding fetal distress or fetal death may occur. Electronic monitoring of the fetal heart rate for signs of fetal distress is thus critical to management. If only slight external bleeding occurs in the absence of uterine pain or rigidity or fetal distress, bedrest and careful observation may suffice temporarily. A hard uterus, usually indicating retroplacental bleeding, and fetal distress suggest severe abruption and the need for rapid delivery.

The route of delivery is determined by obstetric factors and the speed with which vaginal delivery may be anticipated. If there is no contraindication to oxytocin, it should be used together with rupture of the membranes when delivery through the vagina can reasonably be expected within 6 to 8 hours. In all other circumstances cesarean section is required. Severe abruption may be complicated by grave fetal distress or death and by maternal hypofibrinogenemia and acute renal failure.

The primary reason for rapid delivery is to forestall these serious complications, which may increase as the interval between abruption and delivery is prolonged. Aggressive management of abruption, based on the presumptive danger of time-related maternal complications, is not, however, universally practiced. Excellent results have been obtained in many institutions that do not require delivery within eight hours, as long as the maternal blood pressure and renal perfusion remain normal.

Abruptio placentae occurs in about 1% of all pregnancies. The exact frequency depends on the criteria for diagnosis. The precise cause is unknown, although a vascular lesion of the decidua frequently appears to be an underlying factor. Hypertension is associated with abruptio placentae in about one third to one half of cases, chronic hypertension more often than preeclampsia. Maternal mortality should not exceed 1% in well-managed cases, but fetal mortality depends primarily on the extent and acuteness of the separation and the degree of fetal maturity.

Management includes monitoring of maternal blood loss, pulse rate, and blood pressure; typing and crossmatching of blood; monitoring of urinary output and possible use of mannitol as an osmotic diuretic to maintain a urinary flow of 100 ml/hr; monitoring of central venous pressure to avoid overhydration (over 12 cm of water); administration of blood when indicated by prior maternal hemorrhage or a fall in the level of fibrinogen to 100 mg%; and most important, emptying the uterus within 6 to 8 hours by amniotomy and oxytocin or by cesarean section. The use of heparin in treating the consumptive coagulopathy that may occur in the severe forms of this disorder is controversial and potentially dangerous. Effusion of blood within the uterus in cases of severe abruption may produce a bluish discoloration (Couvelaire uterus). It is not necessary to remove the uterus except in the rare event that it fails to contract in response to oxytocin.

Trauma, short cord, and folic acid deficiency are not important etiologic factors. The earlier in pregnancy an abruption occurs, the more it resembles a late incomplete abortion.

The most trivial degrees of separation may include rupture of the marginal sinus. There is about a 10% likelihood of recurrence of abruption in subsequent pregnancies.

Other obstetric conditions in which hypofibrinogenemia occurs include amniotic fluid embolism, fetal death, and severe postpartum hemorrhage. Epsilon-aminocaproic acid is generally contraindicated unless unequivocal excessive activator activity or hyperplasminemia can be demonstrated. Successful management of the renal failure depends on close cooperation with the "dialysis team."

Dystocia: Uterine Dysfunction

Dystocia (difficult labor), or failure to progress in parturition, is caused by one of three main factors or combinations of them:

abnormalities of uterine contractions (uterine dysfunction); abnormalities of size, presentation, or development of the fetus; and abnormalities of pelvic size or architecture. Relative pelvic contraction is often associated with uterine dysfunction. Together they are the most common cause of dystocia.

Management of all forms of dystocia includes clinical assessment of pelvic dimensions and architecture, electronic monitoring of the strength of uterine contractions, careful clinical observation and recording of the progress of labor (effacement and dilatation of the cervix and station of the presenting part), and electronic monitoring of fetal well-being by continuous recording of the fetal heart rate. If the diagnosis of cephalopelvic disproportion is made, stimulation by oxytocin is contraindicated and a cesarean section is performed.

Uterine dysfunction may result from subnormal contractions or abnormal contractions. Subnormal, that is, weak or infrequent, contractions are the most frequent indication for stimulation by oxytocin. In abnormal contractions there is a lack of fundal dominance (gradient from top to bottom of the uterus) or asynchrony of uterine contractions. Uterine dysfunction is most commonly confused with false labor, which requires no treatment. Primary uterine dysfunction is present from the onset of labor. It is essentially a prolongation of the latent phase of the first stage of labor. Prolongation of either the first or the second stage increases perinatal mortality. Secondary dysfunction usually occurs after labor has begun normally. It results from an overdistended uterus, disproportion, premature administration of anesthesia and analgesia, and maternal exhaustion. Secondary dysfunction is usually associated with contractions that are subnormal in amplitude or frequency. It is often designated hypotonic, although the term is physiologically inaccurate. Hypertonic dysfunction is often primary and the contractions are abnormal, with a reversal of gradient or asynchrony of impulses from the cornua. There may possibly be emotional factors in the causation of uterine dysfunction. Graphs of normal and abnormal patterns of labor are shown in Figure III-7.

True labor should not be diagnosed until the cervix has reached at least 3 cm dilatation. During an effective uterine contraction, the uterus cannot be indented. Pain is not a good indication of the effectiveness of labor. In the latent phase, effacement may occur without much cervical dilatation.

Subnormal uterine contractions complicate about 4% of all labors. The strength of a uterine contraction is best measured by means of an intrauterine catheter. Fetal distress occurs late; oxytocin is specific therapy; and rest is of no value.

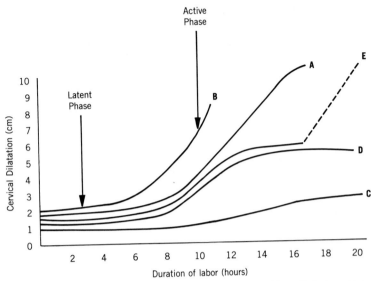

Fɪɢ. III-7. A. Normal labor in primigravida; B. Normal labor in multipara; C. Prolonged latent phase (primary dysfunction); D. Prolonged active phase (secondary dysfunction); E. Effect of oxytocin on secondary dysfunction (dotted line).

Hypertonic uterine dysfunction complicates about 1% of all labors. It involves mostly the latent phase and it may appear to be painful out of proportion to the stage of labor. Fetal distress occurs early. Oxytocin is probably of no value, but rest and sedation for a short period of time may be tried before resorting to cesarean section.

In the management of subnormal uterine contractions it is important to prepare a timetable of action, which includes precise objectives to be achieved by specific points in time. A cesarean section is indicated when these objectives are not met or when disproportion is discovered. The pelvic measurements, cervical dilatation, and fetal station and position must be known precisely. When using oxytocin the physician must remain with the patient, electronically monitoring the fetal cardiac rate and uterine contractions and recording the maternal vital signs. An intravenous infusion of crystalloid and water must be started and the solution of oxytocin (10 units/liter) run into the tubing of the first infusion. The infusion should be started slowly and increased to a maximum of 20 to 30 milliunits per minute, preferably with control by an accurate pump. Higher concentrations are unnecessary and potentially dangerous. When used for proper indications, oxytocin is effective at low concentrations and after only a short period of infusion. The intravenous route is the only accurate, safe, and easily controlled method of administering oxytocin. Prostaglandins also have been used successfully for stimulation of labor in other countries, but ergot alkaloids and other drugs should not be used for this purpose.

A long latent period may be defined as 20 hours in the primigravida and 14 hours in the multigravida. During the active phase the cervix normally dilates at the rate of about 1.2 cm per hour in the primigravida and 1.5 cm in the multipara. A minimal pressure of 15 mm Hg is required for an effective contraction. The pressure exerted during an average uterine contraction is about 50 mm Hg.

Contraindications to oxytocin are absolute and relative. Absolute contraindications include fetopelvic disproportion and transverse lie. Relative contraindications include advanced age (over 35 years), high parity (greater than 5), and overdistension of the uterus (as with twins and hydramnios). If doubt about the propriety of using oxytocin in a particular situation remains, it is safer to avoid using the drug.

Abnormal Presentations

Fetal causes of dystocia include excessive size or malpresentations of a normal-sized infant (for example, transverse lie at term in a normal pelvis). This group also includes fetal anomalies such as hydrocephalus, double monsters, and fetal tumors. Fetal causes of dystocia are managed by cesarean section as soon as the diagnosis is made.

Breech presentation, in which the sacrum or one or both feet may be the presenting part, occurs in 3 to 4% of all pregnancies at term. A breech presentation should be suspected on the basis of physical examination (abdominal and pelvic). The suspicion is usually confirmed sonographically. Since the largest part of the fetus (the head) passes through the pelvis last, the route of delivery (abdominal or vaginal) must be decided early, for there can be no trial of labor. Complications of breech presentation include increased incidence of prolapse of the cord and increased perinatal mortality and morbidity. Cesarean section is indicated in all cases of breech presentation with pelvic contraction or oversized fetus. Sonographic measurement of the biparietal diameter of the fetal head is most useful. Since the breech often does not fit the pelvis well, the likelihood of premature rupture of the membranes is increased. A vaginal examination should be performed immediately after this event to rule out prolapse of the cord. Premature rupture of the membranes should be managed aggressively (p. 135) to minimize intrauterine infection and perinatal morbidity and mortality. Because breech presentation is associated with a 2-fold to 3-fold increase in congenital anomalies, compared with cephalic presentation, it is important that each fetus presenting by the breech be subjected to thorough sonographic examination. If fetal anomalies incompatible with life are found, cesarean section should be performed only for maternal indications.

The most common type of breech is the frank breech (knees extended and thighs flexed on the abdomen). With full, or complete, breech, both knees and hips are flexed. In frank and full breeches, the presenting part is the sacrum. In footlings, one or both hips and knees are extended. The fetal head does not have time to mold and it may be trapped by the cervix if delivery begins before full dilatation. Since the cord is inevitably compressed against the inlet by the fetal head by the time the fetal umbilicus reaches the introitus, delivery must be completed within several minutes of this time to avoid fetal hypoxia.

Although prolapse of the cord commonly occurs with breech presentation, the accident may be associated with any factor that interferes with adaptation of the presenting part to the inlet, such as transverse lie, face presentation, plural gestation, small fetus, or contracted pelvis. Treatment of prolapse of the cord depends upon the dilatation of the cervix. With full dilatation, a forceps delivery of a vertex or a breech extraction may be performed if there are no obstetric contraindications. When the cervix is incompletely dilated and fetus is alive, cesarean section should be performed.

The use of cesarean section for delivery of breeches has increased markedly in recent years. Many obstetricians recommend abdominal delivery of virtually all primigravidas with breech presentations because their pelves are untried. Other indications for cesarean section include footling breeches (to prevent prolapse of the cord), premature breeches (to prevent entrapment of the head by an incompletely dilated cervix), and a hyperextended fetal head (to prevent mechanical difficulties during delivery). Vaginal delivery of a term breech remains an acceptable option for the experienced obstetrician when the fetus weighs less than 3600 g, the pelvis is of normal size and shape, the breech is frank, and the head is not hyperextended. The upper and lower limits for which cesarean section is indicated in breech presentation are still controversial. Many large centers in this country choose cesarean section as the method of delivery for the fetus that weighs between 1000 and 2000 g.

Breech presentation may be associated with hydramnios, hydrocephalus, placenta previa, uterine septa, prematurity, and twinning. Since about 40% of fetuses present by the breech at the twenty-eighth week, whereas only 3 to 4% present by the breech at term, it is evident that 90% turn spontaneously during that third trimester. The perinatal mortality associated with breech presentation at term is three times that of vertex presentation.

External version (p. 183) may be attempted in the last 6 weeks of pregnancy, with tocolysis. The preferred method of delivery is partial breech extraction, or assisted breech delivery. In this procedure the breech delivers spontaneously to the umbilicus. In spontaneous breech delivery the entire fetus is born without assistance, as commonly happens with prematures. Total breech extraction is performed only for difficulties such as fetal distress or a prolonged second stage. The procedure requires deep uterine relaxation and is replaced safely by cesarean section in most cases.

Oxytocin must be used with caution in any breech presentation. Complete breech extraction requires deep uterine relaxation. Fetal injuries associated with breech delivery include fractures of the clavicle, femur, humerus, and spine; injuries to the brachial plexus; hemorrhage in the adrenal, kidney, liver, and spleen; intracranial bleeding; and hypoxia leading to brain damage. The perinatal mortality and morbidity are increased by these factors as well as by prematurity, congenital anomalies, and associated maternal conditions such as placenta previa.

In transverse lie, the long axis of the fetus is perpendicular to that of the mother and the shoulder is the presenting part. This presentation occurs once in about 300 labors. Vaginal delivery of a term-sized fetus in this presentation is usually impossible and cesarean section is therefore required. Transverse lie is associated with a relaxed abdominal wall (high multiparity), pelvic contraction, placenta previa, prematurity, plural gestation, and uterine myomas.

The mother's prognosis in transverse lie is worsened because of spontaneous and traumatic (version) uterine rupture and associated conditions such as placenta previa and advanced age. The fetal prognosis is poor because of traumatic delivery, hypoxia, infection associated with premature rupture of the membranes, and prolapse of the cord. A neglected transverse lie may lead to serious intrauterine infection, which may require cesarean hysterectomy (p. 179).

With face presentations the head is completely extended and the chin is the presenting part. This presentation occurs once in about 400 labors. It should be recognized early and cephalopelvic disproportion, which is frequently associated with face presentation, excluded. A cephalic prominence on the same side as the fetal back suggests face presentation. If the chin is anterior and there is no disproportion, vaginal delivery may be expected. If the chin remains posterior during labor, cesarean section is required for delivery.

Brow presentation is usually transitional from a fully extended (face) to a fully flexed (occiput) presentation. It persists in only 1 in 1000 to 1 in 1500 deliveries. A persistent brow with a term fetus or any cephalopelvic disproportion requires delivery by cesarean section. The perinatal mortality of brow presentation is several times that of vertex presentation.

Occiput posterior is essentially a normal positional variant often associated with anthropoid and android pelves. This position may be associated with a prolonged second stage and incomplete flexion of the head. Most occiput posteriors turn spontaneously to occiput anterior positions. Persistent occiput posteriors may be delivered by rotation (manual or forceps) to an anterior position or as occiput posteriors (face to pubis). Cesarean section should replace difficult midforceps delivery of occiput posteriors.

Pelvic Contraction

Absolute contraction of the pelvic inlet or midpelvis will prevent vaginal delivery of a normal-sized infant. An unusual pelvic configuration even without absolute contraction may necessitate cesarean section. When the major diameters of the pelvis are at or below critical values, oxytocin must be used with great caution in the presence of a normal-sized fetus. Minor degrees of pelvic contraction are often associated with uterine dysfunction.

The critical diameters, in centimeters, of the pelvis are as follows:

	Anteroposterior	Transverse
Inlet	10.0	12.0
Midplane	11.5	9.5

A contracted pelvis may result from malnutrition, injury, or congenital anomalies. Maternal complications include prolonged labor, premature rupture of the membranes, uterine rupture, and fistulas. Fetal complications include infection, prolapse of the umbilical cord, and intracranial hemorrhage.

The ideal obstetric pelvis has a roundish inlet with a broad and deep posterior segment. The lateral walls slope gently toward the symphysis to form a broad and deep forepelvis. The sacrosciatic notch is wide; the pubic arch is wide; and the bones are light. A flat, or platypelloid, pelvis favors a transverse position of the head and a long, or anthropoid, pelvis favors a posterior mechanism of labor.

Plural Gestations

Plural gestations (twins and higher multiples) occur in more than 1% of all pregnancies. The fetuses may lie in any combination of presentations. Initial diagnosis or confirmation of clinical findings may be made by sonography (Fig. III-8). The prevalences of hydramnios, preeclampsia, maternal anemia, and prematurity are increased with plural gestation. The second twin should be delivered within 15 to 30 minutes of the first twin. After delivery of the first infant, the uterine end of its cord should be clamped. Oxytocin and blood should be available in such situations to prevent or combat postpartum hemorrhage.

The rate of monovular twinning is constant in all maternal age groups and races. Dizygotic (binovular, fraternal) twins are more common in the black population. With twins the uterus is usually larger, and more than the usual number of fetal small parts may be palpated. Two fetal heart

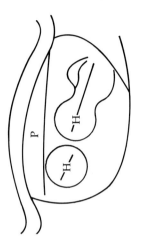

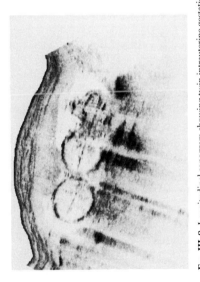

Fig. III-8. Longitudinal sonogram showing twin intrauterine gestation. The two fetal heads (H) are identified. The torso of one fetus and the placenta (P) are also visible.

beats differing by more than 10 beats per minute suggest twins. The infants in plural gestation usually deliver before term. Death of one or both twins during labor or delivery may result from operative interference, prolapse of the cord, or premature separation of the placenta.

When the morula splits during the first 4 days of gestation, dichorionic diamnionic twins develop. The placentas may fuse or remain separate. When the blastocyst splits at a later stage before implantation, during the first week of gestation, the twins develop a common chorion but two separate amnions. The single placenta resulting therefrom is monochorionic diamnionic. When the blastocyst splits after implantation, during the second week of gestation, the amnion will have already differentiated and monochorionic monoamnionic twins develop.

Monochorial twinning may lead to the transfusion syndrome, with the donor twin malnourished and the recipient twin plethoric. Monoamnionic twins may have knotted cords, which may lead to death of one or both fetuses. Twins have a greater prevalence of vasa previa and velamentous insertions of the cord, which may result in injuries to the umbilical vessels and fetal hemorrhage. In vasa previa, the umbilical vessels traverse the lower uterine segment in advance of the presenting part. Rupture of the membranes in cases of vasa previa may result in laceration of the fetal vessels with fetal hemorrhage or death. In cases of velamentous insertion of the cord into the fetal membranes, the umbilical vessels course between amnion and chorion unprotected by Wharton's jelly.

Postpartum Hemorrhage and Obstetric Injuries

Postpartum hemorrhage is defined as loss of more than 500 ml of blood during the first 24 hours after delivery. It is the most common variety of severe hemorrhage in obstetrics and a major factor in maternal mortality. The three principal causes of postpartum hemorrhage are uterine atony, trauma to the genital tract, and retained secundines (placenta and membranes). Uterine atony, the most common cause, may result from any condition that leads to overdistension of the uterus. Injuries result primarily from traumatic deliveries and inadequately repaired episiotomies. Retained secundines usually result in a somewhat more delayed hemorrhage.

Diagnosis and treatment must be performed with minimal delay. As soon as excessive bleeding is recognized, a large-bore needle is inserted into a vein for administration of fluids, and blood is crossmatched and made available. In a healthy young woman the blood pressure and pulse rate may remain almost normal until a great deal of blood has been lost, at which point shock may suddenly develop.

Transfusion should always be instituted before the patient has lost 1000 ml of blood. The first step in management is uterine mas-

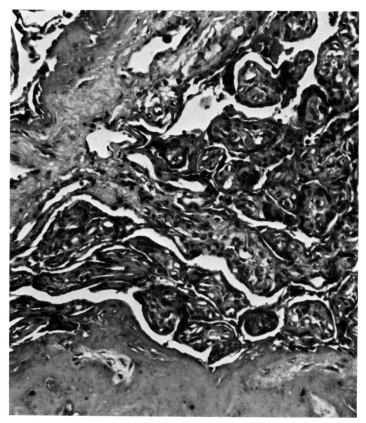

Fɪɢ. III-9. Placenta accreta, showing villi in direct contact with myometrium without an intervening decidual cushion.

sage. An oxytocic agent is administered if the uterus is hypotonic. If bleeding continues from a firmly contracted uterus, injuries to the genital tract are a more likely cause. After any difficult delivery the vulva, vagina (including episiotomy site), and cervix should be inspected and any lacerations repaired. The uterus should be manually explored, especially if the cervix is deeply lacerated, to rule out injury and to remove any placental fragments. Anesthesia provides for a more thorough examination. The delivered placenta should be carefully examined to rule out incomplete removal. In the unusual event of placenta accreta the placenta, or more commonly a part thereof, cannot be separated from the uterus (Fig. III-9). Hysterectomy may then be required to control hemorrhage. The blood should be observed to see whether it clots and to rule out hypofibrinogenemia, which is generally treated by administration of cryoprecipitate. If the uterus is still bleeding after lacerations have been repaired and after oxytocic agents have been administered, the uterus should be compressed bimanually and the patient prepared for laparotomy. The Anti-G, or MAST (military antishock trousers), suit is also a frequently effective means of combating uterine hemorrhage caused by atony. Packing the uterus hides rather than stems the hemorrhage.

Uterine atony accounts for about 90% of all cases of immediate postpartum hemorrhage. It should be anticipated in prolonged labor, high multiparity, and general anesthesia with agents that relax the uterus. It is more common with plural gestation, hydramnios (2000 ml or more amniotic fluid), excessively large infants, and myomas. The likelihood of uterine atony is greatly reduced by the proper use of oxytocic agents. One ampul (10 units) of oxytocin may be administered by intravenous drip after delivery of the infant, but not directly into the vein in a single rapid injection. Methylergonovine maleate (0.2 mg) may be given intravenously after delivery of the placenta.

Trauma to the genital tract results from tumultuous labor, difficult forceps delivery and internal podalic version, injudicious use of oxytocin before delivery, and mismanagement of the third stage (forceful attempts to remove the placenta prematurely). After any difficult labor or delivery the genital tract should be systematically inspected. If a uterine rupture is encountered or suspected, the patient should be transported without delay to the operating room. Ligation of the internal iliac arteries or hysterectomy may be required for hemostasis.

The delivered placenta should be carefully inspected to rule out retention of a cotyledon, as indicated by a defect in the maternal surface. A torn vessel at the edge of the placenta suggests retention of a succenturiate lobe. Retained secundines and subinvolution of the placental site usually lead to postpartum hemorrhage that is delayed (from the second day to a month after delivery). Placental fragments may then be removed by polyp forceps and the subinvoluted site curetted.

Hypofibrinogenemia is a much less common cause of postpartum hemorrhage. It is often associated with severe abruption of the placenta, retention of a dead fetus for more than a month, and amniotic fluid embolism.

Uterine rupture may occur through a scar (usually cesarean section) before and during labor or through an intact organ after difficult labor or delivery. Rupture should be suspected when the uterine contractions cease and the fetal heart tones are lost in the presence of severe abdominal pain. A classical cesarean section scar may rupture early (before the onset of labor), whereas a low-segment scar more often ruptures during labor.

Preeclampsia-Eclampsia

Preeclampsia, characterized by hypertension, edema, and proteinuria, develops after the twentieth week of gestation and appears with increasing frequency as pregnancy progresses. Hypertension and at least one of the other signs are required for the diagnosis. Eclampsia is preeclampsia with convulsions, which may occur ante partum, intra partum, or post partum. The cause of preeclampsia is unknown; the leading, but unproved, hypothesis attributes it to uteroplacental ischemia. It is predominantly a disorder of primigravidas, or more accurately, nulliparas. The diagnosis in multiparas is usually erroneous, and when it does occur there usually is some predisposing factor. Preeclampsia is often confused with essential hypertension or renal disease, either latent and revealed by pregnancy, or frank but unobserved because the patient was not seen until late in gestation. A blood pressure of 140/90 or higher before the twentieth week suggests chronic hypertension antedating pregnancy. Preeclampsia may be superimposed on chronic hypertension. Gestational (pregnancy-induced) hypertension without either proteinuria or edema and with disappearance after delivery is called transient.

Gestational (transient) hypertension is highly likely to recur in some or all later pregnancies and has been the usual basis for the erroneous diagnosis of preeclampsia in multiparas. Gestational hypertension, especially in primigravidas, may occasionaliy be incipient preeclampsia, but more often it is a sign of latent essential hypertension unmasked by pregnancy.

Pregnancy is a screening test for future hypertension. Gestational hypertension indicates a great likelihood of future chronic hypertension, probably of early onset. Normotensive pregnancies are predictive of a greatly reduced likelihood of hypertension; furthermore, if hypertension develops subsequently, it will be less severe because the age of onset will be greater than the average for all women. Preeclamptic and eclamptic hypertension have no remote prognostic significance because women destined to become chronically hypertensive are neither more nor less likely to develop preeclampsia than are women in general.

A major aim of prenatal care is to detect incipient preeclampsia early in its course, for its progression to eclampsia usually can be prevented. Although the only specific treatment is termination of pregnancy, early signs are treated by bedrest. Restriction of sodium, which has been part of the management of preeclampsia for many years, is often recommended although there is no proof that it is beneficial, particularly in the mild forms of the syndrome. The objectives are to prevent convulsions and to salvage the infant with minimal trauma to the mother. With bedrest, the blood pressure, weight, and proteinuria should decrease. If they do not and the patient is within 4 weeks of term, delivery is desirable. If the patient is several weeks from term and the preeclampsia is mild, temporization may be justified. The diagnosis of "mild" preeclampsia must never lead to complacency. Nearly a quarter of women who develop eclampsia have apparently mild preeclampsia until the onset of convulsions and some of them die. The risks of allowing the pregnancy to continue include aggravation of the preeclampsia, fetal death, and abruptio placentae. Signs and symptoms of aggravation call for delivery despite prematurity.

Antihypertensive drugs are used only if the hypertension is so severe as to be dangerous in itself, as with a diastolic pressure sustained at more than 110 mm Hg. Reduction of maternal blood pressure, however, will probably decrease uterine blood flow, which is at most half of normal in hypertensive pregnancies. The fetus will thus be deprived of its supply of nutrition. Hydralazine is the drug of choice in preeclamptic hypertension. An anticonvulsant agent, preferably parenteral magnesium sulfate, is used in the treatment of hyperreflexia, severe preeclampsia, and eclampsia. It is used also in patients with moderately severe preeclampsia at the onset of spontaneous or induced labor. In eclampsia, oxygen should be administered after each convulsion and digitalis given at the onset of pulmonary edema. As soon as the patient is conscious and oriented, labor should be induced or cesarean section performed. Similarly, in patients with severe preeclampsia, pregnancy should be terminated as soon as the clinical condition is stable. Usually the uterus is sensitive to oxytocin and labor can be induced even with an "unfavorable" cervix, but cesarean section may be preferable if vaginal delivery does not appear easy and imminent. Anticonvulsant therapy should be continued for at least 24 hours after delivery. Convulsions are associated with a significant increase in maternal mortality and perinatal loss; a major factor in perinatal loss is prematurity.

Patients with severe preeclampsia are at risk for water intoxication if oxytocin is given in 5% dextrose. The antidiuretic effect of oxytocin is evident even in doses too low to affect uterine contractions. Patients tend to lie supine, furthermore, a position that greatly reduces urinary output.

In superimposed preeclampsia, diagnosed by the specified increases in blood pressure together with proteinuria, the perinatal loss is four times as great as in either preeclampsia or chronic hypertension alone. Low socioeconomic status and geographic and racial differences are alleged to be factors in the development of preeclampsia, although proof is lacking. There is strong evidence that a single recessive gene may determine the development of the disorder.

Hypertension is a sustained rise, over the usual levels, of 30 mm Hg in the systolic or 15 in the diastolic readings, or a sustained pressure of 140/90 or higher. "Sustained" means on at least two occasions 6 or more hours apart. Generalized edema, rather than pedal edema, is a diagnostic sign, although it occurs in many normal pregnant women. Proteinuria means one plus or more.

In differential diagnosis, chronic hypertension rather than preeclampsia is suggested by (1) previous hypertensive pregnancy, (2) multiparity, (3) retinal angiosclerosis, or hemorrhages and exudates, (4) cardiomegaly, (5) exorbitant hypertension, and (6) little or no proteinuria.

Factors predisposing to preeclampsia are (1) nulliparity, (2) familial history of preeclampsia-eclampsia, (3) plural gestation, (4) diabetes, (5) chronic hypertension, (6) hydatidiform mole, with which preeclampsia may occur as early as the fourteenth week, (7) fetal hydrops, and (8) extremes of age.

Inconstant signs of incipient preeclampsia are gains of three or more pounds per week, increasing edema of the hands and face, and a trend to rise in blood pressure. Occasionally the onset of preeclampsia is explosive. The presence of one or more of the following marks preeclampsia as severe: (1) sustained blood pressure of 160/110 or higher, (2) proteinuria of more than 5 g/liter, (3) urinary output of less than 400 ml/24 hours, (4) cerebral or visual disturbances, and (5) cyanosis or pulmonary edema. Others are hemoconcentration, epigastric pain, disseminated intravascular coagulation, and increases of certain hepatic enzymes in the plasma (e.g., SGOT, SGPT, and lactic dehydrogenase). Whether hyperreflexia also indicates severe preeclampsia is not certain.

Magnesium sulfate is given intravenously as an initial dose of 3 or 4 g in 10% solution, followed by either (a) continuous infusion of 1 to 2 g/hour or (b) 10 g in 50% solution by deep intramuscular injection, with later injections of 5 g doses at intervals of 4 hours. The initial dose is safe, but subsequent doses, or the continuous infusion, may not be unless (1) the knee jerk is active, (2) the urinary output is at least 100 ml/4 hours, and (3) the respiratory rate is 12 or more/minute. Calcium gluconate, 10 ml of 10% solution, is an antidote to magnesium toxicity and should always be available. If the urinary output falls below 20 ml/hour, mannitol is infused but not repeated unless the urinary volume rises to about 100 ml/hour. Furosemide may be given intravenously, but it is usually contraindicated, as are all diuretics.

Thiazides are best avoided in pregnancy. Adverse effects of these drugs, particularly in preeclampsia, include further depletion of an already diminished plasma volume, hypokalemia and hyponatremia, hemorrhagic pancreatitis, depression of placental function, and in the newborn, thrombocytopenia.

Complications of preeclampsia and eclampsia include retardation of fetal growth, abruptio placentae, acute renal failure, hypofibrinogenemia, cerebrovascular accidents, hemolysis, disseminated intravascular coagulation, jaundice, and rarely, retinal detachment, hepatic rupture, and trauma incurred during convulsions. The major causes of maternal death in eclampsia are cerebral hemorrhage and cardiac failure.

Anatomic lesions in fatal cases of eclampsia are widespread arteriolitis, thrombosis of small vessels, hemorrhage, and necrosis. A characteristic but not wholly specific renal lesion is found in biopsies from preeclamptic women; the glomerular capillary endothelial cells are swollen, there is an increase in size and possibly number of mesangial cells, and fibrin derivatives are deposited, accounting partially for the reduction in renal blood flow and the still greater decrease in glomerular filtration.

Another characteristic but not entirely pathognomonic lesion is found in the uterine arteries in the placental bed. In preeclampsia, as opposed to normal pregnancy, the "physiologic" dilation of the uterine arteries is restricted to the decidual segments and there is an atherotic change in the vessels. Similar lesions have recently been described, however, in nonpreeclamptic pregnancies complicated by retardation of intrauterine growth.

The fundamental derangements are an abnormally large retention of sodium and arteriolar spasm. There is no good evidence that diuretics and limitations of weight gain and sodium intake prevent preeclampsia; once severe preeclampsia has developed, however, restriction of sodium seems to be beneficial. The arterioles are sensitized to pressor substances, but no such agent has been identified as causing preeclamptic hypertension. Despite the generalized vasoconstriction, the total blood flows to most regions of the body are often normal or nearly so. In normal pregnancy the placenta produces equivalent amounts of thromboxane and prostacyclin, but in preeclamptic pregnancy the placental production of thromboxane is 7 times that of prostacyclin.

Almost the only helpful laboratory tests are serial measurements of proteinuria, which increases with severity, and of the hematocrit as an index to the hemoconcentration occurring in severe preeclampsia and eclampsia. Progressive or irreversible hemoconcentration, low platelet counts, and elevated hepatic enzymes denote a bad prognosis. Hyperuricemia supports the diagnosis of preeclampsia. Significant increases in blood or plasma creatinine point to renal disease.

Ambulatory treatment of severe preeclampsia is unsatisfactory. A patient with minimal signs may be treated at home, but must be seen 2 or 3 times each week. Once the diagnosis seems definite, she should be in the hospital. A convulsion in a pregnant woman must be regarded as eclampsia until proved otherwise. Among conditions to be differentiated are epilepsy, lesions in the central nervous system, and water intoxication. The edema and usually the proteinuria clear within a few days after delivery. In half the cases, the blood pressure returns to normal within 10 days but may be unstable for as long as 6 months. In the other half, the pressure subsides more slowly, but unless the patient has underlying hypertension it will return to normal within a few weeks.

About one third of primigravidas with preeclampsia-eclampsia will have a recurrence of hypertension in later pregnancies, usually without more than mild increases; such women are likely to develop essential hypertension later. The recurrence is usually merely transient hypertension, but roughly 10% may have recurrent preeclampsia or eclampsia. It is improbable that preeclampsia-eclampsia causes so-called residual hypertension.

Hemolytic Disease of the Newborn

Pregnancy may initiate immunologic sensitization of a mother to tissues of her fetus. The usual cause of isoimmunization is the Rh factor. In this situation an Rh-negative mother is sensitized by transfer of fetal erythrocytes to the maternal circulation, usually at the time of delivery but occasionally earlier in pregnancy. The Rh-positive fetal cells enter the maternal circulation through breaks in the placenta. Sensitization may also be produced by transfusion of Rh-positive cells into an Rh-negative mother. In both cases the maternal anti-Rh antibodies are transferred back to the fetus and cause hemolysis. An Rh-negative mother should have serial titers during pregnancy. The antibody titers are not good indications of the severity of erythroblastosis but provide a good screening test. Once the indirect Coombs' test is positive in a titer of higher than 1:16, an amniotic fluid analysis (amniocentesis) must be done to detect the bilirubin levels.

In a sensitized mother obstetric management is directed toward improvement of fetal survival. The management and prognosis of the fetus are related to the amniotic fluid analysis and to the histories of prior pregnancies. The unsensitized Rh-negative mother should receive 300 μg of anti-D (Rho) gamma globulin (RhoGAM) intramuscularly within 72 hours of premature or term delivery if her infant is Rh-positive or if its blood type is unknown. After spontaneous or induced abortion before the thirteenth week, ectopic pregnancy, or amniocentesis, 50 μg of Rh-immune globulin provide adequate protection. After a large transplacental hemorrhage or a mismatched transfusion of blood, more than 300 μg may be required. Whether to use Rh-immune globulin after delivery of a hydatidiform mole is still debatable. All Rh-negative mothers must have fetal cord blood tested after abortion or delivery to assess the fetus' Rh-status and the presence of sensitivity. Administration of Rh-immunoglobulin to Rh-negative women in the third trimester at 28 weeks' gestation will further reduce the likelihood of isoimmunization of the fetus in subsequent pregnancies.

In each pregnancy the mother should have blood group and Rh-type tested and an irregular antibody screen performed as early as practicable. The woman who is Rho(D)-negative but not Rho(D)-isoimmunized should have anti-D antibody tests repeated at 28, 32, and 36 weeks' gestation. If the tests show no anti-D antibody, she should receive Rh-immunoglobulin after delivery; if the tests are positive, she should be managed as an Rho(D)-sensitized mother. The most common cause of Rho(D)-isoimmunization is the delivery of an Rho(D)- or D^u-positive infant by an Rho(D)-negative mother. Rho(D^u)-antigen is a weakly reacting Rh-antigen. When an Rho(D)-negative woman, whether D^u-positive or D^u-negative, delivers an Rho(D)- or D^u-positive infant, she should receive Rh-immunoglobulin after delivery.

The first pregnancy in an Rh-negative woman who has not received a transfusion of incompatible blood usually produces an unaffected child. With each successive pregnancy with an Rh-positive fetus the prognosis becomes worse. A history of prior Rh-disease or a positive maternal antibody titer requires amniocentesis at 26 weeks to detect levels of bilirubin derivatives. An optical density graph of the amniotic fluid is prepared and the peak at 450 mμ is read.

If the graph indicates isoimmunization with hemolysis before 34 weeks, an intrauterine transfusion may be required. Later in gestation early delivery and exchange transfusion are preferable. Because of gross prematurity, intrauterine transfusion is appropriate therapy only after the twenty-fifth week. After the thirty-second week, premature delivery is safer and more appropriate. Intrauterine transfusion thus finds its greatest place between the twenty-fifth and thirty-second weeks of pregnancy.

The terms Rh-positive (DD or Dd) and Rh-negative (dd) refer essentially to the presence or absence, respectively, of the antigen D, although other isoantigens such as C and c or E and e may be involved.

Not all Rh-incompatibility results in hemolytic disease of the newborn (erythroblastosis or isoimmunization). ABO-incompatibility may protect against Rh-disease. Hemolytic disease on the basis of major blood group incompatibilities is uncommon because of the wide distribution of fetal A and B antigens, as a result of which antibodies are bound elsewhere than the erythrocytes. Type O women have anti-A and anti-B antibodies, which hemolyze A and B erythrocytes before maternal sensitization to the Rh-antigens takes place.

Intrauterine death with isoimmunization may occur with cardiac failure, edema (hydrops), and ascites. The neonate may have anemia, hyperbilirubinemia, and kernicterus. The placenta in hydropic forms of erythroblastosis is large. The Langhans layer is prominent, and nucleated erythrocytes are found in fetal vessels (Fig. III-10). The fetus is not jaundiced because the placenta clears its plasma of bilirubin.

In hemolytic disease of the newborn, prompt clamping of the umbilical cord is recommended and the end is left long for possible exchange transfusions. A positive direct Coombs' test on the cord blood means an affected fetus. A hemoglobin level less than 10 g or an unconjugated bilirubin value greater than 5 mg suggests the possible need for exchange transfusion. The bilirubin level should be kept below 20 mg%. Phototherapy is useful to decrease the bilirubin.

Nonimmune fetal hydrops may be caused by cardiovascular disorders (arrhythmias and structural defects), congenital infections, chromosomal

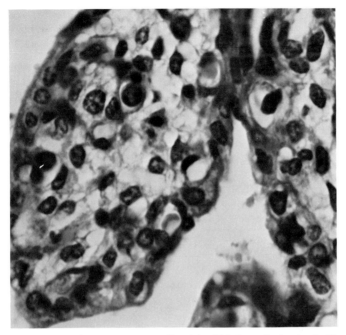

Fɪɢ. III-10. Placenta from pregnancy complicated by Rh-isoimmunization (erythroblastosis fetalis), showing nucleated erythrocytes in fetal vessels.

anomalies, and the twin-to-twin transfusion syndrome. It may result also from pulmonary and renal disorders of the fetus, placental thrombosis and angiomas, and maternal diabetes mellitus or pregnancy-induced hypertension. A significant proportion of nonimmune fetal hydrops is idiopathic. Ultrasound is the key to prenatal diagnosis.

Diabetes Mellitus

Most medical complications do not alter the course of pregnancy and are themselves not altered by pregnancy. A few major exceptions are discussed on pages 157 through 171. Perhaps the most important is diabetes mellitus. Before the introduction of insulin, diabetic patients rarely carried their pregnancies to term or even became pregnant. At present the incidence of this complication of pregnancy is over 1%. The prevalence of insulin-dependent diabetes in the United States is somewhat under 0.5%. The disorder is often first unmasked during pregnancy. Because of the normal gestational changes in carbohydrate metabolism and renal function, the diagnosis must be made with caution. Detection of urinary sugar should be made with a glucose-specific enzyme test to rule out lactosuria. A glucose tolerance test (GTT) should be performed on all pregnant patients with a family history of diabetes, a history of large infants (over 4000 g), prior children with congenital anomalies, unexplained stillbirths, habitual abortions, or significant obesity. If the GTT is normal in early pregnancy in these patients, it should be repeated in each of the subsequent two trimesters.

Pregnancy affects the diabetes and diabetes affects the pregnancy. The effects of pregnancy on the diabetes include an alteration in glucose tolerance. There is hyperinsulinemia in normal pregnancy but a decrease in the effectiveness of insulin. The vomiting of pregnancy may initially lead to insulin shock; later, as a result of starvation, ketoacidosis may be produced. The efforts of labor may deplete the glycogen, and the increased likelihood of infection makes the possibility of acidosis greater in pregnancy. Gestational glucosuria may also stem in part from a change in the filtered load of glucose. Since the level of insulin is higher in pregnancy and its half-life is unchanged, there must be an overproduction of insulin, which may stress the pancreas. Insulin is antagonized by human placental lactogen (human chorionic somatomammotropin); the effect of degradation by insulinases is much less significant. Steroid hormones may further decrease glucose tolerance.

The diabetic pregnancy is complicated by an increased incidence of preeclampsia (perhaps fourfold), hydramnios, large babies, fetal death, and congenital anomalies. There is also an increased incidence of maternal urinary tract infection. In most series, the perinatal mortality rate is increased in insulin-using diabetics, and there is an increase in respiratory distress syndrome (probably related largely to prematurity) and neonatal hypoglycemia, hypocalcemia, hypothemia, and nonhemolytic hyperbilirubinemia. Less common neonatal complications are polycythemia with thrombosis of the renal vein and the caudal regression syndrome.

The best results in management of the pregnant diabetic are provided by an obstetrician with special knowledge of perinatal medicine. The most important factor is medical control of the disease, ideally beginning before conception. The second principle of management is appropriately early delivery. With excellent management the perinatal mortality may be reduced almost to that of normal pregnancy and the maternal mortality essentially to zero.

The nonovert (preclinical, Class A) diabetic is managed obstetrically almost the same as a normal pregnant patient. The class A, or chemical, diabetic has an abnormal glucose tolerance curve, but is maintained free of symptoms without insulin on dietary management alone.

Gestational diabetes occurs in between 3 and 12% of all pregnant women in the United States. The diet of the gestational diabetic should provide 36 to 40 calories/kg of ideal weight/day. It should contain 1.3 g of protein/kg/day and 200 to 500 g of carbohydrate/day. The remainder of the calories should be provided by fat. A typical diet of 2350 calories/day should comprise approximately 15% protein, 45% carbohydrate, and 35% fat.

Uncomplicated Class A diabetics are generally delivered at term. The overt diabetic is managed by an obstetrician or a medical team concerned with maintaining strict control of the diabetes and ensuring timely delivery.

The essence of modern management of the pregnant overt diabetic is control of glucose. The best control is accomplished through intensive education of the patient regarding the relation of glucose to insulin and frequent (several times a day) measurements of blood or plasma glucose. These glucose values are then used to determine the amounts of insulin to be given by frequent injections or continuous infusion with a pump. The blood glucose can be measured simply at home by commercially available techniques. In the best of circumstances, rates of complications in pregnant diabetics who have maintained excellent control of blood glucose before and during pregnancy do not differ significantly from those in nondiabetic pregnant women. Some centers manage the ideally controlled diabetic the same as a normal patient, with respect to timing and route of delivery.

The timing of the delivery depends principally upon two factors: fetal maturity and fetal well-being. Complications to be avoided during pregnancy are infections, acetonuria, and preeclampsia. Dosage of insulin should be regulated according to blood sugars with the aim of maintaining normal glucose levels. It is important to distinguish blood from plasma levels of glucose, for the former are about 87% of the latter. For example, a fasting blood glucose of 90 mg/dl is equivalent to a plasma value of 103 mg/dl.

The patient should be seen at least weekly throughout pregnancy. Overt diabetics are generally delivered between the thirty-fourth and thirty-eighth weeks, depending on the severity of the disease and the degree of control of glucose. Earlier delivery is indicated in more severe diabetes and in the presence of poor control of preeclampsia, repeated ketoacidosis, hydramnios, or advancing retinopathy. Prior intrauterine deaths are another indication for earlier delivery.

Fetal distress may force early delivery despite prematurity. Nonstress tests and oxytocin challenge tests are helpful in detecting fetal distress before the thirty-fourth week. Before that time prematurity may prevent a successful outcome of the pregnancy.

Despite the often large size of the newborn, its fragile condition requires intensive care in the high-risk or premature nursery. Pregnancy should be discouraged in severe diabetics. Therapeutic abortion has been performed for progressive renal disease, retinitis with progressive visual loss, and coronary arterial disease.

Class A diabetics have an abnormal glucose tolerance test, but no clinical signs of diabetes. Class B diabetics are those whose disease began after the age of 20 or has been present for as long as 9 years with no vascular disease. Class C diabetics are those whose disease began between the ages of 10 and 19 or has been present for between 10 and 19 years with no vascular disease. Class D diabetics are those whose disease began before the age of 10 or has been present for 20 years or more, with vascular disease, calcification of the vessels of the legs, or benign retinopathy. Class F diabetics have nephropathy, Class H have cardiac disease, and Class R have proliferative retinopathy. The less severe diabetics often have large babies and placentas, whereas the more severe, namely those with vascular disease, often have undergrown babies and small placentas.

The oral glucose tolerance test is more sensitive and physiologic, but because of variations in absorption from the gastrointestinal tract during pregnancy the intravenous test is often easier to interpret. During labor and delivery, because of the changing requirements for insulin, the crystalline (regular) rather than a long-acting variety should be used. Optimal control is achieved through use of an insulin pump and a glucose infusion.

The criteria for diagnosis of diabetes in pregnancy are far from universally accepted and they differ from those used in the nonpregnant state. If the fasting plasma glucose level is less than 100 mg/100 ml in the intravenous test and if the level at 2 hours is not greater than the fasting level, it is unlikely that the patient has diabetes.

In the intravenous glucose tolerance test, the K value, or the rate of disappearance of glucose from the plasma, expressed as percent per minute, is calculated from the formula:

$K = \dfrac{0.693}{t_{1/2}} \times 100$, where $t_{1/2}$ is the time for the concentration of glucose to decrease 50%.

This value is lower in women with decreased carbohydrate tolerance. Use of the K value allows accurate comparisons of carbohydrate tolerance, with the use of a single number rather than a curve, at various stages of pregnancy.

The patient should be evaluated carefully one week before anticipated delivery in order to regulate her metabolic status and to decide the route of delivery. She should be delivered by cesarean section unless an easy induction can be anticipated. The labor should be monitored and attempts at vaginal delivery abandoned if fetal distress occurs. After delivery, the maternal insulin requirement usually drops.

The problems of the neonate, in addition to those listed on page 158, include birth injuries because of large size and traumatic delivery, and congenital anomalies. The management requires careful regulation of the infant's environmental temperature, oxygen, humidity, and blood glucose. A precipitous fall in neonatal blood glucose may occur if the prior fetal glucose levels, which mirror maternal levels, were elevated as a result of poor control. The fetal prognosis depends on the severity of the maternal diabetes, the medical management and complications of the pregnancy, fetal maturity, and neonatal care. Maternal acidosis may lead to mental retardation in the offspring. The maternal prognosis is influenced by cardiovascular complications, pulmonary emboli, and severe preeclampsia or eclampsia.

During pregnancy oral hypoglycemic agents are not advised. The sulfonylurea compounds may worsen neonatal hypoglycemia. Estrogen replacement is valueless; furthermore, the use of stilbestrol during pregnancy may lead to adenosis of the cervix and vagina and other genital anomalies in daughters and sons years later (p. 239).

The lecithin/sphingomyelin ratio is probably reliable in diabetic pregnancies if a standardized procedure is followed. The dipalmitoyl derivative of lecithin provides an even more reliable index of pulmonary maturity. Phosphatidyl glycerol is the best indicator of pulmonary maturity in the fetus of the diabetic mother. If phosphatidyl glycerol is present in the amnionic fluid, delivery can be accomplished without fear of respiratory distress syndrome in the neonate.

Another means of monitoring the diabetic pregnancy is measurement of glycosylated hemoglobin A_{1c}. An increase in this form of hemoglobin suggests poor control of the diabetes in the weeks prior to its measurement and predicts greater difficulties for the fetus. Optimal control of glucose is associated with normal values of hemoglobin A_{1c}.

Cardiac Disease

More than 1% of all pregnant patients have cardiac disease. Of this group, rheumatic heart disease has long been the most common, but congenital heart disease is forming an increasingly large proportion and in some centers is the most commonly found cardiac disease in pregnancy. Diagnosis of cardiac disease in pregnancy is complicated by the normal gestational changes in the cardiovascular system. The maximal rise in cardiac output during pregnancy occurs as early as the end of the first trimester and is not significantly reduced in the last few weeks unless the patient is kept supine. As a result, the patient may decompensate early and at any time up to term. Cardiac failure occurs most commonly at the time of maximal cardiac output.

A systolic murmur may be functional, but diastolic and presystolic murmurs and precordial thrusts must be considered evidence of organic cardiac disease even in pregnancy. Diagnosis of cardiac disease requires at least one of the following: a diastolic, presystolic, or continuous murmur; unequivocal cardiomegaly; a loud harsh systolic murmur especially with a thrill; or an arrhythmia.

Mild cardiac disease may be managed at home with care to correct anemia and prevent or combat infection promptly. The best results are obtained through combined management by a cardiologist and an obstetrician. Treatment varies according to functional class of the cardiac disease. In general, all patients with cardiac disease should avoid stress and should have increased rest. Preeclampsia, excessive weight gain, and hypertension should be treated vigorously. A cough, rales, or atrial fibrillation should arouse suspicion of impending cardiac failure. Fibrillation should be converted promptly to normal sinus rhythm.

Management of the labor includes well-controlled analgesia and anesthesia (p. 110) to relieve both anxiety and pain. The second stage should be shortened, and antibiotics should be given to prevent subacute bacterial endocarditis. Conduction anesthesia is appropriate for delivery of the patient with cardiac disease. Elevation of the mother's legs from the dorsal lithotomy position may result in an autotransfusion of up to 500 ml of blood and precipitate cardiac failure. Outlet forceps are indicated to shorten the second stage. Hemorrhage is especially dangerous because the patient with cardiac disease often cannot compensate for sudden hypovolemia. Cesarean section must be reserved for obstetric indications.

The puerperium is also a dangerous period for the patient with cardiac disease. The patient with serious cardiac disease is often kept at bedrest for 7 to 10 days after delivery. Tubal ligation should be delayed in these patients. For patients with cardiac disease who refuse tubal ligation or for whom it is not performed for other reasons, effective contraception is mandatory. The patient with severe cardiac disease should be discouraged from becoming pregnant at all.

Abortion is medically indicated for cardiac disease only early in pregnancy, when it can be performed by suction curettage. Later in pregnancy abortion may be as dangerous as carrying the pregnancy to term on bedrest.

Maternal prognosis depends upon the functional capacity of the heart, other complications that increase cardiac work, the quality of medical care, and psychologic and socioeconomic factors, such as the possibility of hospitalization throughout pregnancy.

The anatomic changes in pregnancy that make the diagnosis of cardiac disease more difficult include elevation of the diaphragm, deviation of the heart to the left, and apparent cardiomegaly on chest film. Pulmonic and apical systolic murmurs are often hemic, presumably caused by lower viscosity of the blood during pregnancy. Dependent edema in pregnancy is not necessarily a sign of cardiac disease, nor are tachycardia and palpitations.

The New York Heart Association classification of cardiac disease is as follows:

Class I—No limitation of physical activity.
Class II—Slight limitation of physical activity.
(Ordinary activity produces symptoms.)
Class III—Marked limitation of physical activity.
(Less than ordinary exercise produces symptoms.)
Class IV—Complete limitation of activity.
(Insufficiency at rest, that is, cardiac failure.)

Because decreased cardiac output leads to decreased uteroplacental circulation and function, the fetuses of patients with cardiac disease are often undergrown. Patients in Classes I and II may be managed on an ambulatory basis during the early months of pregnancy. Patients in Classes III and IV should remain at bedrest throughout pregnancy. Although pregnant women in Classes I and II rarely go into failure, they must be watched carefully at frequent antepartum visits.

Warning signs include basal rales, dyspnea, tachycardia, and increasing edema. Optimal management includes bedrest for 10 hours a day, rest for half an hour after each meal, household help, avoidance of respiratory infections, and prompt reporting of any so-called cold. Patients must be taught the early symptoms of decompensation and the conditions that may lead to that serious complication. They must also be instructed to report such symptoms immediately to their physicians. If decompensation occurs, morphine, oxygen, digitalis, rotating tourniquets, and diuretics may be lifesaving.

During the puerperium, hemorrhage, infection, and thromboembolism, which are more serious than in normal patients, must be avoided. Class III patients ideally should not become pregnant. If they do, they must remain in bed throughout the pregnancy. Delivery, by any route, of a patient in failure carries a very high mortality.

Any infection in a woman with valvular heart disease must be treated with massive antibiotics after blood cultures are obtained. If the patient requires anticoagulants, heparin is the drug of choice because it does not cross the placenta.

Maternal hypoxia may lead to abortion, intrauterine death, and prematurity. Kyphoscoliotic heart disease may lead to cor pulmonale.

A cesarean section may be indicated in patients with coarctation of the aorta to prevent rupture of the vessel. There is probably no residual cardiac damage or shortening of life expectancy as a result of pregnancy in any patient with cardiac disease.

Rubella

Rubella (German measles) is the most important of the viral diseases known to cause congenital anomalies in the human fetus. In the mother it is usually a mild disease that causes fever, headache, lymphadenopathy, and a pink, confluent macular rash. The rash appears one week after the viremia. The peak of antibody titer follows the rash by 1 or 2 weeks. The fetus is most severely affected when the mother's viremia coincides with the period of organogenesis, or the first 16 weeks. The congenital rubella syndrome, acquired transplacentally, comprises numerous fetal abnormalities, involving the eye (cataracts, microphthalmia, and chorioretinitis), heart, ear, central nervous system, and other organs. The infants may have microcephaly, deafness, major arterial defects, and low birth weight. In addition, there may be osseous and hematologic changes and mental deficiency. Infants born with the congenital rubella syndrome may excrete the live virus.

The diagnosis of maternal rubella is suspected on the basis of clinical signs and symptoms, but confirmed by a rise in antibody titer as demonstrated by hemagglutination inhibition reactions. There is no effective therapy for the disease, but abortion is often performed to prevent birth of a malformed fetus.

The susceptible female population should be identified and vaccinated with a strain of live rubella virus. Pregnant women, however, must not be immunized with live virus, and pregnancy should be interdicted for at least 3 months after active immunization of the mother.

The earlier in pregnancy the mother contracts rubella, the greater is the likelihood of congenital anomalies in the fetus. Viremia at 4 weeks' gestation is accompanied by a greater than 50% chance of fetal anomalies; by 12 weeks the likelihood has dropped to 10%. The use of gamma globulin in the mother is controversial, because the clinical signs may be masked without affecting the viremia.

If the titer in the first hemagglutination inhibition test is positive in a 1:10 or greater dilution immediately after clinical signs of the disease, the patient may be considered immune. If it is positive only at dilutions of 1:8 or less immediately after the rash and it rises 4-fold or more 10 to 14 days later, the patient very likely has had a viremia even in the absence of clinical signs and symptoms.

The only rubella vaccine currently available in the United States is prepared from the RA 27/3 strain, a live attenuated virus. Vaccination is indicated in adult women shown to be susceptible with a titer of 1:8 or less on hemagglutination inhibition; the woman must not be pregnant and should be on reliable contraception if sexually active. Rubella vaccination is not contraindicated in breastfeeding mothers or in women in the same household with pregnant family members.

Other Perinatal Infections

The incidences of the more common perinatal infections per number of live births are as follows: *Herpesvirus hominis,* 1:6000; toxoplasmosis, 1:1000; streptococcal infections, 1:300; cytomegalovirus, 1:75; and *Chlamydia trachomatis,* 1:35.

The TORCH syndrome may result when the fetus is infected in the first trimester. The etiologic agents are the viruses of rubella, cytomegalovirus, and herpes and a protozoon, toxoplasma. The syndrome comprises microcephaly, chorioretinitis, cerebral calcification, and mental retardation.

Cytomegalovirus is a ubiquitous organism. As the population ages, seropositivity for the virus increases. Diagnosis is made by serologic testing of the mother. Because this is a persistent and latent virus, about 4% of subsequent pregnancies are affected. Of infants who are sick at birth, 5% die early and 85% have neurologic sequelae. Each year in the United States about 6000 infants are born with cerebral damage and 3000 with deafness caused by cytomegalovirus. There is no effective prevention or treatment.

Herpesvirus hominis is described on page 198. This organism makes a small contribution to the TORCH syndrome, but the major infection with this virus occurs at the time of delivery, when the infant contracts the disease during passage through the birth canal. The syndrome includes gingivitis, stomatitis, keratoconjunctivitis, and encephalitis. Approximately half of the affected infants die and 60% of the survivors have long-term neurologic and ocular sequelae. There is no specific prevention or therapy for perinatal herpetic infection, although cesarean section can prevent transmission to the newborn in many but not all patients whose membranes are intact or only recently ruptured.

Toxoplasmosis is caused by the protozoon *Toxoplasma gondii,* an organism that affects many species of animals. The cat is a primary host, but in addition to cat feces, sources of the organism include raw pork, beef, and lamb. Toxoplasmosis, although deleterious to the fetus, causes only a chronic disease of low virulence in the mother. Investigation of an influenza-like syndrome in a pregnant woman should include serologic TORCH titers during both acute and convalescent phases of the illness.

Pyelonephritis

Acute pyelonephritis is the most common renal disease in pregnancy. It is usually bilateral, although the right side appears to be affected more often than the left. The onset, which is frequently abrupt, is heralded by fever, chills, and flank pain. Since it is an ascending infection, it may be preceded by signs and symptoms of lower urinary tract infection, such as dysuria, frequency, and urgency. Diagnosis is made on the basis of leukocytes and bacteria in the urine. Cultures and sensitivity tests determine the choice of therapy. The commonly implicated organisms are *E. coli, Klebsiella, Proteus, Pseudomonas,* and other gram-negative bacilli.

Antibiotic therapy should be intensive and continuous for at least 10 days, since persistent or recurrent pyelonephritis may lead to permanent renal damage. Therapy should not be discontinued until two successive sterile urine cultures are obtained. Ampicillin (0.5 g q.i.d) is frequently the drug of choice. The antibiotics and other antimicrobial drugs cross the placenta and most of them may affect the fetus. If there is no response to antibiotics, a urologic investigation, including cystoscopy, is indicated. An intravenous pyelogram may be indicated post partum to rule out obstructive uropathy or a urologic anomaly.

Dilation of the ureters and renal pelves and decrease in peristalsis, primarily as a result of the hormonal changes of pregnancy, predispose to urinary stasis. Increased renal excretion of glucose and amino acids, furthermore, provides a medium for favorable growth of bacteria. Introduction of bacteria into the bladder (bacilluria) leads to cystitis, which may progress as an ascending infection to involve the ureters and kidneys. Routine catheterization of the bladder in pregnant women is therefore to be avoided.

Bacteriuria is defined as 10^5 or more colony counts per ml of urine in a clean midstream specimen. About 6 to 7% of pregnant patients have asymptomatic bacteriuria, of whom about one quarter, or 1 to 2% of all pregnant women, subsequently develop pyelonephritis. It is now believed that pyelonephritis, but not necessarily asymptomatic bacteriuria, leads to an increase in the rate of prematurity. Despite the cost of screening for asymptomatic bacteriuria, it is recommended so that appropriate antibacterial therapy may be instituted.

Sulfonamides, such as sulfisoxazole, or ampicillin may be used on an outpatient basis for mild urinary tract infections. Sulfonamides, by competing with bilirubin for albumin binding and conjugation by glucuronyl transferase, may cause jaundice and kernicterus in the newborn, particularly the premature. They are not recommended during the first and third trimesters.

Aminoglycosides such as gentamicin and kanamycin may be ototoxic and nephrotoxic to the mother. Tetracyclines administered to the mother in the third trimester may lead to discoloration of the infant's deciduous teeth, and, rarely, may cause jaundice in the mother. Administered in the first trimester, tetracyclines may cause micromelia and other skeletal deformities. Chloramphenicol may produce the "gray baby syndrome" and, rarely, bone marrow depression in the mother (p. 92). Nitrofurantoin should be used only for mild infections or for maintenance after the primary infection has been apparently eradicated by an antibiotic. In patients with a glucose-6-phosphate dehydrogenase deficiency, nitrofurantoin may cause hemolysis. Methenamine mandelate is inadequate therapy for frank pyelonephritis.

Anemia and Thrombocytopenia

Anemia is a condition in which circulating red blood cells are deficient in number or in total hemoglobin content. It may be caused by decreased blood formation or increased blood loss or destruction. In the nonpregnant woman, anemia is defined as a hemoglobin concentration of less than 12 g/100 ml. Since there is normally a decline in hemoglobin concentration in pregnancy because of the relatively greater increase in plasma volume than in erythrocyte mass, anemia in pregnancy is defined as a hemoglobin concentration of less than 10 g/100 ml.

The most common cause (95 to 98%) of anemia in pregnancy is iron deficiency. Its incidence is much higher in lower socioeconomic groups because of poor diet. Most women enter the reproductive age with low iron reserves because of either dietary deficiencies or blood loss from heavy menstruation. Increased requirements of pregnancy will exhaust the reserves of iron and produce anemia. Therefore, supplementary iron is recommended for all prenatal patients.

Maternal complications with severe iron-deficiency anemia include dysphagia, angina pectoris, and congestive heart failure. Perinatal mortality and morbidity are also increased significantly. Diagnosis of iron deficiency depends upon demonstration of a low serum iron content and a high serum iron-binding capacity. Measurement of ferritin provides an even more sensitive index of iron deficiency. In all cases of anemia a direct blood smear should be examined morphologically. In a mild iron-deficiency anemia, erythrocytes may appear normal. In more severe cases, however, hypochromia and microcytosis are demonstrable. Treatment is aimed at increasing the circulating hemoglobin concentration and total reserves of body iron. To this end, supplementary iron is recommended.

Treatment depends on the severity of the anemia. Ferrous sulfate (300 mg) once a day after breakfast is adequate prevention in normal pregnancy. Ferrous sulfate (300 mg) three times a day after meals may be required for anemia. Parenteral iron in the form of iron-dextran may be given if there is an intolerance to oral iron or poor absorption. A blood transfusion is reserved for only the most serious or refractory cases. Therapy is evaluated by monitoring changes in hematocrit, hemoglobin content, structure of the erythrocytes, and reticulocyte count.

Pregnancy requires about 800 mg of iron (p. 64). Since the maximum absorbed from a usual diet is 1 mg a day, supplementary iron is required. The most common cause of failure to respond to oral iron therapy is negligence in taking the daily supplement. Plural gestations require larger supplements. Occult bleeding is a less common cause. Malabsorption without underlying gastrointestinal disease is rare but may be associated with the use of antacids.

Hereditary anemias (hemoglobinopathies) are associated with increased maternal and fetal morbidity and mortality. The most severe complications are found in patients with sickle cell anemia (SS disease) and SC disease. Five percent of American blacks may have the sickle cell trait (SA), but less than 1% have the true disease (SS). Patients with sickle cell disease have an increased prevalence of infections of the urinary tract and of pneumonitis. As the anemia becomes more intense, pain crises become more common and the frequencies of abortions, stillbirths, and neonatal deaths increase.

Advances in restriction endonuclease technology have made possible the molecular analysis and prenatal diagnosis of several human genetic diseases, notably sickle cell disease and other hemoglobinopathies. Pregnant patients with SC or SS disease should receive supplemental folic acid (5 mg daily). The need for supplemental iron should be individualized.

The treatment of a crisis is oxygen, analgesics, and hydration. Patients may benefit from partial exchange transfusion. Optimally, necessary transfusions should be accomplished before delivery and at least a liter of whole blood should be available during delivery. Since serious complications may occur during pregnancy with these hereditary anemias, family size should be limited by either sterilization or effective contraception.

Megaloblastic anemia caused by a dietary deficiency of folic acid is an uncommon cause of anemia in the United States but is reported to be important elsewhere. Signs and symptoms may include fatigue, anorexia, nausea, vomiting, diarrhea, and glossitis. The diagnosis may be made by demonstration of a low hemoglobin, macrocytosis, hypersegmented polymorphonuclear leukocytes, and a low serum folate level. Specific therapy is oral or parenteral administration of folic acid (1 to 5 mg daily). The relation of folic acid deficiency to abruptio placentae has not been demonstrated.

If severe immune thrombocytopenic purpura occurs during pregnancy, prednisone (60 to 100 mg/day) should be given; the dose is then tapered to the lowest amount that will produce the desired effect. Splenectomy may be required if severe thrombocytopenia persists despite administration of steroids.

If the platelet count is greater than $100,000/mm^3$ and no prior splenectomy has been performed, vaginal delivery should be attempted in the absence of obstetric contraindications. Delivery should be by cesarean section if a splenectomy has been performed before delivery or if the maternal platelet count or the fetal platelet count from a scalp sample is less than 100,000/mm^3. Supplemental intravenous steroids should be given during delivery if the patient has received them during pregnancy, and a transfusion of platelets may be required if hemostasis becomes a problem. Splenectomy may be required in certain patients in the course of cesarean section.

The neonate with a normal platelet count should be monitored by daily counts for a whole week. The thrombocytopenia is usually self-limited but prednisone (1-2 mg/kg/day), a transfusion of platelets, or even an exchange transfusion may be required. Splenectomy is contraindicated in the neonatal period.

Thyroid Dysfunction

The normal physiologic changes in the maternal thyroid gland during pregnancy are summarized on page 66. Hyperthyroidism in pregnancy is often caused by Graves' disease, which may be a result of autoimmune phenomena. It is often associated with long-acting thyroid stimulator (LATS), an IgG globulin, which crosses the placenta and may produce hyperthyroidism in the fetus. Signs and symptoms of hyperthyroidism include loss of weight, increased appetite, tremors, increased nervousness, and hyperreflexia. The diagnosis is supported by elevated levels of the free thyroid hormones or the free thyroxine index.

Severe hyperthyroidism during pregnancy must be treated to avoid "thyroid storm" at the time of delivery and possible fetal mortality. Therapy is difficult because antithyroid drugs such as propylthiouracil cross the placenta and may suppress the fetal thyroid. Optimal therapy of hyperthyroidism in pregnancy may be antithyroid medication and iodine to reduce the vascularity of the gland followed by partial thyroidectomy a few weeks later. Radioactive iodine should not be used during pregnancy because it crosses the placenta and is bound in the fetal thyroid.

Hypothyroidism is uncommon in pregnancy and most often results from prior operations on the thyroid or therapy with [131]I. Hypothyroid women may have decreased fertility and high rates of abortion and stillbirth. Diagnosis is made by failure of thyroid hormones to rise as usual in pregnancy and by elevated levels of TSH. Patients are treated with full thyroid replacement. Women who become pregnant while on thyroid hormones should receive full replacement for the duration of pregnancy, with normal levels of TSH as the therapeutic goal.

The easiest and least costly screening tests of thyroid function in pregnancy are TSH and total T_4 (TT_4) and T_3 resin uptake. The product of T_3 and T_4 is termed the free thyroxine index (T_7), which is approximately equal to free T_4 and is unchanged during pregnancy. Because of the striking increase in thyroid-binding globulin in pregnancy (an effect of increased estrogen), the concentrations of total T_3 and T_4 (both bound and free) are similarly elevated and somewhat difficult to interpret. Tests utilizing radioactive iodine are contraindicated in pregnancy. Inasmuch as the thyroid gland in pregnancy is not completely suppressed by exogenous thyroid hormone, the usefulness of thyroid suppression tests is limited.

Rheumatic Diseases

The effect of pregnancy on the rheumatic diseases is variable. The group comprises systemic lupus erythematosus, rheumatoid arthritis, scleroderma, polymyositis and dermatomyositis, Sjögren's syndrome, amyloidosis, necrotizing arthritis, rheumatic fever, relapsing polychondritis, and ankylosing spondylitis. The most important rheumatic diseases that coexist with pregnancy are systemic lupus erythematosus (SLE) and rheumatoid arthritis (RA).

Most patients with SLE have normal fertility, but there is an increased prevalence of abortion, stillbirth, prematurity, and small-for-dates babies, especially in patients with renal disease.

Treatment of SLE must be individualized, but it generally consists of aspirin or corticosteroids. Patients with RA may have clinical remissions during pregnancy with postpartum exacerbations. RA generally has little effect on the pregnancy. Aspirin and corticosteroids are the mainstays of therapy.

Clinical estimates of the prevalence of renal involvement in SLE range from 45 to 75%. The prognosis for pregnancy in patients with lupus nephropathy is best judged by the presence or absence of signs of activity in the 6 months before conception. In the absence of such signs the fetal prognosis is good and two thirds of the mothers will remain in remission. If the SLE has been clinically active within the 6 months before conception, the perinatal loss is about 25%, signs are aggravated in about 50% of the mothers, and few undergo remissions during the pregnancy. Contrary to earlier teaching, when exacerbations occur, they do so predominantly during pregnancy rather than after abortion or delivery. Lupus anticoagulant in the plasma of a pregnant woman identifies her as a patient at high risk for fetal wastage and thrombosis. There is no good evidence that therapeutic doses of prednisone or azathioprine, an immunosuppressant, are teratogenic in human pregnancy.

Thrombophlebitis

Thrombophlebitis complicates only about 1 in 300 to 400 pregnancies, but is more common in the puerperium (p. 172). The patient may present with palpable, indurated tender cords in the lower extremities or vulva. Deep calf tenderness, tachycardia, and fever may also be found. Treatment of superficial thrombophlebitis includes bedrest, elevation of the legs, heat, and anti-inflammatory agents. If the thrombophlebitis fails to improve or worsens with the aforementioned treatment, anticoagulant therapy is indicated, usually in the form of heparin for 10 days. Coumarin derivative, which cross the placenta, are contraindicated during most of pregnancy. In the first trimester they may be teratogenic. In the later stages of pregnancy, particularly during labor and delivery, they may cause fetal hemorrhage, most seriously in the brain. Deep thrombophlebitis of the legs or pelvis requires heparinization. Pulmonary emboli may necessitate ligation or plication of the vena cava and ligation of the ovarian veins.

Disorders of the Puerperium

Puerperal morbidity is any fever of 100.4° F (38° C) or higher on any 2 of the first 10 days post partum, excluding the first 24 hours, as detected with an oral thermometer using a standard technique at least 4 times daily. Unless another cause is found, puerperal infection, often manifested by chills, fever, and tachycardia, is assumed to be endomyoparametritis (often abbreviated to metritis). The other common causes of fever in the puerperium are urinary tract infection, mastitis, thrombophlebitis, and infection of an episiotomy site.

Introduction of bacteria into the genital tract by attendants is one of the main causes of metritis. Another common cause is rupture of the membranes with contamination and colonization of the amnionic cavity by pathologic organisms that are indigenous to the vagina and cervix. The most common pathogens are the anaerobic streptococci, *E. coli* and other coliform bacilli, *Bacteroides fragilis*, beta-hemolytic streptococci, and staphylococci. Confirmation of the diagnosis of metritis is made by cultures of the uterine cavity and blood before administration of antibiotics. When the infection causes a peritonitis, rebound tenderness, malaise, and anorexia generally occur.

Perinatal morbidity and mortality are associated with colonization of the chorionic surface of the placenta by *Ureaplasma urealyticum*, *Mycoplasma hominis*, or both. These organisms are more strongly associated with unfavorable gestational outcomes than are group B streptococci. *Chlamydia trachomatis,* however, does not appear to be an important etiologic agent in reproductive wastage.

Metritis may lead to pelvic abscess or femoral thrombophlebitis. Pelvic abscesses are suggested by manual examination and confirmed by ultrasound. Drainage may frequently be accomplished by transcutaneous aspiration or culdocentesis under sonographic guidance. After pelvic abscess is ruled out, pelvic thrombophlebitis should be suspected in any puerperal patient who does not respond to treatment of presumptive metritis. Thrombophlebitis may first appear seven to ten days after delivery. Pain and swelling of the leg suggest femoral thrombophlebitis. Pelvic thrombophlebitis is suspected on the basis of pain and tenderness on pelvic examination. Pulmonary emboli are occasionally the first signs of deep phlebitis. The treatment usually requires intravenous heparin for 10 days and occasionally ligation of the inferior vena cava. Puerperal infection and its sequelae may be minimized by elimination of infections before labor, correction of anemia, appropriately timed delivery after rupture of the membranes, aseptic technique, restriction of the number of vaginal examinations, and avoidance of trauma and loss of blood during delivery.

Infection of the urinary tract may follow trauma and catheterization superimposed on urinary stasis and bacteriuria. Treatment is discussed on page 166.

Mastitis is treated by heat and antibiotics. Abscesses may require incision and drainage. The most common organism is *Staphylococcus aureus,* which is usually resistant to penicillin; one of the semisynthetic penicillins such as oxacillin is therefore required. Engorgement of the breasts without inflammation may be relieved by support and cold compresses. Analgesics may be required.

Subinvolution of the uterus may be caused by retained secundines, metritis, or myomas. It produces prolonged lochia and occasionally delayed postpartum hemorrhage. Ergot derivatives are useful. If infection supervenes, antibiotics are administered. A curettage is usually required to remove retained tissues or a subinvoluted placental site, but it must be performed gently to avoid removal of excessive endometrium with resulting Asherman's syndrome.

Mortality Statistics

The principles and practice of regionalization of perinatal care have decreased maternal, fetal, and neonatal mortality and morbidity. The concept of regionalization includes levels of obstetric and pediatric services, perinatal centers, and maternal transfers of high-risk patients.

The maternal mortality rate is the number of maternal deaths per 100,000 live births as a direct result of the reproductive process. According to some definitions the term includes all deaths of preg-

nant women from any causes, including those unrelated to pregnancy. The rate for nonwhites is several times that for whites. Although both rates are continuing to fall, the differential is
increasing, primarily as a result of social and economic factors
rather than genetic predisposition. The last full year for which figures are available in the United States reflected a remarkably low
maternal mortality rate of 8.9 per 100,000 live births.

The most common causes of maternal deaths are hemorrhage,
infection, preeclampsia-eclampsia, embolism, anesthesia, and cardiac disease. Deaths associated with abortion continue to account
for significant maternal mortality in jurisdictions where the procedure is governed by restrictive laws. Ectopic pregnancy continues
to account for an increasing number and proportion of maternal
deaths.

Deaths may be related directly to pregnancy or to coincident
diseases that are affected by pregnancy or may be caused by factors
unrelated to pregnancy. Deaths from hemorrhage, preeclampsia-
eclampsia, infections, vascular accidents, and anesthesia may be
considered directly related to pregnancy. Deaths from hemorrhage
have been reduced by blood transfusion and hospital delivery.
Those from infection have been reduced by asepsis, hospital delivery, and antibiotics; and those from preeclampsia-eclampsia have
been reduced by prenatal care and early delivery in the hospital.
Embolism involving amniotic fluid, air, and thrombi may be considered direct results of the reproductive process. Coincident conditions that may be exacerbated by pregnancy include cardiac disease, diabetes, and anemia. Important causes unrelated to
pregnancy include infections and malignant diseases, suicide, and
accidents.

Perinatal mortality is the sum of stillbirths (fetal deaths) and
neonatal deaths (deaths of liveborn infants in the first 28 days of
life). A stillbirth is defined as an infant with no heartbeat who
neither breathes nor cries nor shows any other signs of movement.
The fetal death rate is the number of fetal deaths (deaths of fetuses
weighing 500 g or more) per 1000 births (live births plus stillbirths).
(Five hundred grams corresponds roughly to 20 weeks' gestation.)
The neonatal death rate and the infant mortality rate (deaths under
1 year of age) are calculated per 1000 live births.

Perinatal deaths are divided almost equally between stillbirths
and neonatal deaths. Many stillbirths are caused by maternal diseases such as diabetes, but in a larger percentage of cases there is
no obvious cause. The most common cause of neonatal death is
prematurity. Other causes of perinatal mortality include congenital
malformations, obstetric trauma, intrauterine hypoxia, infection,

hematologic disorders (including Rh-isoimmunization), pulmonary dysfunction (atelectasis and respiratory distress syndrome), and other iatrogenic causes. In many cases there is no sufficient pathologic diagnosis.

Between 1950 and 1980 the total perinatal mortality rate in the United States fell from 40 per 1000 to less than 18 per 1000. The neonatal mortality rate during this period fell from over 20 to less than 8.5 per 1000 live births. The most recent year for which figures are available (1983) reflects a neonatal mortality rate of 7.4. University hospitals and referral centers may have higher mortality rates because of the greater numbers of high-risk patients. Many northern European countries have lower incidences of prematurity and lower perinatal death rates, which may reflect their more stable populations, lower prevalences of poverty, and important possible differences in reporting.

One factor in perinatal mortality, congenital malformations, may be genetically or environmentally induced. Intrauterine hypoxia may result from abruptio placentae; placenta previa; prolapse, knots, or entanglement of the cord; maternal hypotension; anesthesia and analgesia; shoulder dystocia; delayed delivery of the aftercoming head; and prolonged labor.

Infections may be intrauterine or extrauterine and are usually of viral or bacterial origin. Most neonatal viral infections are acquired when the infant passes through the birth canal. Important iatrogenic causes of perinatal mortality include premature and traumatic deliveries. Maternal diseases associated with increased perinatal loss include hypertensive disorders, glomerulonephritis, urinary tract infection, diabetes mellitus, and symptomatic cardiac disease.

IV

Obstetric and Gynecologic
Procedures

Sonography

The application of sonography (diagnostic ultrasound) to obstetrics and gynecology is probably the most important technologic advance in the specialty during the second half of the twentieth century. Although it is not routinely indicated in all pregnancies, there is no documented harm to either mother or fetus when it is used according to accepted guidelines. The most important applications of diagnostic ultrasound are listed in Table 9.

Table 9.   Indications for Diagnostic Ultrasound

1. Estimation of gestational age
2. Evaluation of fetal growth
3. Vaginal bleeding of uncertain cause
4. Diagnosis of fetal presentation
5. Suspected plural gestation
6. Adjunct to amniocentesis
7. Discrepancy between uterine size and clinical dates
8. Pelvic mass
9. Suspected hydatidiform mole
10. Adjunct to repair of incompetent cervix
11. Suspected ectopic pregnancy
12. Adjunct to special procedures
13. Suspected fetal death
14. Suspected uterine anomaly
15. Localization of intrauterine device
16. Surveillance of ovarian follicular development
17. Biophysical evaluation for fetal well-being
18. Observation of intrapartum events
19. Suspected polyhydramnios or oligohydramnios
20. Suspected abruptio placentae
21. Adjunct to external cephalic version
22. Estimation of fetal weight or presentation in premature rupture of membranes or preterm labor
23. Abnormal value of serum α-fetoprotein
24. Follow-up of identified fetal anomaly
25. Follow-up of placental location in identified placenta previa
26. Follow-up of prior congenital anomaly
27. Serial evaluation of fetal growth in plural gestation
28. Evaluation of fetal maturity in patients who register late for prenatal care

Estimation of gestational age in patients with uncertain dates or those who are scheduled to undergo elective repetition of a cesarean section, induction of labor, or other elective termination of pregnancy permits proper timing of delivery and avoidance of the hazard of premature delivery. Monitoring of fetal growth permits assessment of the effect of a complication of pregnancy on the fetus and guides management of the pregnancy. Such monitoring is indicated when there is an identified cause of uteroplacental insufficiency, such as severe preeclampsia, chronic hypertension, chronic renal disease, and severe diabetes mellitus, and in other medical complications of pregnancy in which retardation of intrauterine growth or macrosomia is suspected. In cases of vaginal bleeding, ultrasound often permits assessment of the source of the bleeding and the condition of the fetus. When the identity of the presenting part is not certain, ultrasound permits accurate diagnosis and guides management of the delivery. When plural gestation is suspected by detection of more than one fetal heartbeat, a fundal height greater than expected for dates, or knowledge of prior use of drugs to stimulate ovulation, ultrasound may identify the number of fetuses and guide management.

In the course of amniocentesis, ultrasound permits guidance of the needle to avoid the fetus and placenta, to increase the likelihood of obtaining amniotic fluid, and to decrease the chance of fetal loss. When there is a discrepancy between the size of the uterus and the clinical dates, ultrasound permits accurate dating of the pregnancy and detection of complications, such as oligohydramnios, polyhydramnios, plural gestation, retardation of intrauterine growth, and fetal anomalies. Sonographic examination of a pelvic mass aids in diagnosis of its location, size, and consistency. Ultrasound permits accurate diagnosis of a hydatidiform mole and differentiation of this growth from fetal death. The diagnosis is often suspected on the basis of hypertension, proteinuria, ovarian cysts, or failure to detect a fetal heartbeat with Doppler after 12 weeks (p. 128). Ultrasound aids in timing and proper placement of the stitch or tape in the repair of an incompetent cervix. When ectopic pregnancy is suspected or when pregnancy occurs after surgical procedures on the fallopian tube or prior ectopic pregnancy, ultrasound is valuable for ruling out this complication. Ultrasound facilitates guidance of the appropriate instruments and increases the safety of special diagnostic procedures such as fetoscopy, intrauterine transfusion, placement of shunts, in vitro fertilization, embryo transfer, and sampling of chorionic villi. In cases of suspected fetal death, use of ultrasound provides rapid diagnosis and facilitates optimal management. Sonographic serial surveillance of fetal growth and condition improves fetal outcome in cases of suspected uterine abnormality, such as clinically significant leiomyomata or congenital structural anomalies.

Ultrasound facilitates the removal of an intrauterine device, thus reducing complications that might result from a misplaced contraceptive device. Surveillance of ovarian follicular development by sonography is valuable in the treatment of infertility. Assessment of the volume of amniotic fluid and tone, movements, and breathing of the fetus after 28 weeks of gestation (biophysical evaluation of fetal well-being) assists greatly in the management of high-risk pregnancies. Intrapartum procedures such as version and extraction of a second twin and manual removal of the placenta may be done more safely with ultrasonic visualization. Confirmation of suspected polyhydramnios, as well as identification of the cause of the condition in certain pregnancies, can be accomplished with ultrasound. Confirmation of the diagnosis and extent of suspected abruptio placentae may likewise be accomplished. Visualization provided by ultrasound facilitates external version from breech to cephalic presentation. Information provided by ultrasound facilitates estimation of fetal weight and presentation in premature rupture of membranes and preterm labor and aids management regarding timing and method of delivery.

In evaluation of the significance of abnormal α-fetoprotein values in the serum, ultrasound provides an accurate assessment of gestational age for comparison with standards and identifies several conditions such as twins and anencephaly that may cause elevation of the level of AFP. Ultrasound may be used to follow the change in location of the placenta with respect to the internal os in cases of placenta previa identified earlier in pregnancy. Ultrasound may be employed to assess the progress or lack of change in an identified fetal anomaly and to detect recurrence (or lack thereof) of congenital anomalies in a patient who had an affected fetus in a prior pregnancy.

The psychologic benefits of knowledge that the fetus is normal are obvious. Ultrasound permits recognition of discordant fetal growth in plural gestation, thus aiding management and timing of delivery. Finally, in the case of a patient who registers late in pregnancy for her prenatal care, ultrasound provides accurate knowledge of fetal maturity.

Currently about half of all pregnant women have at least one sonogram. The equipment is available in virtually all hospitals and many obstetricians' offices in the United States. As experience with the technique and knowledge of its safety increase, it seems likely that ultrasound will play an even greater role in obstetrics in the future.

A newer technologic advance is the application of continuous wave Doppler ultrasound to assessment of uterine blood flow. Analysis of waveforms and velocities may predict or detect the growth-retarded fetus at a relatively early stage and thus lead to appropriate clinical management.

Cesarean Section

Delivery of a fetus through incisions in the abdomen and uterus is called cesarean section. The essence of the operation is the hysterotomy. As a result of improvement in surgical technique, antisepsis, blood replacement, and anesthesia, cesarean section has become a safe operation that has replaced difficult vaginal deliveries. The two main types of cesarean sections are the classical, which involves incision of the upper contractile portion of the uterus, and the low-segment operation, which involves incision of the lower uterine segment after dissection of the vesicouterine peritoneum. The low-segment incision is usually transverse, although it may be vertical. Cesarean section may be combined with hysterectomy when it is desirable to remove the uterus for disease.

In the United States today about half of all cesarean sections are primary and half are operations that are repeated because of a uterine scar. Indications for primary cesarean section may be fetal or maternal. A major factor in the perinatal mortality associated with cesarean section is prematurity. Ascertaining fetal maturity (p. 83) before elective or repeated cesarean section will minimize this threat.

Most cesarean operations in the United States are low transverse procedures. The indications for classical section are restricted mainly to certain cases of anterior placenta previa and transverse lies. With premature breeches, because the lower uterine segment is poorly developed, it may be less traumatic to the infant to deliver it through a vertical incision, which may be extended upward if necessary to provide more room. Disadvantages of a classical section include greater likelihood of rupture, especially before the onset of labor, in subsequent pregnancies and a greater incidence of infection, bleeding, and adhesions. Cesarean section-hysterectomy may be indicated for neglected transverse lie with an infected uterus, myomas, carcinoma in situ of the cervix, and postpartum hemorrhage with atony.

Many primary cesarean sections are performed for dystocia related to pelvic contraction or a large fetus. Other important maternal indications include abnormal presentations, uterine dysfunction, placenta previa, abruptio placentae, preeclampsia, hypertension, isoimmunization, diabetes, prior vaginal plastic surgical procedures, and possibly the elderly primigravida (over the age of 35). Fetal indications include prolapsed cord and fetal distress. Fetal monitoring has provided a more logical basis for selection of cesarean section for fetal indications.

The frequency of cesarean section in the United States in the last 17 years has quadrupled, from a rate of a little over 5% in 1970 to about 21% in 1987, or even higher, depending on the proportion of complications in the obstetric population and the local medical attitudes toward repeating all cesarean sections. Complications of the procedure include hemorrhage (the average blood loss during cesarean section is between 800 and 1000 ml), infection, anesthetic accidents, and separation of the uterine wound. Maternal mortality has been reduced to 0.1%, or even less in some series. It is related largely to the indication for the operation, the presence of infection, the duration of labor, and anesthesia. Abdominal delivery per se, nevertheless, involves a distinctly greater risk of maternal mortality and morbidity than does vaginal delivery. Each decision to perform a cesarean section, particularly a primary section, must therefore be made with this increased risk in mind. Perinatal mortality is related to the indication for the operation and in the case of repeated cesarean sections, to the prevalence of prematurity.

The rate of maternal morbidity after cesarean section is approximately 25 to 30%. The prophylactic use of antibiotics in that operation thus seems justified. The drug of choice should be both safe for mother and fetus and effective against the offending organisms. The cephalosporins are appropriate for this purpose. For metritis after cesarean section, clindamycin and an aminoglycoside may be the combination of choice. Other therapeutic regimens include a cephalosporin of the second or third generation or ampicillin together with an aminoglycoside.

In response to concern about the rapidly rising rate of cesarean section in the United States, much attention has been directed to the indications for the procedure and the means of reducing the number of abdominal deliveries. There seems little doubt that the medicolegal climate in the United States has contributed substantially to the high rate of cesarean section. Current emphasis is placed on a careful analysis of dystocia, uterine scars, breech presentation, and fetal distress as the major factors contributing to the rise in the rate of abdominal delivery.

The causes of dystocia are fetopelvic disproportion and dysfunctional labor (p. 140). Disproportion, which should be easily recognized, has not contributed greatly to the rise in cesarean section, but the diagnosis of abnormalities of uterine contraction is the basis for a significant proportion of abdominal deliveries. Before resorting to cesarean section for uterine dysfunction, the obstetrician should consider other methods of treatment such as rest and oxytocin, for abnormal and subnormal contractions, respectively.

The precept of routine repetition of all cesarean sections should be reconsidered. A trial of labor is an option for patients who satisfy all of the following criteria: nonrepetitive indication, uterine incision known to be low-segment transverse, singleton pregnancy, vertex presentation, estimated fetal weight less than 4000 g, and absence of all other contraindications to vaginal delivery. Capability for continuous monitoring of the fetal cardiac rate and uterine activity are prerequisite to attempted vaginal delivery of patients with a uterine scar. The patient must understand that cesarean section may become necessary during the course of labor. Availability of an operating room for immediate cesarean section and appropriate anesthetic and pediatric personnel are required when a trial of labor after cesarean section is attempted. Some centers are now delivering vaginally up to 60% of patients who had prior cesarean section.

Abdominal delivery remains the safest course when the patient has had more than one prior cesarean section and, of course, when the cephalopelvic disproportion is absolute. In each of the last few years about 3.5 million babies have been born in the United States. With a cesarean section rate of about 20%, or 700,000 abdominal deliveries, and a prior uterine incision the indication for about 25% of those operations, almost 200,000 cesarean sections are done each year on that basis alone. If a significant proportion of these 200,000 women can be delivered vaginally with safety, a great medical and economic advantage would result. Nevertheless, the seriousness of uterine rupture for both mother and fetus requires most careful selection of patients for vaginal delivery after cesarean section.

Breech presentation also has contributed to the large increase in the rate of cesarean section. Vaginal delivery of the term breech should remain an option when all of the following conditions are satisfied: fetal weight less than 3600 g, normal pelvic size and shape, frank breech presentation without hyperextended head, and delivery under the supervision of an obstetrician experienced in the technique. The use of external version with tocolysis has reduced the numbers of breech presentations at term and, consequently, of cesarean sections.

The diagnosis of fetal distress should be more carefully documented. Ideally employed, fetal monitoring should not in itself increase the rate of cesarean section, for it may not only identify jeopardized fetuses that require prompt abdominal delivery but may also prevent operations that might otherwise have been unnecessarily performed. With proper surveillance the rate of cesarean section should be kept to 15% or below, with minimal maternal and perinatal mortality and morbidity.

Forceps

The obstetric forceps is an instrument used primarily for traction and rotation of the fetal head. Each pair of forceps consists of two branches. Each branch comprises a handle, a shank, a lock, and a blade. The blade, which may be solid or fenestrated, has two curves. The cephalic curve corresponds to the fetal head, and the pelvic curve corresponds to the pelvic axis. All forceps applications must be cephalic, that is, according to the position of the fetal head.

The forceps may be applied for fetal or maternal indications or electively. Forceps applications are classified as low (outlet), mid, or high. A low forceps operation is performed on a vertex that is on the perineum with the sagittal suture occupying the anteroposterior diameter of the pelvic outlet. Low forceps may be elective (prophylactic) or indicated. A midforceps operation refers to an application to a head that has already engaged but has not yet met the criteria for low forceps. Difficult midforceps operations have been replaced in modern obstetrics by cesarean section. A high forceps operation is performed on an unengaged head. It has no place in modern obstetrics because of its potential dangers to mother and fetus. For several reasons, not least of which is medicolegal, forceps procedures are less commonly employed today than at any other time in the past several decades.

182 · Obstetric and Gynecologic Procedures

About 20% of deliveries in this country entail the use of forceps. The prerequisites to the application of forceps include the following: fully dilated cervix, engaged head, exact knowledge of the position and station, absence of disproportion, ruptured membranes, proper positioning of the patient on the table, appropriate anesthesia, and preferably, empty bladder and rectum. Application of forceps is usually accompanied by an episiotomy.

Maternal indications include a prolonged second stage (often defined as greater than 2 hours), cardiac disease (to shorten the second stage), acute emergencies such as pulmonary edema and abruptio placentae, and anesthesia that prevents voluntary expulsive efforts in the second stage. Fetal indications include prematurity (to prevent trauma to the fetal head on the perineum) and fetal distress (a heart rate lower than 100 or higher than 160 per minute between contractions, irregularity of the fetal heart, or passage of meconium). The use of forceps for fetal distress is justified only when delivery thereby can be accomplished as safely as and more expeditiously than with cesarean section.

Episiotomy

Episiotomy may be midline, or median (from fourchette directly posteriorly through the midline of perineum) or mediolateral, which involves an incision from the fourchette into the perineum at about 45 degrees from the midline. A midline episiotomy is technically a perineotomy. The operation is often performed in first deliveries and in subsequent deliveries after repair of a prior episiotomy. The operation is performed to prevent lacerations of maternal tissues and injury to the fetal head. It is generally used with forceps deliveries. Immediate complications of inadequate repair include hematomas, urinary retention, and shock. Rectovaginal fistula may be a delayed complication of unrecognized or improperly repaired extension of the episiotomy into the rectum.

First-degree obstetric lacerations involve only the vaginal mucosa or perineal skin. Second-degree lacerations involve the underlying muscle and connective tissue but not the sphincter ani. A third-degree laceration involves the anal sphincter in addition. When the rectal mucosa is torn as well, a fourth-degree, or complete, laceration results.

Median episiotomy entails less blood loss, is easier to repair, and is more comfortable for the patient. It may be used in most spontaneous or low forceps deliveries in any patient with an adequate perineum. The main advantage of a mediolateral episiotomy is the decreased likelihood of its extension into the sphincter ani or rectum, a complication that is usually managed easily by an experienced obstetrician. If an extension of the episiotomy occurs, the injury should be repaired immediately by a skilled obstetrician.

Induction of Labor

Labor may be induced medically (by oxytocin) or surgically (amniotomy, or rupture of the membranes). Medical induction is accomplished by means of an infusion containing 10 units of oxytocin/1000 ml of 5% dextrose in Ringer's lactate or isotonic or half-isotonic saline, administered at the same rate and with the same precautions as used for stimulation of labor (p. 142). The hazards of induction with oxytocin include rupture of the uterus, premature separation of the placenta, and fetal hypoxia. Additional complications include prematurity, uterine infection, and prolapse of the umbilical cord. Several clinics have found prostaglandins to be suitable alternatives to oxytocin for medical induction of labor. Vaginally administered prostaglandin has been used successfully to evacuate the uterus in cases of fetal demise toward the end of the second trimester.

A few of the important indications for induction are erythroblastosis fetalis, diabetes mellitus, preeclampsia-eclampsia, and premature rupture of the membranes. Induction of labor in a multipara who lives some distance from the hospital and has a history of rapid labors may be considered obstetrically indicated. When induction of labor is medically indicated, delivery should usually be accomplished within 48 hours after initiation of attempts at induction and within 24 hours after rupture of the membranes.

Strictly elective inductions may appear convenient for the patient and the obstetrician, but their advisability as a routine procedure is at best questionable. Induction is most likely to succeed if rupture of the membranes is accompanied by simultaneous initiation of an infusion of oxytocin. Success of induction is further increased when the cervix is effaced, at least 2 cm dilated, and anterior, and the fetus is mature. An unengaged head is not an absolute contraindication to amniotomy, but before the procedure is performed, the fetal head must be brought as deeply as possible into the pelvis by fundal and suprapubic pressure and facilities for immediate cesarean section should be available to cope with the possibility of prolapse of the umbilical cord.

Version

Version is manual turning of the fetus by the obstetrician from one presentation to another. Cephalic version is turning of the breech or transverse to a head, or a cephalic, presentation. This procedure is done externally without anesthesia under tocolysis before the onset of labor. The fetus may revert to its original position after the maneuver. Podalic version is turning of a cephalic or transverse presentation to breech. It is performed internally during the second stage of labor under deep general anesthesia for delivery of the second twin. Internal version may cause traumatic rupture of the uterus and has been supplanted largely by cesarean section in the United States. Version is contraindicated in the presence of marked oligohydramnios, placenta previa, premature rupture of the membranes, third-trimester bleeding, and possibly a uterine scar.

The Papanicolaou Smear

Because cytologic examination of the cervix should routinely accompany physical examination of the adult woman, the method of obtaining the smear was described under physical examination (p. 52).

The smear may be interpreted as negative, suspicious, or positive for malignant cells. Another popular classification divides the smears into five classes: Class I, or negative; Class II, or atypical but benign; Class III, or atypical and suspicious; and Classes IV and V, or positive for malignant cells, with Class V the more distinctly malignant. In the terminology of cervical intraepithelial neoplasia (CIN), CIN I corresponds roughly to mild dysplasia, CIN II to moderate dysplasia, and CIN III to severe dysplasia and carcinoma in situ.

Schiller Test

In this test the squamous epithelia of cervix and vagina are painted with a solution of iodine and potassium iodide. Abnormal epithelia of various kinds including cancer do not take the mahogany stain because they contain little or no glycogen. This test is not diagnostic of a malignant lesion, but may help to direct the biopsy to a particular site. The Schiller test has been supplanted largely by colposcopically directed biopsy of suspicious lesions of the cervix.

Toluidine Blue

The toluidine blue test helps to identify abnormal areas of squamous epithelium. After the suspicious areas are painted with 1% toluidine blue, they are allowed to dry and are sponged with a 1% solution of acetic acid. The normal epithelium is decolorized. The abnormal areas, which retain the deep blue stain, may then by subjected to biopsy.

Punch Biopsy

This procedure involves the removal of single or multiple pieces of tissue for histologic examination. In gynecology it is performed mainly for lesions of the cervix and may be included in the investigation of irregular uterine or postmenopausal bleeding. This procedure does not ordinarily require anesthesia and is generally performed in the office.

Colposcopy

This is a technique for examination of the cervix at a magnification of 10 to 40 times. The procedure discloses epithelial abnormalities and suggests areas for directed biopsies. After 3% acetic acid is applied, the cervix is inspected to detect abnormal findings, such as white epithelium, punctation, mosaics, and atypical vessels. Colposcopy may be used as a means of improving the rate of detection of cervical cancer in conjunction with exfoliative cytology. Satisfactory colposcopy requires visualization of the entire squamocolumnar junction. When colposcopically directed biopsies are performed to investigate an abnormal Papanicolaou smear (one with dysplastic cells), they should be accompanied by endocervical curettage to detect lesions in the canal. The accuracy of a directed biopsy varies from 85 to 95%. If the site of biopsy continues to bleed, hemostasis may often be achieved by careful application of Monsel's solution (ferric subsulfate).

Four-quadrant cervical punch biopsy has been supplanted largely by colposcopically directed biopsy. It involves biopsy of the cervix at the 3, 6, 9, and 12 o'clock positions around the external os. The squamocolumnar junction should be included in as many specimens as possible. Biopsy at the 6 o'clock position is often performed first to avoid contamination of the operative field by bleeding from above.

Cone Biopsy

This is an excision of a cone of cervical tissue for histologic diagnosis. It is required to rule out invasive carcinoma when the Papanicolaou smear is positive and colposcopy has not been performed or has been unsatisfactory. The number of cone biopsies performed has been greatly reduced by the successful use of colposcopy. This procedure is done in the hospital or ambulatory surgical facility. The base of the cone surrounds the external os and the apex is at or near the internal os. The cone thus includes essentially all of the endocervical canal.

Dilation and Curettage

A therapeutic curettage, as performed for incomplete abortion, serves as both diagnosis and treatment of the condition. A diagnostic curettage is performed to identify a lesion in the endocervix or endometrium. It is best performed fractionally; that is, endocervix and endometrium are curetted in sequence and the specimens placed in separate containers for orientation and identification of the site of the lesion. For ordinary diagnostic curettage the cervical canal is scraped with a small curette before it is dilated. The size and configuration of the uterine cavity are first ascertained by sounding before the curettage. The endometrium is systematically curetted and polyp forceps are inserted to ensure that large lesions such as polyps have not been missed by the sharp curette.

Complications of dilatation and curettage include cervical laceration and uterine perforation. Curettage should therefore be done in a day surgery center or hospital, where accidents may be promptly treated. The procedure is indicated for diagnosis of irregular uterine bleeding except in very young girls. Contraindications include intrauterine pregnancy and acute pelvic inflammatory disease. Suction curettage is the removal of the uterine contents by means of a hollow curette attached to a vacuum pump. Suction curettage usually requires little cervical dilatation. Because it can be safely performed in an outpatient facility, emergency room, or doctor's office, it is gradually replacing sharp curettage as a diagnostic and therapeutic procedure.

Endometrial Biopsy

This procedure involves removal of a small fragment of endometrium by means of a small sharp curette or a suction curette. It is usually performed as part of the investigation of infertility to ascertain ovulation or adequacy of the luteal phase of the endometrial cycle. This procedure may not be adequate for the detection of endometrial carcinoma or atypias.

Culdoscopy

This is endoscopic visual examination of the female pelvic viscera through the posterior vaginal fornix. It is used most often in the investigation of infertility and endocrine problems. It is best performed in a hospital or day surgery center but does not necessarily require general or regional anesthesia. This technique has been supplanted for most purposes by laparoscopy. Contraindications to culdoscopy are fixed cul-de-sac and adherent uterine retroversion.

Laparoscopy

This an endoscopic procedure performed by introduction of a telescope through a stab incision in the abdominal wall after creation of a pneumoperitoneum. The laparoscope is used for a variety of diagnostic procedures such as the detection of tubal patency, the visualization of adnexa in cases of infertility and endocrine syndromes, and the elucidation of obscure pelvic pain. In addition, it serves many therapeutic purposes such as tubal interruption. Laparoscopy may be performed using open or closed techniques. Current improvements in the instrument have extended the range of its possible diagnostic and therapeutic uses and increased its safety.

Culdocentesis

This procedure is the aspiration of fluid from the rectouterine pouch by puncture of the posterior vaginal fornix. It may be used to identify peritoneal fluid, blood, or pus. It is performed in certain cases of suspected intraabdominal hemorrhage and abscess in the cul-de-sac.

Colpotomy

This is an incision of the posterior vaginal fornix into the rectouterine pouch to visualize pelvic structures, perform surgical procedures on the adnexa, and drain pelvic abscesses.

The Rubin Test

This is an office procedure for the investigation of tubal patency. It has been supplanted largely by hysterosalpingography and laparoscopy. Carbon dioxide is introduced into the cervix and the pressure is monitored with a manometer. If the tubes are patent, a rush is heard by means of a stethoscope over the abdomen when a pressure of between 60 to 90 mm Hg is reached. At that time the pressure in the manometer drops. Shoulder pain indicates gas under the diaphragm, which provides another criterion of tubal patency.

Hysterosalpingography

This is a radiologic procedure for investigation of tubal patency and visualization of congenital anomalies and deformities of the uterine cavity and tube. Both water-soluble and oily contrast media have been successfully employed. The definitive sign of tubal patency is spill of contrast medium into the peritoneal cavity, not merely the presence of contrast medium in the fallopian tube. The radiologically visualized defects may be caused by space-occupying lesions such as polyps and myomas or extrinsic pressure. This examination is now generally performed under fluoroscopy with image intensification and may be combined with laparoscopy for maximal diagnostic information.

Hysteroscopy

Hysteroscopy is an endoscopic technique for visualization of the endometrial cavity. It can be used for diagnosis and, in some countries, sterilization by electrocoagulation of the uterine ostia of the oviducts or placement of plugs in the ostia. It may also be used to remove small myomas and polyps, divide septa, retrieve intrauterine contraceptive devices, and obtain biopsies.

Cauterization, Cryosurgery, and Laser

Cauterization is the induction of cellular necrosis by means of physical or chemical agents. In gynecology it is usually performed upon the cervix.

Cryosurgery is the technique of freezing by means of special probes cooled with either liquid nitrogen, Freon gas, or carbon dioxide. It is most often employed in gynecology for treatment of benign lesions of the cervix after a negative Papanicolaou smear has been obtained.

The laser is another accepted technique for ablation of many lesions of the cervix, vagina, and vulva. Properly employed it may produce less destruction of tissue and better cosmetic results than do electrocautery and cryosurgical techniques. A drawback of the laser is the high cost of the equipment.

Hysterectomy

Total hysterectomy is removal of the entire corpus and cervix uteri. It may be performed through the abdominal route (abdominal hysterectomy) or through the vagina (vaginal hysterectomy).

Supravaginal hysterectomy, performed through a laparotomy incision, leaves the vaginal portion of the cervix. It is almost synonymous with supracervical hysterectomy, which leaves the entire cervix, or with partial, incomplete, or subtotal hysterectomy. None of these procedures implies removal of the tubes and ovaries, as in complete hysterectomy with bilateral salpingo-oophorectomy. Subtotal hysterectomy is performed today only in emergencies or special circumstances in which continuation of the operation would pose a serious hazard to the patient. The total hysterectomy is preferred because it eliminates the risk of subsequent cervical carcinoma and distressing leukorrhea.

Abdominal hysterectomy is generally preferred for large myomas, ovarian tumors, endometriosis, pelvic inflammatory disease, endometrial cancer, and some cases of carcinoma in situ of the cervix. It is the procedure of choice when exploration of the upper abdomen is required.

Vaginal hysterectomy is indicated for various degrees of uterine prolapse and other forms of pelvic relaxation (often in conjunction with anterior colporrhaphy or operations for the vaginal correction of stress incontinence), small mobile uteri that are bleeding, and certain small myomas. Several conditions may by treated satisfactorily by either vaginal or abdominal hysterectomy.

A major complication of hysterectomy is hemorrhage, immediate or delayed. Formation of a hematoma is manifested by a fall in hematocrit, a rise in temperature, and a palpable mass in the cul-de-sac or parametria. Urologic complications of hysterectomy include pyelonephritis, ligation or transection of the ureter, urinary tract fistulas, and urinary retention. Bowel complications include paralytic ileus, mechanical obstruction, and rectovaginal fistula. Other serious complications are atelectasis and pneumonia, local infection, evisceration, and pulmonary embolism.

Between 1970 and 1982 about 5.2 million women aged 15 to 44 underwent hysterectomy in nonfederal facilities in the United States. The rate, which dropped slowly from 1970 to 1982, appears to have reached a plateau of about 7.5 hysterectomies per 1,000 women.

Other Major Gynecologic Operations

Radical hysterectomy includes removal of the uterus, upper vagina, and parametria, with mobilization of the ureters. The radical hysterectomy, when performed for invasive carcinoma of the cervix (virtually its sole indication), is usually combined with pelvic lymphadenectomy, which removes en bloc bilaterally the iliac, hypogastric, obturator, and periaortic lymph nodes.

Exenteration is the complete surgical removal of the pelvic viscera including rectum, or bladder, or both, together with all the structures removed during radical hysterectomy and pelvic lymphadenectomy. Its primary indication is persistent or recurrent cervical carcinoma. Anterior exenteration is complete surgical removal of the pelvic viscera anterior to the rectum, including pelvic lymphadenectomy, with urinary diversion. Posterior exenteration is complete removal of the pelvic viscera posterior to the bladder and urethra, including pelvic lymphadenectomy and colostomy. Total pelvic exenteration is complete removal of the pelvic viscera with ureterointestinal anastomosis and colostomy.

Simple vulvectomy, performed for benign disease, is the superficial removal of vulvar structures including skin, mucosa, and superficial fat and connective tissue.

Radical vulvectomy, performed for cancer involving the vulva, is the wide removal of all structures of the vulva together with adjacent skin, a portion of the mons, and subcutaneous fat down to the deep fascia and muscles. It is usually accompanied by regional lymph node dissection through single or separate incisions.

Anterior colporrhaphy is the repair of a cystocele, or relaxation of the anterior wall of the vagina.

Posterior colporrhaphy is the repair of a rectocele, or relaxation of the posterior wall of the vagina.

Kelly plication is usually accompanied by anterior colporrhaphy. It is a plication of the connective tissue around the bladder neck and urethra for the relief of urinary stress incontinence.

Retropubic suspension of the bladder neck for stress incontinence of urine is performed through the space of Retzius. In the standard operation, sutures attach the periurethral tissue to the posterior surface of the pubic symphysis. Many simplifications of the procedure based on the same anatomic principles are currently employed, including attachment of the periurethral tissues to Cooper's ligament.

V

General Gynecology
and
Gynecologic Oncology

Gynecologic Infections

Infections of the breast, except those related to pregnancy and lactation, are not customarily treated by gynecologists in most parts of this country. Postpartum mastitis is a pyogenic cellulitis usually caused by staphylococci or streptococci. The mainstay of treatment is the appropriate antibiotic, as determined by culture and sensitivity tests. Analgesics and heat provide symptomatic relief. Treatment of an abscess is best accomplished by incision and drainage (p. 300).

Vulva

The vulva includes all the structures visible from the lower margin of the pelvis to the perineum: the mons veneris, labia majora, labia minora, clitoris, vestibule, hymen, external urethral orifice, and various glandular and vascular structures (Fig. V-1). Each labium minus is a thin fold of connective tissue devoid of fat and covered on both surfaces with a keratinized, stratified squamous epithelium. The labia minora have no hair, but a few sweat and sebaceous glands are found on their lateral surfaces. The labia majora are covered by typical skin with pilosebaceous complexes and sweat glands. After puberty they are covered with hair, particularly on the lateral surfaces. A digital process of fat below the surface of the skin creates the typical contour of the adult vulva.

The clitoris, its crura, and the bulbs of the vestibule contain erectile tissue. The crura and clitoris are surrounded by a tunica albuginea. The bulbocavernosus and ischiocavernosus muscles covering the bulbs of the vestibule and crura of the clitoris, respectively, consist of skeletal muscle, as do the other muscles of the superficial and the deep perineal pouches (p. 28). The greater vestibular glands (Bartholin's glands) are of the tubulo-alveolar variety.

The vulva is subject to the same diseases that affect the skin of other parts of the body. Vulvitis often causes pruritus, which leads to scratching and secondary trauma. Vulvitis may be associated with vaginitis; the inflammation is then designated vulvovaginitis.

General dermatologic conditions that may affect the vulva include eczema, herpes, and psoriasis. Vulvar eczema is treated by removal of the irritant, steroid creams, and antihistaminics. The vulva is subject to intertrigo because of the moisture of the labia and inguinal areas. Seborrhea and folliculitis may also involve the vulva. Infestations include pubic pediculosis (phthiriasis pubis, or "crabs"), fleas (pulicosis), bed bugs (cimicosis), and scabies.

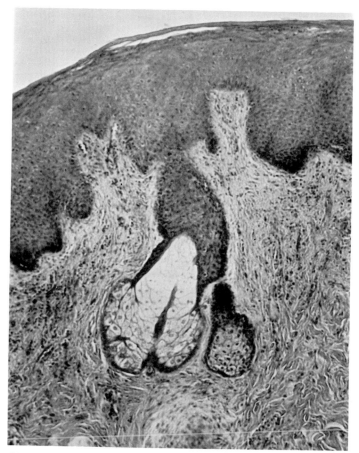

Fig. V-1. Normal vulva, showing keratinized stratified squamous epithelium and epidermal appendages.

The recommended treatment for pediculosis pubis (lice and nits) is lindane (1%), lotion or cream, applied in a thin layer to the infested and adjacent hairy areas and thoroughly washed off after eight hours or lindane (1%) shampoo applied for 4 minutes and thoroughly washed off. Lindane is not recommended for pregnant or lactating women. Alternatively, pyrethrins and piperonyl butoxide may be applied to the infested and adjacent hairy areas and washed off after 10 minutes.

Scabies is also treated with lindane (1%), 1 oz. of lotion or 30 g of cream applied thinly to all areas of the body from the neck down and washed off after 8 hours. Alternative therapies are crotamiton (10%) and sulfur (6%) in petrolatum.

Syphilis

The primary lesions of sexually transmitted (venereal) diseases are often found on the vulva. The primary lesion of syphilis is a painless chancre, which appears three to four weeks after exposure. The ulcer has indurated edges with a depressed center. There is edema of the surrounding skin and inguinal adenitis. The initial lesion regresses in about a month. Darkfield examination of the serous exudate from a chancre reveals the spirochete. The serologic test for syphilis is usually not positive until several weeks after the appearance of the primary lesion. Serologic tests for syphilis (STS) include the VDRL, which may be falsely positive in several systemic disorders.

Greater specificity may be obtained by use of the fluorescent treponemal antibody absorption (FTAA) test or the *Treponema pallidum* immobilization (TPI) test. The secondary lesions of syphilis include condylomata lata and mucous patches. The condyloma latum is a slightly raised, flat, ovoid structure that appears in clusters. It must be distinguished from condyloma acuminatum (see p. 196). Condyloma latum produces an exudate, the darkfield examination of which is positive, as are serologic tests for syphilis at this stage. The tertiary lesion, or gumma, is an uncommon finding today. The treatment of choice for primary syphilis is 2.4 million units of benzathine penicillin in a single intramuscular injection.

The treatment of choice for early syphilis (primary, secondary, or latent syphilis of less than 1 year's duration) is benzathine penicillin G (2.4 million units intramuscularly in one dose) because it provides effective treatment in a single visit.

Syphilis of more than 1 year's duration, except neurosyphilis (latent syphilis of indeterminate or more than 1 year's duration, cardiovascular, or late benign syphilis) should be treated with benzathine penicillin G, 2.4 million units, intramuscularly, once a week for 3 successive weeks (7.2 million units total). Patients who are allergic to penicillin should be treated with tetracycline or erythromycin, 500 mg., by mouth, four times a day for 30 days. Neurosyphilis requires treatment with 12 to 24 million units of aqueous crystalline penicillin G, intravenously, per day for 10 days, followed by benzathine penicillin G, 2.4 million units, intramuscularly, weekly for 3 doses; or aqueous procaine penicillin G, 2.4 million units, intramuscularly, daily with probenecid, 500 mg, by mouth, four times a day, both for 10 days, followed by benzathine penicillin G, 2.4 million units, intramuscularly, weekly for 3 doses.

For patients who are allergic to penicillin, tetracycline hydrochloride (500 mg four times a day by mouth for 15 days) or erythromycin stearate, ethylsuccinate, or base (500 mg four times a day by mouth for 15 days) may be used. These antibiotics appear to be effective but have been evaluated less extensively than penicillin.

All pregnant women should have a nontreponemal serologic test for syphilis, such as the VDRL or RPR test, at the time of the first prenatal visit. The treponemal tests such as the FTA-ABS should not be used for routine screening. In women suspected of being at high risk for syphilis, a second nontreponemal test should be performed during the third trimester and the cord blood should be tested for antibody to syphilis. Seroreactive patients should be evaluated promptly, by history and physical examination as well as by a quantitative nontreponemal test and a confirmatory treponemal test. Both of these tests should be repeated within 4 weeks. If there is clinical or serologic evidence of syphilis, the patient should be treated. Patients for whom there is documentation of adequate treatment for syphilis need not be retreated unless there is clinical or serologic evidence of reinfection, such as darkfield-positive lesions or a fourfold rise in titer of a quantitative nontreponemal test.

Patients at all stages of pregnancy who are not allergic to penicillin should be treated with the same doses of the drug as are used for nonpregnant patients. For patients who are allergic to penicillin, erythromycin (stearate, ethylsuccinate, or base) should be used in the doses recommended for nonpregnant patients. Although these dosages of erythromycin appear safe for mother and fetus, their efficacies are not proven. Tetracyclines are not recommended for syphilitic infections in pregnant women because of potential adverse effects on mother and fetus.

Congenital syphilis may occur if the mother has syphilis during pregnancy. If the mother has received adequate penicillin during pregnancy, the risk to the infant is minimal, but all infants should be examined carefully at birth and at frequent intervals thereafter until nontreponemal serologic tests are negative. Infants should be treated with penicillin at birth if maternal treatment was inadequate or unknown or with drugs other than penicillin, or if adequate follow-up of the infant cannot be ensured.

Chancroid

Chancroid produces a lesion known as a soft chancre, which unlike the hard chancre of syphilis is very painful. It occurs ten times more frequently in men than in women. The causative organism is the *Hemophilus ducreyi*, a gram-negative coccobacillus, which may be found in a smear or scraping of the primary lesion. A pustule appears 3 to 10 days after exposure. The primary lesion is a progressive ulcer of the vulva. Because it is difficult to culture this organism, material from the lesion must be placed in a sterile tube containing the patient's own blood and sent to the laboratory without delay. Treatment is erythromycin, 500 mg, by mouth, four times a day, or double-strength trimethoprim (160 mg) and sulfamethoxazole (800 mg), by mouth, twice a day. Both treatments should be continued for a minimum of 10 days and until ulcers and lymph nodes have healed. In 1985 the Centers for Disease Control added ceftriaxone, a long-acting, third-generation cephalosporin, as another option for treatment of chancroid.

Lymphogranuloma venereum

Lymphogranuloma venereum (lymphopathia venereum), or LGV, is a sexually transmitted disease caused by a serotype of *Chlamydia trachomatis,* an obligate intracellular organism that is now classified as a bacterium rather than a virus. The short period of incubation of the infection results in a lesion 1 to 3 weeks after exposure. The primary infection is accompanied by fever and malaise. A suppurative inguinal adenitis (a bubo that may drain) appears 2 to 3 weeks later. Vulvar edema may progress to elephantiasis.

Complications include draining sinuses and pseudoepitheliomatous hyperplasia of the affected skin. The lymphatics of the genital, inguinal, and anal areas are involved, and rectal strictures may form. The Frei test becomes positive 2 to 6 weeks after the initial lesion and may remain positive for life. Because the complement fixation test has greater sensitivity, it has replaced the Frei test. Since squamous cell carcinoma may complicate this lesion, biopsy should be performed before treatment is initiated. Strictures of the large bowel and fistulas may require surgical intervention. The treatment of choice is tetracycline, 500 mg, by mouth, four times a day for at least 2 weeks. Alternatives, effective in vitro but not evaluated extensively in cases confirmed by culture, are doxycycline, 100 mg, by mouth, twice a day for at least 2 weeks; erythromycin, 500 mg, by mouth, four times a day for at least 2 weeks; and sulfamethoxazole, 1 g, by mouth, twice a day for at least 2 weeks.

Granuloma inguinale

Granuloma inguinale (donovanosis) is a tropical disease that is common in the Caribbean but rare in the United States. The primary lesion is a papule, which may undergo extensive ulceration and necrosis. Unlike lymphogranuloma venereum, this disease does not produce suppurative lymphadenopathy. The pathognomonic finding is the Donovan body, an inclusion in the mononuclear cells. *Calymmatobacterium granulomatis,* the etiologic agent, is a heavily encapsulated, gram-negative bacterium. Biopsy may be required to rule out carcinoma. The treatment of choice is tetracycline, 500 mg every 6 hours, by mouth, continued preferably for 3 weeks. Failures of therapy with tetracycline may require gentamicin, 1 mg/kg, twice a day, intramuscularly, or chloramphenicol, 500 mg, every 8 hours, by mouth. Both these drugs require use for 3 weeks.

Condyloma acuminatum

Condylomata acuminata (venereal warts) appear in the form of multiple papillary warty growths on the vulva, vagina, perineum,

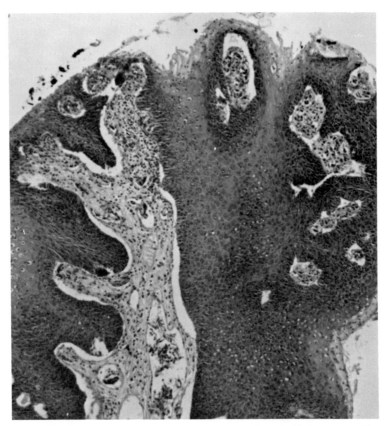

Fig. V-2. Condyloma acuminatum of the vulva, showing hyperplastic stratified squamous epithelium with hyperkeratosis and parakeratosis and vascular core of connective tissue.

cervix, and external urethral meatus (Fig. V-2). They are caused by a virus and produce a profuse, irritating vaginal discharge, often associated with *Trichomonas vaginalis*. These anogenital lesions have been linked to the development of cancer (p. 243). Unlike the condyloma latum, condyloma acuminatum has a narrow base. The diagnosis is made by biopsy. Darkfield examination for spirochetes, culture for the gonococcus, and a Papanicolaou smear should be done at the same time. External and perianal warts may be treated with 10 to 25% podophyllin in tincture of benzoin. Normal surrounding tissue should be protected and the solution washed off in 1 to 4 hours. Podophyllin should not be used during pregnancy. Alternative treatments are cryotherapy and electrocautery for lesions of moderate size, and surgical excision with the scalpel or ablation with the laser for larger condylomata.

Lymphoblastoid interferon has been used successfully on an experimental basis to treat resistant condylomas. Vaginal-cervical condylomas may be treated with 5-fluorouracil. Infants delivered through a vagina involved in condylomata may develop lesions in the larynx.

Herpes

Infection with genital herpes simplex virus (*Herpesvirus hominis, Herpes genitalis,* or *H. progenitalis*) causes a chronic and recurring infection for which there is no known cure. The organism is found in smegma and cervical secretion and is sexually transmitted. The isolates are Type II in 85% of cases and Type I in 15%. In addition to the vulvitis and vaginitis, the infection produces a cervicitis in 75% of cases. The primary lesion is a group of vesicles with surrounding erythema and edema.

For the treatment of initial genital herpes, one 200 mg capsule of acyclovir is prescribed every 4 hours, while the patient is awake, for a total of 5 capsules daily for 10 days (total 50 capsules). Acyclovir does not prevent recurrences and has not been tested in pregnant and lactating women. Patients should abstain from sexual contact when the lesions are present. The risk of transmission of the herpes virus during asymptomatic periods is unknown. Use of acyclovir for recurrent disease may decrease the severity of the recurrence. The intermittent therapy involves use of one 200 mg capsule every 4 hours while awake for a total of 5 capsules daily for 5 days (total 25 capsules). Therapy should be initiated at the earliest sign or symptom (prodrome) of recurrence. Although there is no proof of the etiologic relation between herpetic infection and cervical dysplasia and carcinoma (p. 243), women with a history of this disease should have annual Papanicolaou smears. As early as possible in pregnancy women should advise their obstetricians of a history of herpetic infection so that appropriate management of labor and route of delivery may be planned. The differential diagnosis of herpes genitalis includes herpes zoster and erythema multiforme.

Chlamydia trachomatis

Infections caused by *Chlamydia trachomatis,* an obligate intracellular parasite, are the most prevalent sexually transmitted diseases in the United States today. The Centers for Disease Control (CDC) have estimated the new cases of chlamydial infection in the United States for 1986 as 4,600,000, as compared with 1,800,000 for gonorrhea, 1,000,000 for condylomata acuminata, 500,000 for herpes, 90,000 for syphilis, and 15,000 for the acquired immunodeficiency syndrome (AIDS). Chlamydial organisms may be isolated from 10 to 30% of sexually active adolescent girls and approximately 5% of women in college. Infections caused by the various serotypes of *Chlamydia trachomatis* include hyperendemic blinding trachoma and lymphogranuloma venereum (LGV), which are uncommon in the United States; and the prevalent inclusion conjunctivitis; nongonococcal urethritis, cervicitis, endometritis, proctitis, and epididymitis; and pneumonia of the newborn.

Populations of pregnant women have a prevalence of *Chlamydia trachomatis* of 10 to 20%, as compared with 1 to 2% for gonorrhea. Infants born through a vagina infected with *C. trachomatis* may contract conjunctivitis or pneumonia. A positive diagnosis of chlamydial infection requires culture or detection by means of a fluorescein-labeled monoclonal antibody. Screening for both chlamydial and gonococcal infections may be accomplished by solid-phase enzymatic immunoassays (chlamydiazyme and gonozyme, respectively). Oral contraceptives, which have been alleged to offer some protection against gonococcal pelvic inflammatory disease, do not offer similar protection against chlamydial infection.

For culture-proven infections caused by non-LGV strains of *C. trachomatis* the following recommendations have recently been made by the CDC. Similar treatment is appropriate for nongonococcal urethritis caused by *Ureaplasma urealyticum*. Uncomplicated urethral, endocervical, or rectal infections in adults are best treated with tetracycline hydrochloride, 500 mg, by mouth, four times a day for at least 7 days or doxycycline, 100 mg, by mouth, twice a day for at least 7 days. For patients in whom tetracyclines are contraindicated or not tolerated, erythromycin, 500 mg, by mouth, four times a day for at least 7 days may be used. For pregnant women with chlamydial infections, the preferred regimen is erythromycin, 500 mg, by mouth, four times a day on an empty stomach for at least 7 days or, for women who cannot tolerate this regimen, a decreased dose of 250 mg, by mouth, four times a day for at least 14 days.

Gonorrhea

Gonorrhea is still a major bacterial disease in the United States. Acute gonorrhea may represent an initial infection or an exacerbation of a chronic infection. The signs and symptoms in the woman occur three to five days after exposure, but the primary infection may go unnoticed, rendering her an asymptomatic carrier. The gonococcus causes a purulent, malodorous discharge from the urethra, Skene's glands, cervix, and anus. All of these sites and the throat should be cultured in the attempt to make the diagnosis.

The infection is suspected when the gram-negative intracellular diplococci are demonstrated on smear and is confirmed by culture. Thayer-Martin agar plates are often used for culture of gonococci. A change from opaque to transparent colonies is associated with greater virulence. The treatment of gonococcal infections is discussed in the section dealing with upper genital tract gonococcal infections (p. 211).

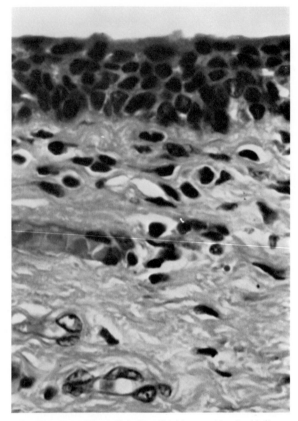

FIG. V-3. Cyst of Bartholin's duct, lined by transitional epithelium.

Bartholinitis is often of gonococcal origin but it commonly represents a secondary infection with coliform organisms or polymicrobial pathogens. In 15% of cases, *Bacteroides fragilis* may be recovered. Treatment of the acute infection includes antibiotics, analgesics, and heat. An abscess of the Bartholin gland presents as a painful, ovoid, tender mass in the inferior portion of the labia. Treatment is incision and drainage. An abscess may subside to form a cyst (Fig. V-3), which may be treated by marsupialization (evacuating the contents of the cyst and suturing its edges to those of the external incision), or occasionally excision.

Vagina

The vagina is lined by nonkeratinized, stratified squamous epithelium (Fig. V-4). Its lamina propria consists of dense connective tissue. The vagina lacks glands, but the large vessels that supply it

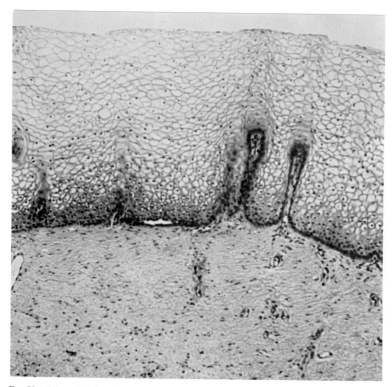

FIG. V-4. Normal adult vagina, showing nonkeratinized stratified squamous epithelium and absence of cutaneous appendages.

dilate during sexual excitation and produce the vaginal lubrication that was formerly thought to arise from the cervical and greater vestibular glands. Thickening of the lamina propria creates the anterior and posterior rugal columns with their transverse ridges, as seen in the nullipara. The muscularis is arranged longitudinally and is covered by adventitia except over the posterior fornix, which is coated with peritoneum for about 1 cm.

The vagina also responds to changing levels of hormones. During the estrogenic (proliferative) phase, its epithelium is thick and the mature squamous cells that desquamate have small, pyknotic nuclei. Because progesterone inhibits maturation, the cells sloughed during the secretory phase appear intermediate or immature. In postclimacteric years, when the vagina undergoes atrophy, the desquamated cells are of the parabasal type.

Vaginitis is often secondary to vulvitis or cervicitis. Atrophic vaginitis occurs after natural or surgical menopause as a result of a deficiency of estrogens. It produces an irritating discharge, with pruritus, edema, and often dyspareunia. The pale, thin, smooth vaginal mucosa may be secondarily infected with *Gardnerella vaginalis* or trichomonads, which may cause a purulent or sanguineous discharge. Women who continue regular coitus are less likely to have atrophic vaginitis. Treatment is local application of estrogen cream.

The main causes of adult vaginitis are *Trichomonas, Candida, Gardnerella vaginalis,* and anaerobic bacteria. Infections may be caused by combinations of these organisms.

Trichomonas

Trichomonas produces a thin, watery, yellowish-green, foamy, malodorous discharge. The organism is a flagellated protozoon, which may be identified in a hanging-drop preparation. It is transmitted primarily through sexual contact. The hyperemic vaginal mucosa may exhibit petechiae (strawberry-like appearance) and cause pruritus and soreness. Manifestations of trichomoniasis are often aggravated after a menstrual period. The best treatment is metronidazole (Flagyl). The drug is effective as a single oral dose of 2 g. An alternative regimen is 250 mg, by mouth, three times a day for 7 days. The male partners of women with trichomoniasis should be treated with the single oral dose of 2 g of the drug. Metronidazole is contraindicated in the first trimester of pregnancy and is best avoided throughout pregnancy. Lactating women may be treated with metronidazole, 2 g, by mouth, in a single dose, but breastfeeding should be interrupted for at least 24 hours after therapy.

Candida

Candida (Monilia) produces a thick, white, cheesy, curdlike discharge. On microscopic examination or culture the yeastlike buds and hyphae are seen. The infection may produce vulvar irritation, burning, and pruritus. Exacerbation of the infection is often noted in pregnancy, in diabetes, and with the use of oral contraceptives or antibiotics. The usual therapy is intravaginal insertion of nystatin (Mycostatin), miconazole nitrate, or clotrimazole in the form of cream or tablet, daily for 7 days. Intravaginal tablets may be used in conjunction with externally applied creams for vulvar and perianal lesions. Ketoconazole is also effective against *Candida albicans* but is contraindicated during pregnancy. Another imidazole, butoconazole, has proved highly effective.

Gardnerella

The new suggested term for Gardnerella vaginitis is bacterial vaginosis. *Gardnerella vaginalis,* formerly called *Hemophilus vaginalis* or *Corynebacterium vaginale,* produces a nonirritating, odoriferous, thin grayish-white vaginal discharge associated with an elevated vaginal pH (greater than 4.5) and the formation of a fishy odor (amines) when the fluid discharged is alkalinized with 10% potassium hydroxide. The normally acidic environment of the vagina is the result of lactic acid produced by the action of lactobacilli (Döderlein bacilli) on glycogen. The acidic pH of the vagina may protect against many infections. Microscopic examination reveals absence of gram-positive rods and presence of small coccobacillary organisms attached to squamous epithelial cells ("clue cells"). Gardnerella acts synergistically with anaerobic bacteria to produce this syndrome. Treatment is metronidazole, 500 mg, by mouth, twice a day for 7 days. An alternative regimen is ampicillin, 500 mg, by mouth, four times a day for 7 days. Ampicillin is less effective treatment for Gardnerella but is recommended for pregnant patients or other women for whom metronidazole is contraindicated.

In the investigation of a vaginal discharge, foreign bodies should be sought and removed. Although any severe vaginal infection may lead to a bloody discharge, carcinoma must be excluded by appropriate diagnostic techniques.

Pediatric vaginitis or vulvovaginitis is commonly initiated by a foreign body. Additional predisposing factors are poor hygiene and labial agglutination, which is treated by separation followed by estrogen cream. The organisms frequently involved are *Enterobius vermicularis* (pinworm), *Trichomonas vaginalis,* gonococci, and coliform bacilli. Pinworms may be identified by examination of a preparation made with scotch tape and are treated with piperazine citrate.

The cervix of the uterus, unlike the corpus, consists primarily of connective tissue rather than muscle. The mucosa of the endocervical canal is composed of a single layer of high columnar cells filled with mucoid material. Many of the epithelial cells are ciliated and the glands are thrown into a complicated system of clefts. The vaginal portion of the cervix is covered by squamous epithelium (Fig. V-5). The squamocolumnar junction is normally a sharp line near the external os. In older women the stratified squamous epithelium extends into the cervical canal. When the junction occurs on the portio vaginalis outside the external os, an ectropion results.

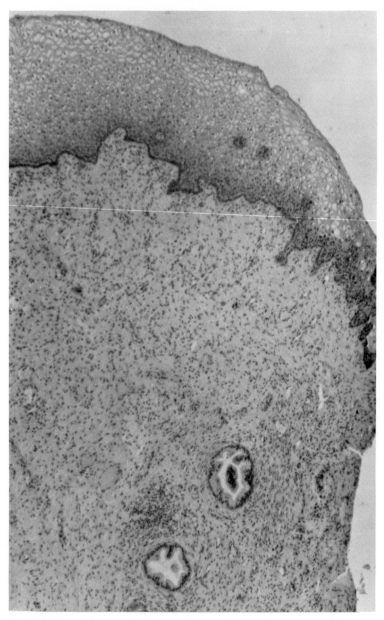

Fig. V-5. Normal adult cervix, showing nonkeratinized stratified squamous epithelium and glands with mucinous columnar endothelium.

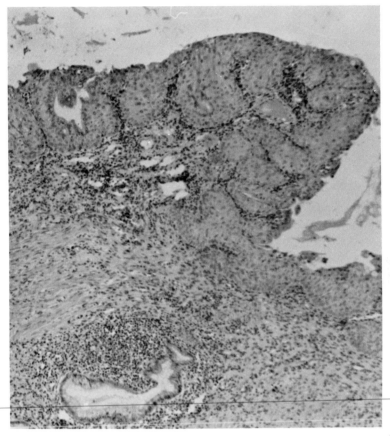

FIG. V-6. Chronic cervicitis with squamous metaplasia.

Microscopic demonstration of chronic inflammatory cells in the adult human cervix is a normal finding. Gonorrhea produces an acute cervicitis, which may cause a profuse purulent discharge as well as a chronic infection; the frequently associated urethritis causes dysuria and frequency.

Cervix

Cervicitis may be related to erosion (ulceration of the everted columnar epithelium of the endocervix and the squamous epithelium of the portio vaginalis) or eversion (rolling out of the endocervical mucosa onto the portio). Epidermidalization (covering or replacement of columnar epithelium by stratified squamous epithelium) and plugging of endocervical glandular ducts may cause retention cysts (nabothian follicles). Chronic cervicitis is the

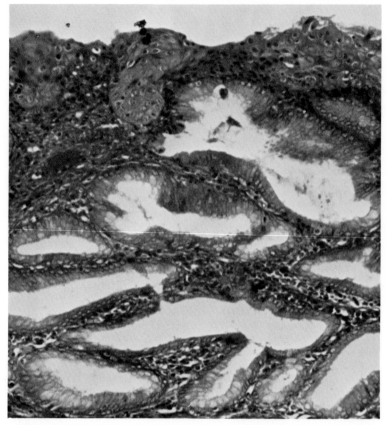

Fig. V-7. Squamous metaplasia of the cervix, showing columnar epithelium overgrown by squamous epithelium.

most common cause of leukorrhea (Figs. V-6 and V-7), which is an increase in secretions of the endocervical mucus-producing cells, vaginal effusion, and endometrial debris. Less common causes of cervicitis include secondary infection of a cervical chancre, a tuberculous or herpetic lesion, or a condyloma acuminatum.

Before treatment is begun for any cervicitis, a Papanicolaou smear should be obtained. A mucopurulent endocervical exudate suggests cervicitis caused by gonococcal or chlamydial infection. Gonorrheal cervicitis is treated by systemic penicillin or an alternative antibiotic (p. 211). Because infections with N. gonorrhoeae and C. trachomatis are frequently concurrent, it is currently recommended that in addition to penicillin, tetracycline or erythromycin be given to treat the chlamydial component. Other forms of cervicitis may be treated by locally applied antibiotics, cauterization, or removal of infected tissue by cryosurgery or laser.

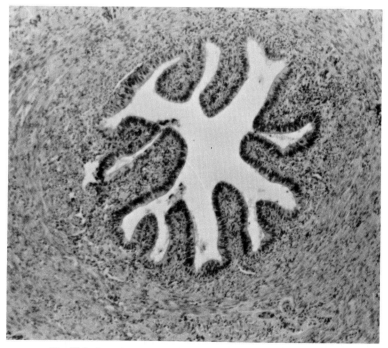

Fig. V-8. Cornual end of fallopian tube, showing simple rugal pattern.

Endometritis usually points to an underlying cause. The principal associated lesions are submucous myomas, endometrial polyps, carcinoma of the endometrium, fragments of retained placenta, or a foreign body. The inflammatory reaction associated with an intrauterine device does not usually produce a clinical endometritis.

Pelvic Inflammatory Disease

Pelvic inflammatory disease (P.I.D.), acute or chronic, is most commonly polymicrobial. The principal etiologic organisms are listed on p. 212. Less common infections are pyogenic and granulomatous. Gonococcal and chlamydial pelvic inflammatory diseases are ascending infections that spread along mucous membranes from the vulva to the adnexa.

In the adult, gonococcal infection skips from Skene's glands, the urethra, and Bartholin's glands to the cervix, because the stratified squamous epithelium of the adult is rather resistant to the infection. In infants, however, gonococcal vaginitis may be a rapidly progressive and highly contagious infection. Since the endometrium usually resists chlamydial and gonorrheal infection, the

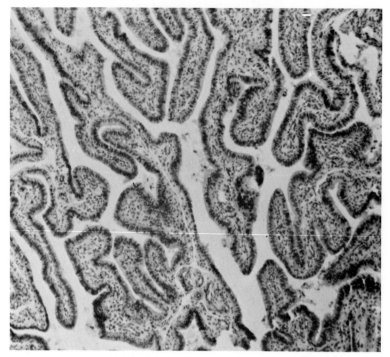

Fig. V-9. Infundibular end of fallopian tube, showing complex rugal pattern.

disease skips from the cervix to involve the tube, the main site of serious P.I.D.

The oviduct (uterine tube, or fallopian tube) is lined by a low columnar epithelium, comprising both secretory and ciliated cells. The mucosa is thrown into a series of complicated branching folds that are oriented in a longitudinal direction (Figs. V-8 and V-9). These folds are most complex in the infundibulum, slightly lower and less complex in the ampulla, still lower in the isthmus, and least complex in the intramural (interstitial) part of the oviduct. The lamina propria is typical connective tissue and a submucosa is lacking. The muscularis, which consists of an inner circular and an outer longitudinal coat, is poorly developed.

If untreated, the course of tubal infection is as follows: acute, subacute, and chronic salpingitis (Figs. V-10 and V-11), which may progress to a pyosalpinx as the fimbriated end is blocked. Resorption of the pus converts the pyosalpinx to a hydrosalpinx (Fig. V-12). In advanced infection, the ovary, which may be adherent to the tube, is involved in a perioophoritis. In the final stages of the disease a tubo-ovarian abscess may form, in which a pus-filled cavity is surrounded by a common wall of tubal and ovarian tissue.

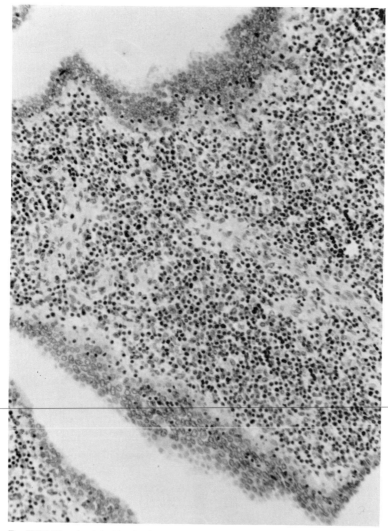

Fig. V-10. Chronic salpingitis, showing lamina propria infiltrated by numerous lymphocytes and plasma cells.

When the diagnosis of gonorrhea is made or suspected, a serologic test for syphilis should be performed at the same time and repeated several weeks later.

In patients with acute pelvic inflammatory disease, temperature, leukocyte count, and sedimentation rate are elevated. A marked rise in temperature requires a blood culture. Radiologic examination of the abdomen may be required to rule out ileus or mechanical intestinal obstruction. In pelvic inflammatory disease the pain and tenderness are usually located lower than in an acute

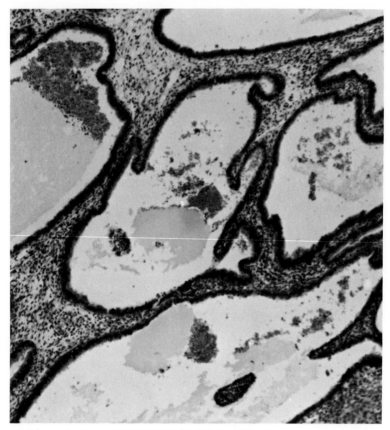

FIG. V-11. Chronic follicular salpingitis.

abdomen of other cause and the gastrointestinal signs and symptoms are less prominent. Tachycardia, rigidity, and rebound are nonspecific, but an adnexal mass and pain on motion of the cervix suggest pelvic inflammatory disease, which in gonococcal salpingitis is often exacerbated during the menses.

The differential diagnosis of salpingitis includes all causes of the acute abdomen. With salpingitis the pain is more likely bilateral and there is less nausea and vomiting than with appendicitis, for example. With ectopic pregnancy the leukocyte count and temperature are lower and the patient usually shows some signs of pregnancy (p. 128). When the peritonitis is caused by salpingitis the patient appears less ill than when the acute abdomen is a result of appendicitis or pancreatitis, for example.

In the diagnosis of the acute abdomen it is most important to distinguish pelvic inflammatory disease from the other causes, since acute salpingitis (like acute pyelonephritis) is a nonsurgical

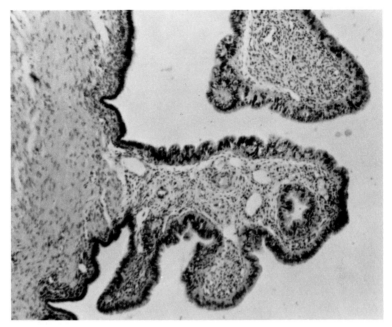

Fig. V-12. Hydrosalpinx, showing blunted rugae projecting into distended lumen.

disease, which responds to antibiotic therapy, as opposed to ectopic pregnancy, appendicitis, and torsion of an adnexal mass, for example. If doubt about a "surgical abdomen" persists, laparoscopy, or if necessary, laparotomy must be performed. If the diagnosis proves wrong and acute salpingitis is found, the abdomen should be closed without further procedures.

Because of the rapid spread of pelvic inflammatory disease, it is appropriate to treat infection of the lower genitourinary tract before confirmation of the diagnosis is obtained. A standard treatment for gonorrhea of the lower genitourinary tract is aqueous procaine penicillin, 4.8 million units in a divided dose, half in each buttock, with 1 g of probenecid by mouth. An alternative regimen is amoxicillin, 3 g, or ampicillin, 3.5 g, by mouth, with 1 g of probenecid. The oral regimen is ineffective against anorectal and pharyngeal gonococcal infections, and both the oral semisynthetic penicillins and intramuscular aqueous procaine penicillin are ineffective against chlamydial infections, which may coexist with gonorrhea in as many as 45% of cases. A combined regimen that may be effective against gonorrheal and chlamydial infections is the aforementioned dose of amoxicillin or ampicillin together with tetracycline, 500 mg, by mouth, four times a day for 7 days, or doxycycline, 100 mg, by mouth, twice a day for 7 days.

Tetracycline or aqueous penicillin G is the preferred therapy for pharyngeal gonococcal infection, which is not effectively treated by amoxicillin, ampicillin, or spectinomycin. Patients with proven penicillinase-producing *Neisseria gonorrhoeae* (PPNG) infection should receive 2 g of spectinomycin, intramuscularly, in a single injection. Tetracycline may be added to treat coexistent chlamydial infection. Patients with positive cultures after treatment with spectinomycin should be given cefoxitin, 2 g, intramuscularly, in a single injection together with 1 g of probenecid, by mouth, or cefotaxime, 1 g, intramuscularly, in a single injection without probenecid. A daily dose of 9 tablets containing 80 mg of trimethoprim and 400 mg of sulfamethoxazole for 5 days should be used to treat pharyngeal gonococcal infection caused by PPNG.

All pregnant women should have endocervical cultures for gonococci during their first prenatal visits (p. 95). A second culture late in the third trimester should be obtained from women at high risk of gonococcal infection. The treatment of choice is amoxicillin or ampicillin with probenecid. Women allergic to penicillin or probenecid should be treated with spectinomycin, 2 g, intramuscularly. Erythromycin in the doses previously recommended may be added to treat coexistent chlamydial infection. Tetracycline should not be used in pregnant women because of possible adverse effects on the fetus.

The revised guidelines of the CDC published in 1985 recommended, as an additional option for treatment, ceftriaxone for uncomplicated gonorrhea of the lower genital tract, failures in treatment of gonorrhea with other drugs, PPNG, disseminated gonococcal infections, and ambulatory therapy of acute pelvic inflammatory disease.

Acute pelvic inflammatory disease refers to the endometritis, salpingitis, parametritis, and peritonitis caused by the ascending spread of microorganisms from the vagina and endocervix. The principal etiologic agents are *N. gonorrhoeae*, *C. trachomatis*, anaerobic bacteria including *Bacteroides* and gram-positive cocci, facultative gram-negative rods such as *Escherichia* coli. *Actinomyces israelii*, and *Mycoplasma hominis*. The most appropriate treatment includes agents active against the broadest range of these pathogens. The CDC recommends hospitalization of patients with acute pelvic inflammatory disease (PID) in the following circumstances: when the diagnosis is uncertain, when surgical emergencies such as appendicitis and ectopic pregnancy are to be excluded, when a pelvic abscess is suspected, when severe illness precludes management as an outpatient, when the patient is pregnant, when the patient cannot follow or tolerate the regimen as an outpatient, when the patient has failed to respond to therapy as an outpatient, and when clinical follow-up after 48 to 72 hours following the start of antibiotic treatment cannot be arranged.

A useful clinical staging of acute salpingitis has recently been proposed. State I is acute salpingitis without peritonitis. It is divided into monomicrobial and polymicrobial with or without N. gonorrhoeae. Stage II is acute salpingitis with peritonitis (including all patients with intrauterine devices). Stage III is acute salpingitis with evidence of tubal occlusion or tubo-ovarian complex. Stave IV is ruptured tubo-ovarian complex.

No treatment of choice has been determined and no single agent is effective against the entire spectrum of pathogens, but several antimicrobial combinations are recommended because of their activity against the major pathogens in vitro. Doxycycline, 100 mg, intravenously, twice a day together with cefoxitin, 2 g, intravenously, four times a day, should be continued for at least 4 days and at least 48 hours after fever subsides. Doxycycline should be continued in doses of 100 mg, by mouth, twice a day after discharge from the hospital to complete 10 to 14 days of therapy. The combination of doxycycline and cefoxitin provides optimal coverage for N. gonorrhoeae, including PPNG, and C. trachomatis, but may not provide optimal treatment for anaerobes, a pelvic mass, or PID associated with an intrauterine device.

Another regimen is clindamycin, 600 mg, intravenously, four times a day, together with gentamicin or tobramycin, 2 mg/kg, intravenously, followed by 1.5 mg/kg, intravenously, three times a day in patients with normal renal function. The drugs should be continued intravenously for at least 4 days and at least 48 hours after fever subsides. Clindamycin should be continued in a dose of 450 mg, by mouth, four times a day after discharge from the hospital to complete 10 to 14 days of therapy. The combination of clindamycin with gentamicin or tobramycin provides optimal activity against anaerobes and facultative gram-negative rods, buy may not provide optimal activity against C. trachomatis and N. gonorrhoeae.

When the patient is not hospitalized, use of one of the following regimens is recommended: cefoxitin, 2 g, intramuscularly; amoxicillin, 3 g, by mouth; ampicillin, 3.5 g, by mouth; or aqueous procaine penicillin G, 4.8 million units, intramuscularly (half in each buttock), each along with probenecid, 1 g, by mouth. Each of the aforementioned drugs is to be followed by doxycycline, 100 mg, by mouth, twice a day for 10 to 14 days, or tetracycline, 500 mg, by mouth, four times a day for 10 to 14 days. Tetracycline is less active than doxycycline against certain anaerobes. Cefoxitin or an equivalently effective cephalosporin together with doxycycline or tetracycline provides activity against N. gonorrhoeae, including PPNG, and C. trachomatis. PPNG-associated P.I.D. is not adequately treated with the combination of amoxicillin, ampicillin, or aqueous procaine penicillin and doxycycline.

Sexual partners of patients with P.I.D. should be examined for STD and promptly treated with a regimen effective against uncomplicated gonococcal and chlamydial infections. All women treated as outpatients should be reevaluated clinically in 48 to 72 hours and admitted if a favorable response is not detected.

Rape

A patient who has been raped or claims to have been raped may be at risk for both pregnancy and sexually transmitted diseases. The duty of a physician in such cases is to record the history as accurately as possible, preferably in the patient's own words, and to record objectively the physical findings. The first examiner should describe the condition of the clothing and record whether there are bruises or lacerations on the patient's body. The gynecologic consultant should perform an examination of the lower abdomen, buttocks, and external genitalia to record injuries. The throat and rectum should be examined as well. The condition of the hymen is then recorded. A speculum should be inserted, if possible, to expose the cervix, and a specimen of fluid from the vagina should be examined to detect spermatozoa. The possibility of STD and pregnancy should be discussed with the patient and appropriate treatment instituted. If the patient is not already pregnant, stilbestrol, 50 mg per day for 5 days may be given as a postcoital contraceptive (p. 355). Ideally a counselor should be available to minimize the likelihood of adverse psychologic sequelae.

The initial examination of the rape victim should include cultures for *N. gonorrhoeae* from any potentially infected sites; cultures, if possible, for *C. trachomatis* from those sites; examination of vaginal specimens for *T. vaginalis* by wet mount; a serologic test for syphilis; and a single sample of serum that is frozen and saved for future testing.

The risk of infection is thought to be low but prophylaxis may be administered with tetracycline, 500 mg, by mouth, four times a day for at least 7 days, or doxycycline, 100 mg, by mouth, twice a day for at least 7 days. Patients who are allergic to tetracycline and those who are pregnant should be given amoxicillin, 3 g, or ampicillin, 3.5 g, each in a single oral dose preceded by 1 g of probenecid. Medical follow-up is indicated in 7 days and the aforementioned studies, except for the serologic test for syphilis, should be repeated. The STS should be repeated 6 weeks after the incident.

Any sexually transmitted infection in a child should be considered evidence of sexual child abuse until proved otherwise. Such cases should be reported promptly to the appropriate authorities. These children should be evaluated for STD as described for victims of rape, but with particular care to avoid physical and psychologic trauma. Treatment is indicated when disease is found, but prophylaxis is usually not administered unless there is evidence that the assailant is infected.

Chronic pelvic inflammatory disease is often suspected on the basis of a history of repetitive acute infections. If the disease is untreated, the tubes are ultimately occluded and the mucosa and fimbriae are destroyed. The patient is thus rendered infertile. When antibiotic therapy is inadequate to eradicate the inflammation, a follicular salpingitis may result. This lesion predisposes to ectopic pregnancy (p. 126). In exacerbations of pelvic inflammatory disease and in the chronic form, polymicrobial infections with anaerobic organisms are found.

The signs and symptoms of chronic pelvic inflammatory disease are referable primarily to the adnexal disease. Exacerbation of the infection leads to adhesions, more or less constant pelvic pain, and dyspareunia. A palpable mass and recurring spikes of temperature suggest a tubo-ovarian abscess or a pelvic abscess.

The important surgical decision in chronic pelvic inflammatory disease is whether or when to operate rather than what procedure to perform, for in many cases total abdominal hysterectomy with bilateral salpingo-oophorectomy is the operation of choice for the advanced lesion. The decision to operate therefore depends upon the symptoms and the degree of incapacitation. With the advent of in vitro fertilization and embryo transfer, patients with advanced pelvic inflammatory disease have been managed with antibiotics and conservative surgical procedures, retaining the uterus. The possibility that an adnexal mass is an ovarian neoplasm must be excluded by the appropriate diagnostic method. The differential diagnosis of chronic pelvic inflammatory disease also includes ectopic pregnancy and endometriosis.

The sudden disappearance of a mass accompanied by softening of the abdomen suggests rupture of a tubo-ovarian abscess. This emergency is usually best treated by total hysterectomy and bilateral salpingo-oophorectomy and administration of broad-spectrum antibiotics. An abscess that points in the cul-de-sac may occasionally be drained by colpotomy, but a true tubo-ovarian abscess cannot be approached safely through that route. Pelvic inflammatory disease is occasionally accompanied by septic shock. The management is the same as that of septic shock of other causes (p. 125).

Particularly in the young patient, conservative surgical procedures are often attempted. Rarely, however, can a tube seriously damaged by gonococcal salpingitis be reconstructed sufficiently to ensure fertility, especially if the fimbriae are destroyed.

Active gonococcal infection in the mother may lead to gonococcal ophthalmia in the newborn. For prophylaxis, silver nitrate, penicillin, or occasionally another antibiotic is placed in the conjunctival sacs of all newborn infants as a routine.

Pyogenic infections caused by streptococci and staphylococci were formerly more common complications of abortion and delivery. Unlike gonorrhea, they spread by lymphatic and hematogenous routes. The infection extends directly through the endometrium and the myometrium into the parametria and broad ligaments, causing a pelvic cellulitis and

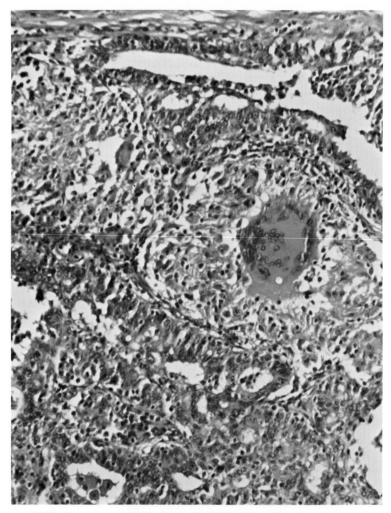

Fig. V-13. Tuberculous salpingitis, showing typical Langhans giant cell and microtubercle.

involving the tube from the outside. In these infections also, the involved organs are occasionally secondarily invaded by coliform organisms and anaerobes. The pyogenic salpingitides usually respond to large doses of penicillin.

Tuberculosis

The granulomatous salpingitides are exemplified by tuberculosis, which still accounts for a small percentage of all pelvic inflammatory disease in the United States. The infection is almost always secondary to pulmonary tuberculosis. Tuberculous pelvic inflammatory disease is a hematogenous infection that involves the tube as the primary site in the pelvis. The abdominal end of the tube may remain open, although the fimbriae are often destroyed and peristalsis is abolished. Histologically the highly proliferative lesions may superficially resemble carcinoma (Fig. V-13). Peritoneal tuberculosis may be accompanied by ascites.

The infection involves primarily women between the ages of 20 and 40 and is characterized by malaise, a low-grade fever, and nagging abdominal pain. Menstrual disorders and infertility are common. Tuberculosis should be suspected in a case of salpingitis that does not respond to penicillin and in pelvic inflammatory disease in virgins. A granuloma on endometrial biopsy directs suspicion to the lesion, and the presence of acid-fast bacilli on a Ziehl-Neelsen stained preparation of the tissue is confirmatory. Final diagnosis is made by inoculation into guinea pigs.

When surgical extirpation was the mainstay of treatment, postoperative complications such as fistulas were common. Antituberculous drugs are now the treatment of choice. The drugs are usually continued for 9 to 18 months, with surgical treatment reserved for an adnexal mass (to rule out carcinoma of the ovary) and for unresponsive pain or fever.

The primary drugs used for treatment of pelvic tuberculosis are rifampicin, ethambutol, and isoniazid (INH). Streptomycin and para-aminosalicyclic acid (PAS) are less commonly used today.

An unusual form of chronic salpingitis is salpingitis isthmica nodosa, which causes fibrosis of the tubal wall with nodular thickenings and obstruction at the cornual end (Fig. V-14). The cause of this lesion is poorly understood.

Toxic Shock Syndrome

The toxic shock syndrome (TSS) includes fever of at least 102° F, a diffuse macular erythema, desquamation (particularly of the palms and soles), hypotension, and involvement of three or more of the following organs or systems: gastrointestinal (vomiting or diarrhea), muscular (myalgia or elevated creatine phosphokinase), mucous membranes (vaginal, oropharyngeal, or conjuctival hyperemia), renal (elevated blood urea nitrogen or creatinine, or pyuria in the absence of infection of the urinary tract), hepatic (elevated bilirubin, serum glutamic oxaloacetic transaminase, or serum glutamic pyruvic transaminase), hematologic (decrease in platelets), and central nervous system (disorientation or alterations in consciousness without focal neurologic signs when fever and hypotension are absent). Cultures from blood, throat, and cerebrospinal fluid, if obtained, must be negative as must serologic tests for Rocky Mountain spotted fever, leptospirosis, and measles.

Toxic shock syndrome has been related to the use of tampons during the menstrual period, particularly brands that are highly absorbent. TSS has also been described in women who did not use tampons, particularly those using the contraceptive sponge, and even in men. The organism most frequently implicated is *Staphylococcus aureus*. It is now believed that an exotoxin is the causative agent and that lysogeny, or the presence of temperate bacteriophage, characterizes the virulent strains of the bacterium.

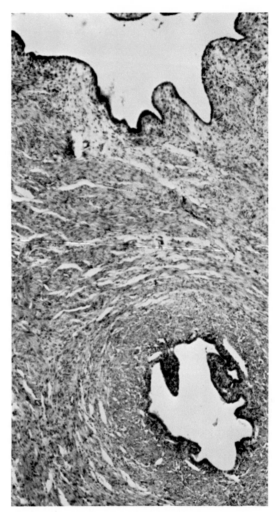

Fig. V-14. Salpingitis isthmica nodosa, showing central lumen and cleft-like glandular spaces in myosalpinx.

Acquired Immunodeficiency Syndrome

Although most cases of acquired immunodeficiency syndrome (AIDS) in the United States occur in homosexual men and users of intravenous drugs, the proportion heterosexually transmitted and involving women is increasing. By the end of 1986 about 25,000 cases of the syndrome had been reported in the United States with a mortality rate of slightly over 50%. Counseling and testing should be offered to all women who have evidence of HTLV-III infection; who have used intravenous drugs for nonmedical purposes; who were born in countries where heterosexual transmission is thought to play an important role in the spread of the virus, such as Haiti or Central Africa; who have been prostitutes; or who have been sexual partners of users of intravenous drugs, bisexual men, men with hemophilia, men born in high-risk countries, or men who otherwise have evidence of infection with HTLV-III virus.

If the woman tests positive for AIDS she should be advised to delay pregnancy until more is known about the perinatal transmission of the virus. Infected women who are already pregnant may need additional medical services to reduce the risk of contracting opportunistic infections and should be advised against breastfeeding. Abortion may be offered to the infected woman to prevent perinatal transmission. The virus appears to be transmitted primarily prior to labor and delivery; in this respect the infection differs from that caused by the herpes virus.

Late in 1986 azidothymidine (AZT) was released for use in modifying the course of AIDS. The drug, which blocks the action of reverse transcriptase in translating the code of RNA into that of DNA, although not a cure for AIDS has prolonged the lives of many patients with the disease. Additional promising antiviral agents have more recently undergone clinical trials.

Pelvic Relaxation and Gynecologic Injuries

Pelvic relaxation refers to a group of anatomic, sometimes symptomatic, defects including uterine prolapse (descensus), relaxation of the anterior vaginal wall (urethrocele and cystocele), relaxation of the posterior wall (rectocele), herniation of the peritoneum of the cul-de-sac (enterocele), and laceration of the perineum. These disorders are usually related to childbirth or aging and are rarely congenital. Prolapse of the vagina may occur after hysterectomy.

The principal weakness is in the endopelvic fascia and the muscular levator sling. Attenuation of the vesicovaginal (anterior) portion of the endopelvic fascia, between bladder and anterior vaginal wall, results in prolapse of the bladder into the anterior vaginal wall (cystocele). Weakening of the connective tissue between the urethra and vagina produces a urethrocele. Weakening of the rectovaginal (posterior) portion of the endopelvic fascia causes bulging of the anterior wall of the rectum into the vagina (rectocele).

Laceration or attenuation of the condensed pericervical areolar tissue (endopelvic fascia), laceration of the perineum, and injury to the levator sling usually result from obstetric injuries or the atrophy of aging. Attenuation of the cardinal and uterosacral ligaments contributes to the relaxation. Herniation of small bowel through the hiatus between the uterosacral ligaments produces an enterocele, which is a true hernia. The components of pelvic relaxation occur in various degrees and combinations. The best prevention is good obstetric care.

The syndrome of pelvic relaxation is related in part to the anatomic changes associated with the bipedal condition. Women with pelvic relaxation are more likely than the general population to develop hemorrhoids, hernias, and varicose veins. Racial factors also play a role in susceptibility to pelvic relaxation. Black women, for example, are less likely than white women to develop uterine prolapse.

The greater prevalence of pelvic relaxation in many foreign countries as compared with the United States, however, is more likely related to differences in obstetric practice. Prophylactic obstetric measures include the appropriate use of outlet forceps and episiotomy, shortening of the second stage, and anatomic repair of lacerations. These maneuvers protect the perivaginal connective tissues and the muscles of the pelvic floor.

The relative roles of the pelvic musculature and the connective tissue ligaments in the prevention of pelvic relaxation remain somewhat controversial. The levator ani, which consists of the pubococcygeus, iliococcygeus, and ischiococcygeus, forms the deep support. The perineal muscles form a second line of defense; they comprise the ischiocavernosus, bulbocavernosus, and superficial and deep transverse perineal muscles, together with the urogenital diaphragm and external anal sphincter. The broad ligament provides no support, but the condensed connective tissue in the cardinal and uterosacral ligaments helps to maintain the uterus in its normal position.

The signs and symptoms of pelvic relaxation depend on the combination and degree of anatomic defects. Uterine prolapse usually produces merely a sagging sensation in the pelvis. Severe degrees of prolapse are associated with other symptomatic components of pelvic relaxation.

In first-degree prolapse, the uterus descends, but the cervix remains within the vagina. In second-degree prolapse, the cervix appears partially or totally outside the vaginal orifice. In third-degree prolapse (procidentia), the entire uterus is outside the vaginal orifice. In a prolapsed uterus the cervix is often hypertrophied and ulcerated, but is not more frequently subject to carcinoma.

A cystocele may reach large size without becoming symptomatic. Problems referable to a cystocele include frequency of urination, a sensation of pelvic pressure, and a predisposition to recurrent urinary tract infections. The cystocele does not, however, produce stress incontinence (the involuntary loss of urine upon increase in intraabdominal pressure).

A rectocele causes a sensation of a mass in the vagina and difficulty in evacuating the rectum except by placing a hand in the vagina to reduce the bulge. The enterocele is subject to all the complications of hernias elsewhere in the body. The relaxed perineum may lead to unsatisfactory intercourse.

The most serious complaint in patients with pelvic relaxation is stress incontinence, which results from a urethrocele, or a funneling of the bladder neck.

Differential diagnosis of pelvic relaxation usually presents few problems. A prolapsed uterus must be differentiated from a normally situated uterus with an elongated cervix. An enterocele must be differentiated from a high rectocele, a urethrocele from a suburethral diverticulum, and a cystocele from a large midline mesonephric ductal cyst.

The treatment of pelvic relaxation depends on correction of the fascial and muscular defects. The cystocele is repaired by plication of the anterior portion of the endopelvic fascia (anterior colporrhaphy, p. 190). Care must be taken to avoid overcorrection, thereby obliterating the posterior urethrovesical angle and producing stress incontinence. An extensive anterior colporrhaphy should be accompanied by a plication of the bladder neck (Kelly plication, p. 190) to maintain the urethrovesical angle.

The rectocele is repaired by plication of the posterior portion of the endopelvic fascia (posterior colporrhaphy, p. 190). In complete pelvic repairs, it is desirable to perform only minimal posterior colporrhaphy in a young woman in order to preserve sexual function. A relaxed perineum may be reconstructed to provide normal support by the operation known as perineorrhaphy. An enterocele is repaired by excision of the hernial sac and obliteration of the hiatus between the uterosacral ligaments.

Retroversion, except possibly the adherent variety found in endometriosis (p. 227), is a normal variant of uterine position. It does not require surgical therapy.

The abdominal approach to correction of pelvic relaxation is anatomically illogical and therapeutically unsuccessful. The principal treatment of uterine prolapse is vaginal hysterectomy. This procedure in itself, however, does not correct the often accompanying cystocele and rectocele or the stress incontinence. These problems are managed by colporrhaphy and Kelly plication (p. 190). The advantages of vaginal hysterectomy are the prevention of pregnancy, which could break down a previously successful repair, and after the menopause, removal of a functionless organ, which could be the site of benign or malignant disease.

Before vaginal hysterectomy and repair of a cystocele it is desirable to eradicate local infections of the vagina, cervix, and bladder. For minor degrees of pelvic relaxation, exercises to strengthen the perineal muscles may be helpful.

Pessaries are infrequently used today, except for temporary replacement of a prolapsed uterus during preoperative healing of an infected cervix. They may be used also as a therapeutic test to ascertain whether repositioning of the uterus will relieve the patient's symptoms. Pessaries are used for definitive treatment only in the aged patient or the woman who is too sick to tolerate a surgical procedure. Pessaries are associated with an increased incidence of discharge, ulceration, and rarely, vaginal carcinoma, unless they are periodically removed and cleaned and unless the atrophic vagina is treated with exogenous estrogen.

Urinary Incontinence

Stress incontinence of urine is the most troublesome result of pelvic relaxation. It may become sufficiently serious to render the patient a social invalid. Urinary continence depends on maintenance of normal detrusor function and support by the muscles of the pelvic floor. Normally the posterior urethrovesical angle is 90 to 100 degrees; in stress incontinence it is usually blunted. The basic anatomic defect is weakness of the musculofascial supports of the bladder and upper urethra. As a result, the bladder is constantly in the state of prevoiding, or first-stage voiding. With stress, such as coughing or other increases in intraabdominal pressure, urine descends through the lower two thirds of the urethra and escapes.

Urination begins with relaxation of the muscles of the pelvic floor and the urethral sphincter, followed in 2 to 5 seconds by contraction of the detrusor and funneling of the bladder neck. With voluntary increase in intravesical pressure, urination occurs.

Type I stress incontinence results when the bladder neck prolapses (loss of posterior urethrovesical angle) but the urethral axis retains its normal relation to the vagina. Further descent of the anterior wall of the vagina causes descent of the base of the bladder and rotation of the urethral axis backward and downward. When these anatomic changes are superimposed on prolapse of the vesical neck, Type II stress incontinence results.

The differential diagnosis of urinary incontinence includes stress, urgency, overflow, and total incontinence. With stress incontinence, usually a small amount of urine escapes from the urethra when intraabdominal pressure is increased, as with coughing or sneezing. Total incontinence most often results from a urinary tract fistula, which causes more or less constant loss of urine. Urgency incontinence (detrusor instability, or detrusor dyssynergia) results from involuntary and uninhibited contractions of the detrusor. With urgency (classical detrusor instability) large amounts of urine may be voided. Urgency may be produced by urinary tract infection and vaginitis (infectious or atrophic). Eradication of the infection and local estrogen may be beneficial. Overflow incontinence results from overdistension of the bladder. Underlying causes include neuropathies, as with diabetes mellitus; syphilis; multiple sclerosis; and spinal injuries. Many women with urinary incontinence have a combination of stress incontinence and detrusor instability.

Accurate diagnosis of urinary incontinence, which is essential to successful therapy, requires a careful history of the symptoms, pelvic and neurologic examinations, and urinary cultures and sensitivities. Additional diagnostic studies include measurement of residual urine to rule out inadequate emptying or neuropathy involving the bladder. Urethrocystoscopy and cystometrograms provide objective evidence of intrinsic lesions of the urinary tract and of the relations of the bladder neck and urethra to the vagina and symphysis pubis. Intravenous pyelography may be required to rule out an ectopic ureter and other lesions higher in the urinary tract. Urodynamic evaluation of the lower urinary tract uses multiple simultaneous measurements of pressure and flow to assess the functional status of the urinary system at rest and under conditions of stress. Such an evaluation is particularly useful in patients with complicated clinical problems.

Although perineal exercises and estrogen therapy for patients with estrogenic deficiency may be helpful in the management of patients with mild stress incontinence, more severe degrees of the disorder usually require surgical treatment. A Kelly plication (p. 190) is often the first procedure employed, whereas retropubic suspension of the vesical neck through the abdominal route (p. 190) is frequently required for more severe or Type II lesions. The rate of cure after 5 years may be as high as 80% with either procedure, if properly chosen and performed.

When conventional vaginal and abdominal operations are unsuccessful, one of the many "sling" operations may be effective. In these procedures a sling of rectus fascia, fascia lata, or synthetic material is passed under the urethra through the space of Retzius and reattached to the anterior abdominal wall. Other operative procedures include implantation of an artificial sphincter and urinary diversion. Reduction in weight and treatment of a chronic cough may improve the results of surgical management of stress incontinence.

Total incontinence of urine may be caused by fistulas between the vagina and the urinary tract. These lesions are the result of the close anatomic relation of the female reproductive and urinary organs. The obstetric causes have decreased relatively as a result of technical improvements and the avoidance of difficult vaginal deliveries and long labors, but the gynecologic injuries have increased relatively as a result of more extensive surgical and radiologic treatment.

Vesicovaginal fistulas may result from unrecognized injury during hysterectomy or colporrhaphy. If not repaired immediately, these fistulas are most successfully closed, usually by the vaginal route, after a delay of 4 to 6 months. Other causes are injury from radiation and direct involvement by carcinoma.

A vesicovaginal fistula may be demonstrated by the appearance of dye in the vagina after instillation of methylene blue into the bladder. A ureterovaginal fistula may result from a radical (p. 189) or difficult total hysterectomy in which the ureter is ligated or cut. This fistula may be demonstrated by the appearance of dye in the vagina after intravenous injection of indigo carmine or by pyelography. A urethrovaginal fistula in the distal third of the urethra is unlikely to result in urinary incontinence and ordinarily requires no treatment.

The surgical principles of repair of a vesicovaginal fistula are as follows: adequate dissection and mobilization of the involved organs without injury to adjacent structures; excision of the scarred, epithelialized fistulous tract; separate closure in layers of the vesical and vaginal walls without tension on the suture lines; minimization of infection by good hemostasis, use of fine sutures, obliteration of dead space, and administration of appropriate antibiotics; and postoperative drainage of the bladder.

Vaginal fistulas may involve the bowel as well as the urinary tract. A rectovaginal fistula may result from unrecognized obstetric injuries, gynecologic operations, radiation therapy, or direct growth of a carcinoma. A small rectovaginal fistula may result only in incontinence of gas, whereas a larger fistula usually causes fecal incontinence as well. The principles of closure are similar to those of vesicovaginal fistulas.

Adenomyosis and Endometriosis

Adenomyosis and endometriosis are frequently discussed together although they are etiologically different disorders, which require different treatments.

Adenomyosis is a condition in which endometrial tissue penetrates the myometrium by direct extension from the lining of the uterine cavity. The circumscribed lesion is termed an adenomyoma and the diffuse form, adenomyosis (Fig. V-15).

Endometriosis is a disorder in which endometrial tissue occurs outside its normal intrauterine location not connected with the endometrial surface. It also may be a circumscribed (endometrioma) or diffuse (endometriosis) lesion.

Diagnosis of adenomyosis can be made only by examination of the excised tissue and requires the finding of endometrial glands or stroma a specified distance from the base of the endometrium. The distance varies,

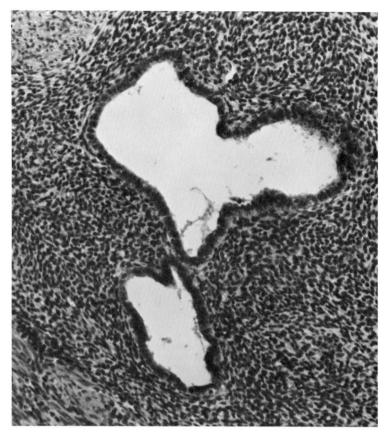

FIG. V-15. Adenomyosis, showing endometrial gland and stroma.

according to different authorities, from one high-power to two low-power fields. One low-power field, however, is a commonly accepted definition.

Adenomyosis comprises endometrial tissue surrounded by myometrium. In special circumstances, gland or stroma may predominate or occur exclusively. Since the tissue is composed largely of basal endometrium, it is not fully responsive to the endocrine changes of the endometrial cycle or to exogenously administered hormones.

Adenomyosis, unlike endometriosis, is most common in multiparas in the fourth to sixth decades. It may be associated with myomas and endometrial hyperplasia and occasionally with endometriosis and carcinoma of the endometrium. Grossly, the myometrium is irregularly thickened on cut surface.

The characteristic symptoms and signs of adenomyosis are progressive dysmenorrhea, menorrhagia, and an enlarging tender uterus. Additional findings include dyspareunia and a premenstrual syndrome that resembles pelvic congestion (p. 373). The diagnosis is often made incidentally at the time of laparotomy. The differential diagnosis includes carcinoma of the corpus, endometrial polyps, and myomas. The gross pathologic differential diagnosis includes sarcoma and myoma. Unlike the myoma, neither the adenomyoma nor the sarcoma has a pseudocapsule that allows easy enucleation from the surrounding myometrium.

A special form of the lesion is stromal adenomyosis, or endometrial stromatosis. This disease may clinically resemble a low-grade endometrial sarcoma.

The etiologic factors in adenomyosis are unknown, although an estrogenic imbalance may be influential.

The prevalence of the disease is difficult to assess, although it is commonly found in uteri removed for other causes. Since hormonal treatment is generally unsatisfactory, the symptomatic lesion is most often treated by hysterectomy. In women near the menopause, after malignant disease has been excluded, temporization may be logical, for the lesion regresses with cessation of ovarian function.

The prevalence of endometriosis is difficult to ascertain because it also is often discovered as an incidental finding at laparotomy. Endometriosis, unlike adenomyosis, is most commonly found in nulliparas between the ages of 25 and 40. The widespread use of laparoscopy has resulted in the detection of many more examples of endometriosis recently. It is said to occur more commonly in the white, middle-class, high-income patients who marry late. These differences most likely reflect socioeconomic rather than racial factors. Private patients, furthermore, are more likely to register minor complaints, thereby creating the impression of a greater prevalence of the disease in that group.

Endometriosis is rarely if ever found in the prepuberal girl or in the postmenopausal period and often seems to be improved during pregnancy. Early childbearing plays a role in preventing endometriosis.

Several etiologic concepts are still being debated. One hypothesis favors retrograde menstruation, with the resulting implantation of endometrial tissue on the ovaries and peritoneum. A retroverted uterus, which is commonly found in patients with endometriosis, may predispose to retrograde menses. A second etiologic hypothesis is celomic metaplasia, by which celomic derivatives are transformed into tissues of endometrial type. A third concept, which combines retrograde menses with metaplasia, is induction, by means of which a chemical substance from sloughed endometrial tissue leads to transformation of other tissues to the endometrial type. Hematogenous and lymphatic spread probably plays only a small role in the histogenesis of endometriosis.

Several studies suggest that the peritoneal fluid in women with endometriosis contains higher than normal levels of thromboxane B_2 and 6-keto-prostaglandin $F_{2\alpha}$. Thus, the relation between endometriosis and infertility may be based in part on the action of prostaglandins on oviductal function. Current research, furthermore, suggests an increase in activated macrophages in the peritoneal fluid and an autoimmune response to endometrium in patients with endometriosis.

Endometriosis usually comprises both gland and stroma, although one or the other element may be predominant or exclusively present. The gross lesions may resemble "powder burns" on the peritoneum and serosal surfaces. Large hemorrhagic cysts of the ovary containing dark blood are referred to as "chocolate cysts," although not all such hemorrhagic ovarian cysts are the result of endometriosis.

When the wall of a hemorrhagic cyst contains hemosiderin but the epithelium of origin is unidentifiable, the diagnosis should be hemorrhagic cyst rather than endometrial cyst.

Rupture of an endometrial cyst may lead to extensive adhesions, denser that those of pelvic inflammatory disease. Intraperitoneal bleeding or pain resulting from rupture of an endometrioma may create a surgical emergency. The resulting adhesions may cause fixed retroversion of the uterus, involvement of adjacent organs, and strictures of the bowel. In extreme cases, a "frozen pelvis" may result.

The structures involved in endometriosis, in order of frequency, are the ovary (Fig. V-16), the posterior cul-de-sac, the uterosacral ligaments, the rectovaginal septum, the oviducts, the rectosigmoid, and the bladder. Distant organs are rarely involved. Endometriosis of the lymph nodes, pleura, and extremities is difficult to explain on the basis of the common histogenetic theories.

Carcinoma may develop in ovarian endometriosis, but unless a clear transition from normal endometrium to malignant tissue is seen within the ovary, the origin of the tumor from endometriosis cannot be proved.

The endometriotic tissue is usually responsive to the hormones of the menstrual cycle and to externally supplied hormones. This endocrine dependence explains the progress of the disease as well as the response to treatment.

The accuracy of preoperative diagnosis of endometriosis is relatively low. The lesion is often found incidentally in patients oper-

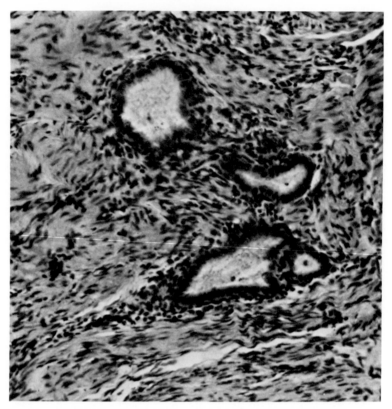

FIG. V-16. Endometriosis of the ovary, showing endometrial glands and stroma.

ated upon for other reasons. The number of false-positive and false-negative diagnoses will be reduced by preoperative laparoscopy. Definitive diagnosis is made only after histologic examination of a biopsy specimen.

Endometriosis characteristically presents with acquired dysmenorrhea, acute and chronic pelvic pain, and abnormal uterine bleeding. Infertility may become a major problem. The dysmenorrhea, which usually begins after age 25, is progressive. As the disease continues, pain and bleeding occur in increasingly greater portions of the menstrual cycle. Dyspareunia may result from involvement of the uterosacral ligaments and implants in the cul-de-sac and fornices. The abnormal bleeding may result from ovarian dysfunction, which together with dense adhesions may lead to infertility.

Less common manifestations of endometiosis include pain, bleeding with bowel movements or tenesmus (as a result of involvement of the rectovaginal septum and rectum), and dysuria and cyclic hematuria (as a result of involvement of the bladder). A less specific but more common manifestation is dull pain radiating to the thighs.

A careful rectovaginal examination is essential for the clinical diagnosis of endometriosis. Highly suggestive findings include nodules in the cul-de-sac, the posterior fornix, and the uterosacral ligament; fixed retroversion of the uterus; and obliteration of the cul-de-sac by dense adhesions. Differential diagnosis includes chronic pelvic inflammatory disease and ovarian neoplasms. Additional diseases to be considered are carcinoma of the rectum or sigmoid, diverticulitis, and tuberculosis.

With endometriosis a greater degree of fixation of organs is found than with other diseases that are considered in differential diagnosis. Laboratory data are not diagnostic, but a normal white count points to endometriosis rather than pelvic inflammatory disease.

Pelvic examination under anethesia may differentiate endometriosis from the pelvic congestion syndrome, because in endometriosis the thickening and nodularity of the uterosacral ligaments, for example, will not decrease or disappear. The diagnostic workup, depending on signs and symptoms, may include barium enema, cystoscopy, and intravenous pyelography.

Treatment of endometriosis is influenced by the patient's age and parity. The three methods of management are supportive, hormonal, and surgical. Supportive therapy entails careful observation, reassurance, and analgesics. A trial of pregnancy, where possible, should be recommended, for it may be curative. Observation is contraindicated in the presence of an undiagnosed adnexal mass.

Surgical and hormonal techniques of management of endometriosis are complementary. Prolonged hormonal therapy, which is time-consuming and expensive, should be reserved for patients who have a histologic diagnosis of endometriosis.

Surgical therapy is indicated for failure of medical management, persistent infertility for 1 year after hormonal treatment, and ovarian masses greater than 6 cm in diameter. Surgical therapy may also be the modality of choice when the patient has completed her family or is near the menopause. Surgical management may range from conservative procedures, such as excision of small implants, to total abdominal hysterectomy and bilateral salpingo-oophorectomy with removal of as many of the implants as possible.

Total abdominal hysterectomy and bilateral salpingo-oophorectomy are often curative even when not all of the implants are removed. It is unwise to attempt excision of every implant when adjacent organs would thereby be jeopardized. The laser may be used to advantage in removal of small foci of endometriosis that are in intimate relation to easily damaged structures. Hysterectomy without removal of the adnexa may be performed in a young patient who has completed her family. After hysterectomy and removal of the adnexa and implants it is possible to provide hormonal supplementation, since there is no longer a proliferating endometrial mucosa to generate additional endometriotic implants.

In connection with conservative operations, uterine suspension and presacral neurectomy may be performed for symptomatic relief. Further decrease in pain may be achieved by interruption of the nerve tracts in the uterosacral ligaments.

The hormonal therapy of endometriosis is often the treatment of choice. It may be adjunctive to conservative operations and is indicated in patients who refuse operations. Estrogens, androgens, and progestins have all been used to interrupt the ovarian cycle and control endometriosis. Danazol has been used both preoperatively and in cases of residual endometriosis, postoperatively.

Almost any estrogen may be employed successfully. Androgens are also effective but they carry the danger of masculinization. Methyl testosterone in doses of 5 mg every day for three to six months, however, rarely produces permanent side effects.

The mainstays of current hormonal therapy of endometriosis are danazol and the synthetic steroids used commonly as oral contraceptives. The progestins produce a pseudopregnancy, characterized by atrophy of the endometrial glands and decidual transformation of the stroma.

Almost any of the currently used oral contraceptives may be employed for treatment of endometriosis, but excellent results have been achieved over long periods of time with norethynodrel and ethinyl estradiol. The initial dose of 10 mg/day is gradually increased at two-week intervals to a maximum of 20 to 40 mg/day. Such therapy continued for 9 months has resulted in cures or remissions in 80% of cases of endometriosis.

Estrogen-progestin therapy is commonly complicated by nausea, edema, irregular uterine bleeding, and possible growth of myomas. The hormones have also been used preoperatively to "soften" the adhesions in a patient about to undergo surgical treatment.

Danazol, a derivative of ethisterone, is an orally effective agent that inhibits the anterior pituitary. It is anabolic and weakly androgenic. Its main side-effect is weight gain. The drug is required in doses of up to 800 mg/day for 6 months. The considerable expense of this form of therapy is its major drawback. Unlike the progestational agents, which stimulate parts of the endometrium and produce a pseudopregnancy, danazol does not stimulate the target organ but produces a pseudomenopause. It is not contraindicated in patients who are susceptible to thrombophlebitis.

Progestins alone, either by mouth or intramuscular injection, have also been used successfully. Medroxyprogesterone acetate (Depo-Provera) is currently approved by the F.D.A. for use in endometriosis but not routine contraception. The injection may be given every 2 weeks in doses of 50 or 100 mg. If breakthrough bleeding occurs, the progestin is supplemented with estrogen by injection or by mouth.

Radiotherapy, which was formerly used to effect castration, plays no role in the modern management of endometriosis.

A new and promising approach to suppression, if not complete eradication, of endometriosis is a long-acting gonadotropin-releasing hormone (GnRH) agonist. Treatment with this drug is associated with menopausal but not androgenic side-effects.

Gynecologic Neoplasms

Breast

Although neoplasms of the breast are treated by general surgeons in most parts of this country, the obstetrician-gynecologist has excellent opportunities to detect these lesions during prenatal visits, at the time of the annual Papanicolaou smear, and during examinations for contraception. The details of history of mammary disease and physical examination of the breast are given on pages 49-50. Because mammary carcinoma is the most common cancer in women, every mass in the breast must be viewed with suspicion. Fixation, retraction, and asymmetry of the breasts, as well as discharge from the nipple, require further diagnostic investigation. Aspiration of a cyst and needle biopsy may be performed in a properly equipped office and excisional biopsy in an outpatient surgical facility. Further details of mammary disease are presented on pages 294-308.

Current recommendations regarding mammography are as follows:

1. Mammographic screening should be available to women over 50.
2. For asymptomatic women between the ages of 40 and 49, physical examination of the breast should be performed annually and mammography should be performed at intervals of 1 to 2 years.

3. For women between the ages of 35 and 39, mammography should be used only if the woman has previously had cancer in one breast.
4. The examination of the breast by heat (thermography) has proved to be less valuable than that by radiography.
5. Mammography should not be used to screen women under the age of 35.
6. Mammography should be used for women of any age to aid in the diagnosis of suspected tumor.

The recommended dosage of radiation has been reduced to less than one rad to the midbreast for a two-view examination.

The gynecologist is likely to encounter three benign diseases of the breast. An intraductal papilloma is the tumor that most commonly causes bleeding from the nipple. A fibroadenoma presents as a firm, discrete mass that requires biopsy to distinguish it from carcinoma. Fibrocystic disease poses diagnostic difficulties. The lesion presents as diffuse nodularity associated with increasing tenderness immediately before the menses. A nodule that does not regress postmenstrually may require biopsy.

Vulva

Benign tumors of the vulva include those of the skin in general and a few special growths. Condyloma acuminatum is viral rather than primarily neoplastic and is discussed among infections (p. 196). Abscesses and cysts of Bartholin's gland are discussed under inflammatory lesions (p. 200). Solid benign epithelial tumors include papillomas, adenomas, and nevi. Sebaceous cysts and hidradenomas are also found on the vulva.

The hidradenoma may be highly cellular and therefore mistaken for an adenocarcinoma, but it is rarely malignant, as shown in Figure V-17. Benign connective tissue tumors of the vulva include lipomas, fibromas, hemangiomas, and lymphangiomas. Varices of the vulva may be mistaken for neoplasms.

Any suspicious lesion of the vulva, and any lesion that does not respond quickly to conservative treatment, particularly in older women, should be subjected to biopsy.

The International Society for the Study of Vulvar Disease has suggested a logical and succinct classification of the vulvar dystrophies (Table 10). Included among the vulvar dystophies are disorders formerly described as leukoplakia, kraurosis, atrophic dys-

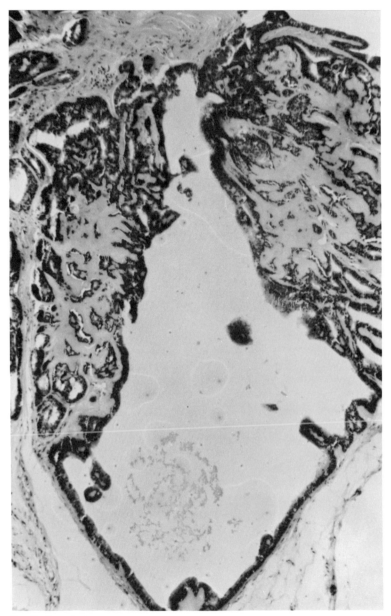

FIG. V-17. Hidradenoma of the vulva with papillary glandular proliferation but no cytologic atypia.

tophy, hyperplastic vulvitis, leukoplakic vulvitis, and neurodermatitis. Additionally, the following terms are no longer recommended: lichen sclerosus et atrophicus, leukokeratosis, Bowen's disease, erythroplasia of Queyrat, and carcinoma simplex.

Table 10.   The Vulvar Dystrophies

I. Hyperplastic Dystrophy
   A. Without atypia
   B. With atypia
II. Lichen Sclerosus
III. Mixed Dystrophy (lichen sclerosus with foci of epithelial hyperplasia)
   A. Without atypia
   B. With atypia

Dystrophic lesions are important because they are sometimes precursors of carcinoma of the vulva. "White lesions" of the vulva include a variety of disorders, only some of which are premalignant. The greater the cellular atypia, the more likely is a white lesion to be a precursor of carcinoma.

In hyperplastic dystrophy there is epithelial hyperplasia, acanthosis, hyperkeratosis, and chronic inflammation (Fig. V-18). In lichen sclerosus there is thinning of the squamous epithelium with loss of the rete pegs (Fig. V-19). The dermis just beneath the squamous epithelium appears acellular and homogeneous. In mixed dystophy, areas of lichen sclerosus and hyperplastic dystrophy are found in the same lesion. The atypia accompanying any of the dystrophies may be classified as mild, moderate, or severe. Hyperkeratosis and parakeratosis may be found in all grades of atypia.
Atrophic lesions of the vulva may cause pruritus, which leads to scratching and secondary infection. Dystrophic lesions with cellular atypia may be precursors of vulvar carcinoma. Suspicious lesions should be subjected to biopsy. Widespread dysplastic lesions may be managed best by prophylactic vulvectomy.

Carcinoma of the vulva accounts for about 5% of all gynecologic cancers. The invasive lesion may be preceded by dysplasia and carcinoma in situ.

The typical vulvar carcinoma in situ is of the squamous cell variety. Another intraepithelial form, Paget's disease, which may be of apocrine origin, usually involves postmenopausal women. Pathognomonic Paget cells with clear, vacuolated cytoplasm are found, initially in the basal layers of the epidermis and later throughout the epithelium (Fig. V-20). Papanicolaou smears are unreliable for diagnosis of vulvar carcinoma because of the frequently associated hyperkeratosis. Toluidine blue and colposcopy may aid in selecting a site for the biopsy. Because these lesions are often multifocal, multiple biopsies are required to rule out invasion. The preinvasive lesion may be treated safely be simple vulvectomy or vaporization by laser. Paget's disease may recur in the vulva after local excision and may involve anus, cervix, and breasts.

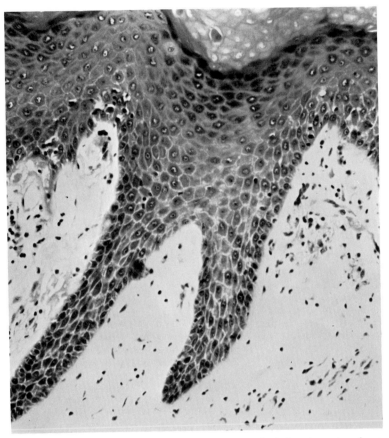

Fɪɢ. V-18. Hyperplastic dystrophy of the vulva, showing acanthosis, hyperkeratosis, and parakeratosis.

Invasive carcinoma of the vulva is of the squamous cell variety in 95% of cases (Fig. V-21). It most frequently occurs in postmenopausal women but is occasionally found in younger women as well. About 40% of vulvar carcinomas are preceded by identifiable dysplastic lesions and intraepithelial carcinoma. Etiologic factors include chronic infections (such as lymphogranuloma venereum) and poor hygiene.

The most common sites of carcinoma of the vulva, in order of frequency, are the labium majus, the posterior commissure, the clitoris, and the labium minus. Spread occurs locally and lymphatic drainage is first to inguinal and femoral nodes and later to deep pelvic nodes.

Carcinoma of the vulva may present as a persistent asymptomatic exophytic mass or ulcer or may cause pruritus, a foul-smelling bloody discharge, or pain on urination or defecation. Diagnosis

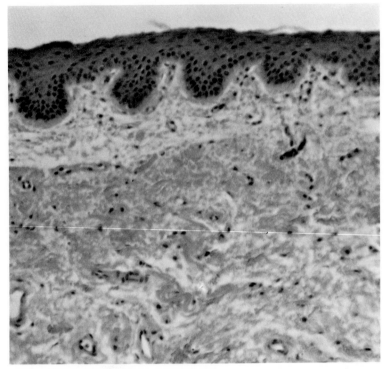

FIG. V-19. Lichen sclerosus of the vulva, showing atrophic epithelium and homogenization of subepithelial connective tissue.

is provided by biopsy, which is the only means of distinguishing an intraepithelial from an early invasive lesion. Use of toluidine blue and colposcopy may aid in directing biopsy to the most abnormal areas. Because treatment of the two lesions varies greatly, multiple biopsies should be performed to rule out invasion. Differential diagnosis includes syphilis and other granulomatous sexually transmitted lesions.

Stage 0 is carcinoma in situ. Invasive carcinoma of the vulva, like other pelvic cancers, may be staged. Stage I lesions are confined to the vulva and are less than 2 cm in diameter. Inguinal nodes may or may not be palpable but are not enlarged or fixed. Stage II lesions are also confined to the vulva but are greater than 2 cm in diameter. Nodes may or may not be palpable but are not enlarged or fixed. Stage III lesions include tumors of any size with adjacent spread to the urethra, vagina, perineum, or anus; or palpable nodes in the groin that are enlarged, firm, and mobile (clinically suspect for metastases). Stage IV lesions include tumors of any size that infiltrate the mucosa of the bladder or rectum, are fixed to bone, or have distant metastases.

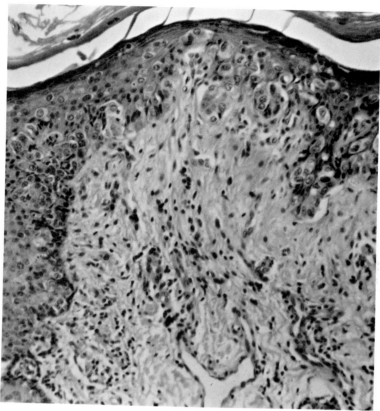

FIG. V-20. Paget's disease of the vulva, showing typical large, pale cells adjacent to basal layer and in underlying epidermal appendages.

Standard surgical treatment of carcinoma of the vulva is radical vulvectomy (p. 190) with en bloc removal of inguinal and femoral lymph nodes. If the superficial nodes are positive, the deep pelvic nodes are dissected. An alternative to dissection of the deep pelvic nodes is megavoltage radiation therapy to the whole pelvis postoperatively.

Carefully selected patients with microinvasive lesions (less than 2 cm in diameter and less than 5 mm in depth and without vascular involvement) may be treated with simple vulvectomy and ipsilateral dissection of the superficial femoral lymph nodes.

Megavoltage therapy is occasionally used for inoperable lesions or recurrences. Radium needles and external irradiation may occasionally be appropriate in carefully selected cases. The 5-year survival rate in Stages I and II is about 75%. In Stage III it is 40%, and in Stage IV it is close to zero.

Basal cell carcinoma may be treated by wide local excision or simple vulvectomy without node dissection.

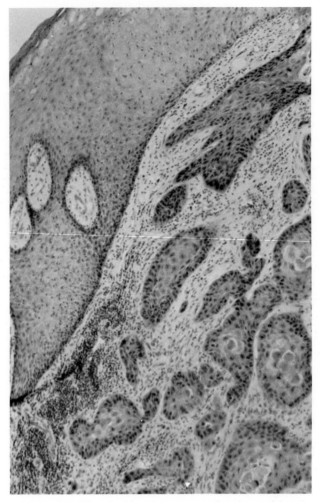

Fɪɢ. V-21. Well differentiated invasive squamous cell carcinoma of the vulva.

An adenocarcinoma of the vulva may arise rarely from Bartholin's gland. Secondary carcinomas of the vulva may be metastatic from a primary cancer of the uterus or rectum. Uncommon malignant tumors of the vulva include melanoma (pigmented and unpigmented), lymphoma, and fibrosarcoma.

Vagina

Symptomatic benign lesions of the vagina are uncommon. Inclusion cysts are commonly 1 to 2 cm in diameter. They usually result from burial of tags of squamous epithelium under a suture line after episiotomy or repair of a laceration. Myomas and fibromas are rare lesions that produce no characteristic clinical findings. Cysts of Gartner's duct (mesonephric duct) may form in the upper portion of the vagina. Endometriosis of the vagina may produce dysmenorrhea and dyspareunia (p. 228).

Adenosis of the vagina develops from müllerian remnants. Administration of diethylstilbestrol (DES) to the mother during pregnancy has been associated with adenosis and rarely with adenocarcinoma of the vagina in the offspring. For this reason, DES is contraindicated in pregnancy. Children of mothers who have received the drug during pregnancy should be examined carefully to detect vaginal lesions.

Palpation and the Schiller test are the main methods of detecting DES-induced lesions. The likelihood of induction by DES of clear cell carcinoma of the upper vagina and cervix is between 0.14 and 1.4 per thousand, but benign anomalies of the genital tract are far more common. Abnormalities of the female upper genital tract include a T-shaped uterus, a small uterine cavity, fundal constrictions, filling defects, and synechiae. Abnormalities of the lower genital tract include transverse vaginal and cervical ridges (collars, rims, cockscombs, or pseudopolyps). The male progeny of DES-exposed women may also be affected. Abnormalities in the male include cysts of the epididymis, hypoplastic testes, cryptorchidism and microphallus.

The most important carcinoma of the vagina is of the squamous cell variety (Fig. V-22), although it accounts for only 2% of female genital cancers. It usually occurs in women 60 years of age or older. Spread occurs locally and by lymphatics. An intraepithelial form resembling that of the cervix often precedes invasive cancer. A positive Papanicolaou smear after hysterectomy suggests carcinoma of the vagina. Diagnosis is made by biopsy, usually aided by Schiller's test and colposcopy.

The most common site for vaginal carcinoma is the posterior wall of the upper third of the vagina. The lesion may be exophytic or ulcerative. In advanced stages the vaginal tube may be fixed to the pelvic wall. Carcinomas of the upper vagina may behave like those of the cervix, whereas those of the lowermost vagina spread like those of the vulva. Death is commonly from uremia.

Staging of carcinoma of the vagina resembles that of the cervix. Stage 0 is carcinoma in situ. Stage I carcinoma is limited to the vaginal wall. Stage II carcinoma extends into the paravaginal connective tissue but does not reach the pelvic side wall. A Stage III lesion reaches the pelvic side wall. Stage IV carcinoma involves the mucosa of the bladder or rectum (IVa) or has spread to distant organs (IVb). If squamous cell carcinoma is found in both cervix and vagina, it should be considered primary cancer of the cervix with extension.

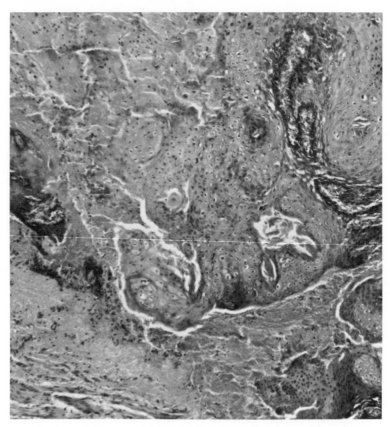

Fig. V-22. Infiltrating well differentiated squamous cell carcinoma of the vagina.

The usual treatment for carcinoma of the vagina is irradiation of the whole pelvis combined with intravaginal radium. Radical surgical therapy may be indicated for selected young patients with Stage I disease. Exenteration may be beneficial in highly selected patients with involvement of the bladder or rectum. For all stages combined the 5-year survival remains about 35%, although survivals of 65% to 80% have been reported for Stage I lesions. The rates of survival for clear cell adenocarcinoma are higher: for Stage I the rate is 90%, compared with 78% for all stages combined.

Carcinoma in the vagina is more often secondary than primary. The vagina is involved by direct spread from the cervix or by metastases from the ovaries, oviducts, choriocarcinoma, and occasionally carcinoma of the breast or hypernephroma. The vagina is involved by metastases, direct extension, or recurrence in about 10% of carcinomas of the corpus.

Sarcoma botryoides is a rare, highly malignant, usually fatal tumor that involves the vagina and is ordinarily found in infants.

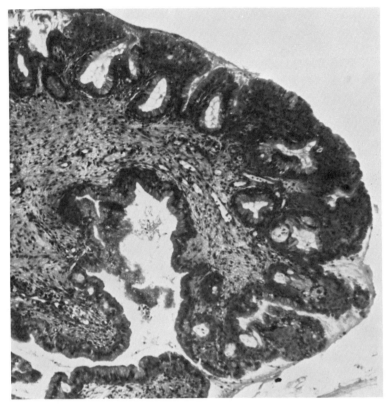

FIG. V-23. Endocervical polyp, showing covering of mucinous columnar epithelium and connective tissue core with vascular congestion and inflammatory cells.

Cervix

Benign lesions of the cervix include polyps and condylomata acuminata (p. 196). Polyps, which may be single or multiple, have a core of connective tissue and an epithelial covering (Fig. V-23). They are usually glandular, arising from the endocervix, but are occasionally squamous, arising from the portio. They range in size from minute to several centimeters in length. They may cause no symptoms or may produce irregular bleeding or increased vaginal discharge. They very rarely undergo malignant change. A large polyp may be confused with a prolapsed myoma. The treatment is polypectomy, followed by fractional curettage.

Occasionally hyperplasia of the endocervical epithelium may result from the use of oral contraceptives. This change should not be confused with adenocarcinoma. This form of hyperplasia may produce contact bleeding but will regress after discontinuation of oral contraception.

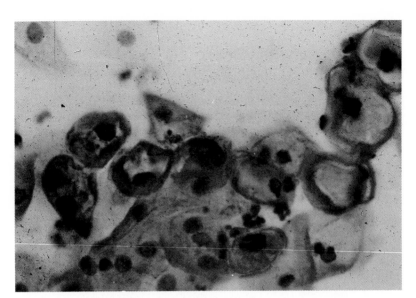

Fɪɢ. V-24. Asymptomatic infection with human papilloma virus, detected on cytologic smear of cervix.

Benign tumors of the cervix include leiomyomas, hemangiomas, and squamous papillomas. In addition, endometriosis and adenomyosis, as well as cysts and adenomas arising from mesonephric remnants, may involve the cervix. Adenosis and adenocarcinoma of the cervix, as well as of the vagina, have been reported in the children of mothers who received stilbestrol during their pregnancies (p. 239).

Invasive carcinoma of the cervix accounts for about 30% of all deaths from gynecologic cancer. The estimated number of new cases of invasive cancer of the cervix for 1986 is 14,000 and the number of deaths is 6,800. Invasive cancer is usually preceded by an intraepithelial form, which in turn is preceded by various degrees of increasing dysplasia. Cervical intraepithelial neoplasia (CIN) is a term that includes epithelial changes ranging from mild dysplasia to carcinoma in situ (CIS). All forms of cervical intraepithelial neoplasia may regress, but the earlier stages do so more commonly. The etiologic factors in dysplasia, carcinoma in situ, and invasive carcinoma are similar. The disease is more common in lower socioeconomic classes and in women who begin coitus and childbearing early in their lives. It is also more common in prostitutes and other women with multiple sexual partners. Contact

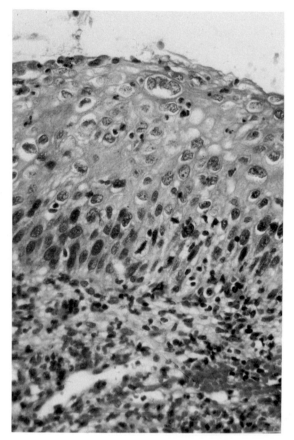

FIG. V-25. Histologic section of cervix infected with human papilloma virus, showing typical koilocytes.

with *Herpesvirus hominis* type II (p. 198) is no longer considered an important etiologic factor, but exposure to the human papilloma virus (HPV) is attracting greater attention in the genesis of cervical cancer. The concentration of histones in the semen is positively correlated with the risk of cervical carcinoma. Cigarette smoking has been associated with an increase in both dysplasia and carcinoma of the cervix.

There is a close and probably causative relation between human papilloma virus and both cervical intraepithelial neoplasia and invasive cancer of the cervix. Virtually all women with CIN and invasive cancer demonstrate DNA of HPV by techniques of in situ hybridization. Subclinical, asymptomatic HPV infection is detected on cytologic screening (Fig. V-24).

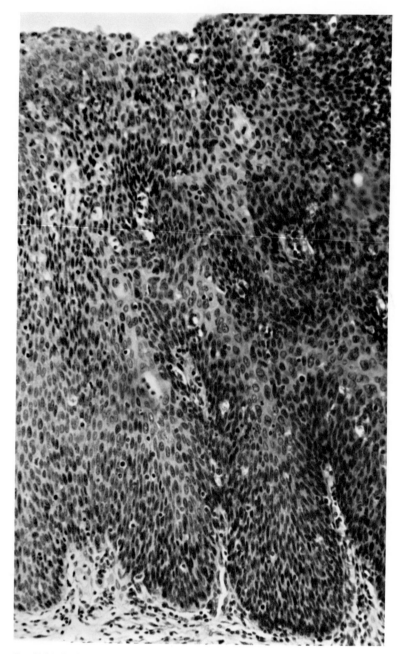

FIG. V-26. Carcinoma in situ of the cervix (CIN III), showing replacement of entire epithelium by dysplastic cells.

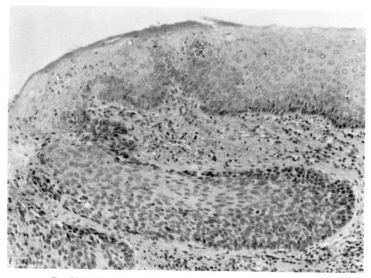

Fɪɢ. V-27. Carcinoma of the cervix, showing early stromal invasion.

Careful colposcopic examination will demonstrate features of HPV in the vulvas, vaginas, and cervices of most patients with abnormal cytologic smears. Typical koilocytes are seen on histologic examination (Fig. V-25).

HPV types 6 and 11 are less likely and types 16, 18, and 31 are more likely to be associated with lesions that progress to cancer. Atypical mitotic figures in the biopsy are associated with higher rates of progression and more commonly with HPV type 16. Patients with condylomas and atypical mitotic figures and those with condylomas and CIN should be treated promptly with laser, cryotherapy, conization, or hysterectomy. About 80 to 90% of the male partners of women with condylomas will demonstrate similar lesions on the penis when examined with the colposcope.

Dysplasia connotes nuclear atypia of the cervical epithelium without involvement of its entire thickness. True carcinoma in situ (intraepithelial, or preinvasive, cancer) usually involves the entire thickness of the cervical epithelium (Fig. V-26). The histologic changes include loss of polarity, hyperchromatism, abnormal mitoses, and increase in nuclear size and number of nucleoli.

The essential feature of intraepithelial carcinoma is the limitation of the abnormal cells by the basement membrane of the cervical epithelium. Involvement of the endocervical glands does not constitute invasion, because the glands are part of the cervical epithelium.

Microinvasion represents the transition between intraepithelial carcinoma and the invasive lesion (Fig. V-27). The definition and the treatment of this stage of the disease are still somewhat contro-

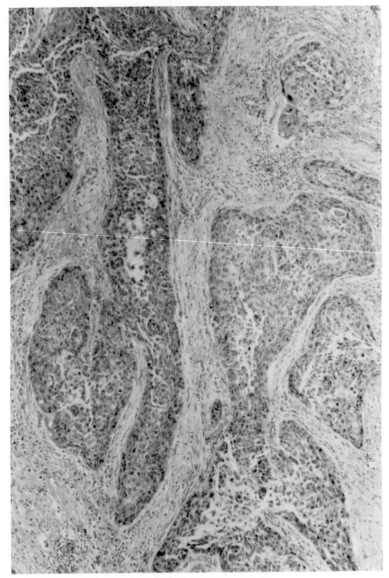

Fig. V-28. Invasive epidermoid carcinoma of the cervix. This lesion is often designated squamous cell carcinoma.

versial, although the earliest forms are now often managed in the same manner as carcinoma in situ.

Histologically most carcinomas of the cervix (about 95%) are epidermoid (Fig. V-28). About 5% are adenocarcinomas (Fig. V-29); carcinomas of mesonephric origin are rare. The tumor most commonly arises at the squamocolumnar junction. Chromosomal

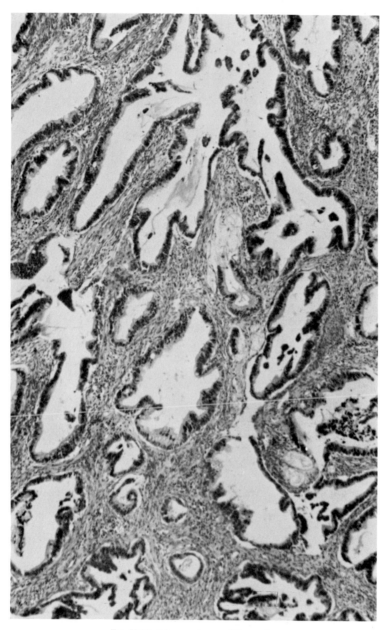

FIG. V-29. Adenocarcinoma of the cervix.

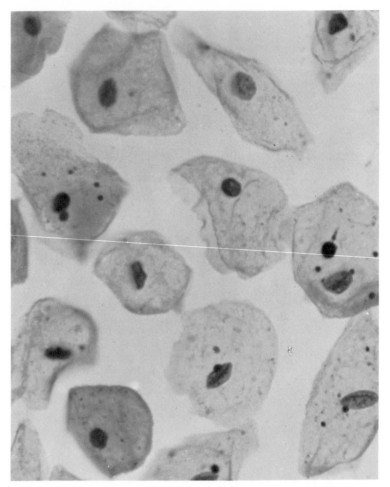

Fɪɢ. V-30. Negative Papanicolaou smear, showing superficial squamous cells with normal nuclei and abundant cytoplasm.

aneuploidy is found with increasing frequency as the lesion progresses from dysplasia through intraepithelial carcinoma to frankly invasive cancer. The tumor spreads locally into the vagina and parametria and then by regional lymphatics. A cervix that harbors an invasive lesion may be grossly normal, ulcerated, or replaced by a bulky exophytic tumor.

The peak incidence of carcinoma in situ occurs at about 37 years, whereas that of invasive cancer occurs about 10 years later (45 to 48 years). Because clinical signs of cervical cancer occur relatively late, success in the early detection and cure of this tumor depends on its identification in the preclinical stages. The most important means of achieving this goal is the routine use of the Papanicolaou smear (exfoliative cytology) (Fig. V-30 and V-31).

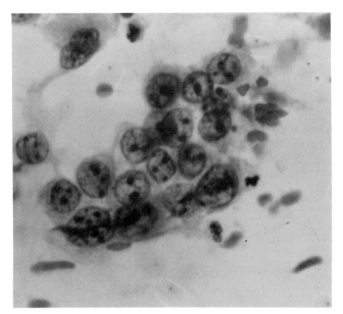

Fig. V-31. Positive Papanicolaou smear, showing malignant cells with nuclei containing abnormal clumps of chromatin and increased nucleocytoplasmic ratio.

The earliest clinical signs of carcinoma of the cervix are blood-tinged leukorrhea and postcoital or contact bleeding. Pelvic pain, edema of the lower extremity (lymphatic involvement), irritability of the bladder, and rectal discomfort are late signs. Cachexia and genital tract fistulas indicate advanced disease. The tumor ultimately obstructs the ureters, producing uremia, the most common cause of death from carcinoma of the cervix. In advanced cases infection is often superimposed.

Successful management of carcinoma of the cervix depends on the detection of the preinvasive lesion, for intraepithelial carcinoma is curable in virtually 100% of cases. Once frank invasion occurs, the 5-year cure rate drops to about 85%. The mainstay of detection of the earliest stages of cervical cancer is the Papanicolaou smear. A single Papanicolaou smear is about 80% effective in detecting desquamated malignant cells from the cervix and vagina. The specimens should be obtained from the endocervical canal and portio vaginalis of the cervix. The squamocolumnar junction should be adequately sampled. Any clinically suspicious lesion should be subjected to biopsy regardless of the cytologic findings, even during pregnancy.

The possibility of rendering carcinoma of the cervix a preventable disease is still far from realized because many women in the United States are not routinely screened cytologically. These women, furthermore, often belong to groups with a high prevalence of cervical carcinoma. A larger group of women may be screened through the use of irrigation smears, which the patient obtains herself. Disadvantages of that method include greater error in collection of the specimen and the lack of a simultaneous pelvic examination.

The Papanicolaou smear may be reported by Class (I through V); by narrative description; or simply as positive, suspicious, or negative. Class I is negative (no suspicious cells); Class II shows benign reactive changes or minimal cellular atypia; Class III shows mild to moderate atypia; Class IV shows severely atypical or malignant cells; and Class V shows unequivocally malignant cells.

Cervical intraepithelial neoplasia I (CIN I) means minimal or mild dysplasia; CIN II means moderate dysplasia; and CIN III means severe dysplasia or carcinoma in situ.

Because cytology is only a screening method, no therapy is to be based on the cytologic findings alone. Instead, a suspicious or positive smear must be investigated further. Treatment is based only on a histologic diagnosis. The management of the abnormal Papanicolaou smear is diagrammed in Table 11. A suspicious smear without a clinical lesion may be repeated before histologic investigation, but a frankly positive smear should be confirmed without delay. Any gross lesion must be subjected at once to biopsy. A clinically normal cervix should be investigated by colposcopically directed biopsy (p. 185) or cone biopsy. Iodine-negative areas that do not contain glycogen may indicate epithelial atypia and suggest the areas for punch biopsy. The number of diagnostic cone biopsies performed has been greatly reduced by the wide use of colposcopy.

The colposcope provides a magnification of 6 to 40 times and helps determine the site for biopsy. Because colposcopy cannot detect a lesion in the endocervical canal, endocervical curettage or conization is required to rule out a lesion in that location. If the entire squamocolumnar junction cannot be visualized, conization is necessary to exclude invasive carcinoma. Colposcopy depends largely on the interpretation of vascular and epithelial patterns. A satisfactory colposcopic examination requires complete visualization of the entire squamocolumnar junction and all suspicious lesions.

If the punch biopsies reveal invasive cancer, it is not necessary to perform a diagnostic cone. If they reveal a lesion less extensive than invasive cancer, a satisfactory colposcopy or a cone is required to rule out the coexistence of a more advanced lesion.

The complications of conization (p. 185) include bleeding, parametritis, and injury to the internal os. Where no other method of exclud-

Table 11. Management of the Abnormal Papanicolaou Smear

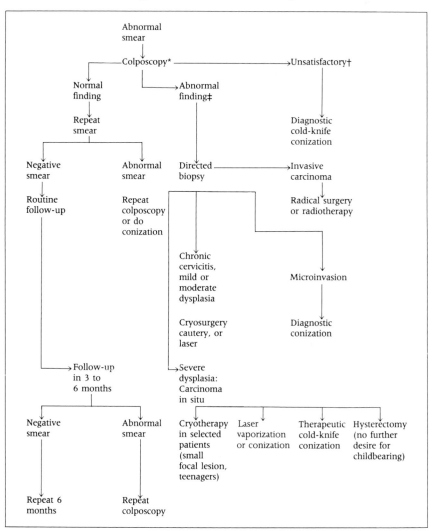

*If colposcopy is not available, conization may be required at this point if patient cannot be referred.
†Satisfactory colposcopy requires that entire squamocolumnar junction be identified and entire lesion seen.
‡Biopsy is performed in presence of clinical lesion regardless of cytologic findings.

ing invasion is available, however, the cone is still required for diagnosis and treatment.

Staging of carcinoma of the cervix is crucial for decisions about treatment and for comparison of the results of treatment in various centers.

Stage 0 is carcinoma in situ, preinvasive carcinoma, or intraepithelial carcinoma.

Stage I is invasive carcinoma confined to the cervix. (Extension to the corpus should be disregarded in staging.) Stage Ia is preclinical carcinoma (diagnosed only microscopically). Stage Ia1 refers to a lesion that has minimal microscopically evident stromal invasion. Stage Ia2 lesions are also detected microscopically but can be measured. The upper limit of the measurement should not have a depth greater than 5 mm from the base of the epithelium from which it originates, and the horizontal spread should not exceed 7 mm.

Stage Ib lesions are those of greater dimensions than described for Stage Ia2, whether seen clinically or only microscopically.

Stage II involves the vagina (exclusive of the lowest third), the parametria (but not to the side walls of the pelvis), or both vagina and one or both parametria.

Stage IIa lesions involve the vagina but not the parametria.

Stage IIb lesions involve the parametria with or without the vagina.

Stage IIIa lesions involve the lowest third of the vagina, and Stage IIIb lesions reach one or both pelvic side walls. Hydronephrosis or a nonfunctioning kidney relegates the lesion to Stage III.

Stage IV lesions involve the mucosa of the bladder or rectum (Stage IVa) or have distant metastases (Stage IVb).

Any patient with a cervical carcinoma that may require radical surgical procedures or radiotherapy should have a diagnostic investigation that includes as a minimum the following: complete blood count, chest roentgenogram, intravenous pyelogram, cystoscopy, proctoscopy, and hepatic and renal function tests.

Although the involvement of lymph nodes does not affect the staging of carcinoma of the cervix, it does affect the prognosis. The frequencies of involvement of the lymph nodes in the various stages of cervical carcinoma are as follows: Stage I, 15%; Stage II, 30%; Stage III, 45%; and Stage IV, 60%.

The treatment of carcinoma of the cervix depends on the stage of the lesion. Severe dysplasias and carcinoma in situ (Stage 0) may be treated with therapeutic cone with close follow-up in the woman who desires children. Other conservative treatments include cryosurgery, electrocautery, and the CO_2 laser. In older women and multiparas the treatment of choice is often total hysterectomy (vaginal or abdominal) with a large vaginal cuff. Invasive cancer is treated by radical surgical procedures or radiation, depending on the stage.

Surgical treatment is required for radioresistant lesions and for recurrences after full radiation. Radiation is employed in patients who present poor operative risks and for some recurrences after surgical treatment. In most cases almost identical cure rates are obtained by surgical or radiotherapeutic means.

Stage I lesions may be treated by radical hysterectomy and pelvic lymphadenectomy or by radiation. Because the likelihood of lymph node involvement is Stage Ia lesions is less than 2%, it may be safe to treat these minimally invasive lesions as though they were intraepithelial carcinomas. Some Stage IIa lesions may be treated by radical hysterectomy, but most Stage IIb lesions are better treated by radiation. Stage III lesions are treated best by radiation. Stage IV lesions are occasionally cured by ultraradical surgical procedures such as exenteration (p. 189). This drastic treatment should be employed in advanced lesions or recurrences only for cure and not for palliation.

Radiation therapy of cervical carcinoma usually involves an internal and an external source. The internal treatment typically consists of intrauterine and intravaginal radium, cesium, or other radioactive sources. [60]Cobalt or gamma radiation is used for the external source to increase the dose to the pelvic side walls. In certain circumstances the external therapy is delivered before the intravaginal radiation.

Radiation therapy is frequently administered by afterloading techniques. Hollow applicators designed to carry a radioactive source are implanted or inserted into the area to be treated. Their position is checked before any of the radioactive material is inserted. The advantage of this technique is the minimization of exposure of the personnel to the radiation.

Understanding the principles of radiotherapy of gynecologic cancer, particularly carcinoma of the cervix, requires definition of certain terms. A curie is a special unit of radioactivity equal to 3.70×10^{10} disintegrations per second. The curie (Ci) is based on the rate of disintegration of one gram of radium. A gamma ray is a photon emitted from the nucleus of a radioactive atom, differing from an x-ray photon only with respect to origin. A roentgen (R) is a special unit of the radiation quantity "exposure," equal to an electrical charge (produced by ionization) of 2.58×10^{-4} coulomb/kg of air. A rad is a unit of the radiation quantity "absorbed dose." One rad is equal to an energy absorption of 0.01 joule/kg. The rem (Roentgen-Equivalent-Man) is a special unit of the radiation protection quantity "dose equivalent." Dose equivalent is obtained by multiplying absorbed dose by a "quality factor." When dose is expressed in rads, dose equivalent is in rems.

Point A is an imaginary point lying 2 cm lateral to the cervical canal and 2 cm above the external cervical os. Point B lies 3 cm lateral to point A and is used as a means of evaluating the dosage to the pelvic wall.

Complications of radical surgical procedures include fistulas, hemorrhage, and immediate operative death. Blood volume should be measured before any radical procedures and the central venous pressure monitored during and after operation. Complications of radiation include urinary frequency (cystitis), diarrhea (frequently bloody), and bowel fistulas. Stenosis of the vagina and dyspareunia may also result.

Carcinoma of the cervix complicated by pregnancy requires special consideration. Carcinoma in situ may be managed conservatively, provided every effort has been made to rule out invasion. The pregnancy may be carried to term and the patient delivered vaginally. Definitive treatment may be performed post partum. Invasive cancer must be treated during pregnancy as in the nonpregnant state. In the first trimester the patient may be subjected to radical hysterectomy or radiation treatment (which produces abortion). In the third trimester maximal delay of a few weeks to ensure reasonable likelihood of fetal survival may be justified before cesarean section and definitive treatment are performed. In the second trimester it is usually necessary to treat the carcinoma despite the nonviability or immaturity of the fetus.

The survival in carcinoma of the cervix depends on the staging, which in turn is influenced by the success of the screening program. A successful program will result in a higher proportion of intraepithelial and early invasive lesions. The 5-year prognosis by stage is as follows: Stage 0—almost 100%; Stage I—85–90% (approximately equal by radiation or radical surgery); Stage II—65–75%, and Stage III—35–40% (these stages are generally better treated by radiation); and Stage IV—approximately 5–15% (by ultraradical surgical procedures).

Corpus

The uterine corpus has a thick muscularis, the myometrium. Its internal surface is lined by mucous membrane, the endometrium, composed of columnar epithelium and simple tubular glands that extend deep into the lamina propria. Under the influence of the hypothalamus, the hypophysis, and the ovary, the endometrium undergoes the changes of the menstrual cycle.

The lamina propria of the uterus consists of three layers: a superficial stratum compactum, a middle stratum spongiosum, and a deep stratum basale. The compactum and spongiosum are made of cellular connective tissue and are nourished by coiled arteries. The stratum basale is made of dense cellular connective tissue and is vascularized by straight arteries. The stratum compactum and stratum spongiosum together form the stratum functionale, most of which is sloughed during the menstrual pe-

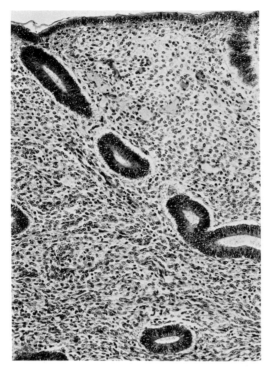

Fig. V-32. Early proliferative endometrium, showing short, straight, narrow glands.

riod. During menses pieces of the endometrium are discarded irregularly; the entire endometrium does not slough simultaneously. While parts of it are degenerating, other areas already have begun to regenerate.

At the time of menstruation the hypothalamus signals the hypophysis to secrete FSH, which initiates the development of immature follicles and stimulates the production of estrogen. Under the influence of estrogen, the regenerative phase begins with proliferation of the epithelium lining the glands embedded in the stratum basale. The epithelium spreads over the surface denuded by the sloughing of the stratum functionale. Initially it is flat, but later in the cycle it changes to low cuboidal and then simple columnar, with some of the cells ciliated and others secretory.

As levels of estrogen rise, the hypothalamus secretes luteinizing hormone releasing hormone (LHRH), which stimulates the adenohypophysis to produce and release LH. The midcyclic surge of LH and FSH appears to trigger ovulation. LH stimulates the resulting corpus hemorrhagicum to develop into the corpus luteum.

If implantation does not occur, the high titers of progesterone cause the pituitary to stop producing LH; as a result, the corpus luteum degenerates. As the blood level of progesterone falls, the coiled arteries that sup-

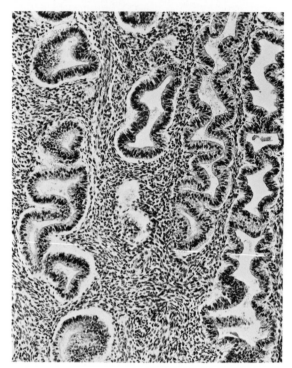

FIG. V-33. Late proliferative endometrium, showing elongated, tortuous glands with pseudostratified nuclei.

ply the stratum compactum and stratum spongiosum contract, with resulting ischemia and endometrial sloughing (menstruation). The falling levels of estrogen stimulate the hypophysis to secrete FSH, and a new group of immature follicles begins to develop.

In the early proliferative phase the mucosa is low and the glands are short, narrow, and straight (Fig. V-32). As the proliferative phase advances, the glands become longer, thicker, and more tortuous (Fig. V-33). Mitotic figures are seen in the endometrial epithelium throughout the proliferative but not in the secretory phase. The first sign of ovulation that can be detected with the light microscope is the subnuclear vacuole, on approximately the sixteenth day of a typical 28-day cycle (Fig. V-34). During the first few days of the postovulatory (secretory) phase, the subnuclear vacuoles move past the nuclei to reach the lumina of the endometrial glands. By about day 21 (midsecretory phase) the glandular epithelium has become low and the endometrial secretions and stromal edema have provided an ideal bed in which the ovum may implant (Fig. V-35). By day 25 (late secretory) the cytoplasmic borders of the glandular cells have become ragged and secretory exhaustion occurs (Fig. V-36). The second half of the secretory phase, or the last week of the menstrual cycle, is concerned with changes in the stroma. In a cycle in which pregnancy does not occur, the secretory (premenstrual) endometrium regresses and menstrua-

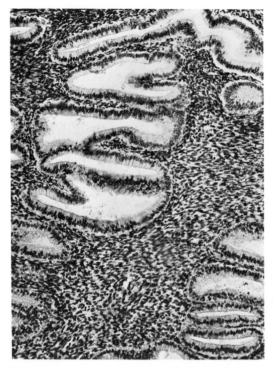

FIG. V-34. Endometrium, day 17 (early secretory), showing subnuclear vacuoles.

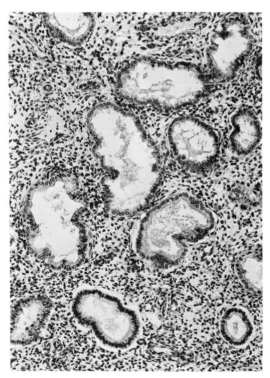

FIG. V-35. Endometrium, day 21 (midsecretory), showing glands with intraluminal secretion and loose stroma.

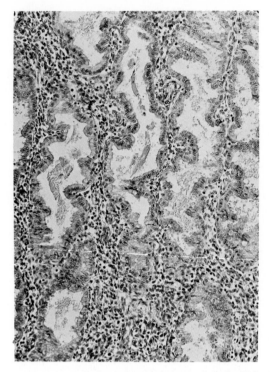

FIG. V-36. Endometrium, day 25 (late secretory), showing serrated glands with inspissated secretion.

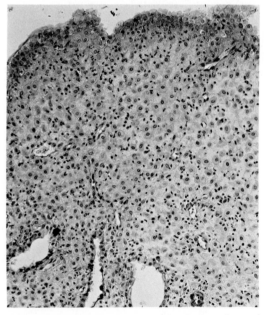

FIG. V-37. Decidua parietalis, showing round and polygonal stromal cells.

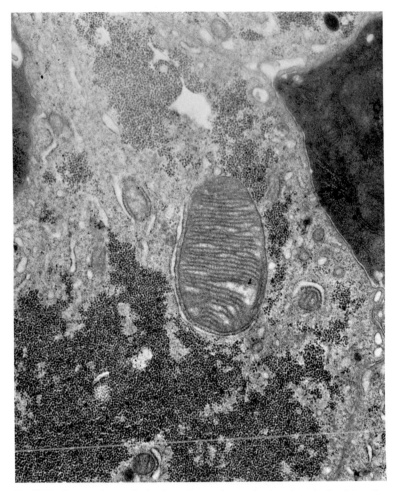

FIG. V-38. Electron micrograph of endometrium on day 17, showing giant mitochondrion adjacent to deposit of glycogen.

tion follows. If pregnancy occurs, the stromal changes progress to form a decidua, which begins first around the endometrial arteries (Fig. V-37).

Morphologic signs of ovulation can be detected with the electron microscope almost 2 days earlier than with the light microscope. A subnuclear accumulation of glycogen is ultrastructurally evident on day 14. Additional electron microscopic features of the early postovulatory endometrium are the giant mitochondria (Fig. V-38) and the characteristic nucleolar channel system (Fig. V-39).

Myomas are the commonest benign tumors of the uterus. About 25% of women over the age of 30 have palpable myomas.

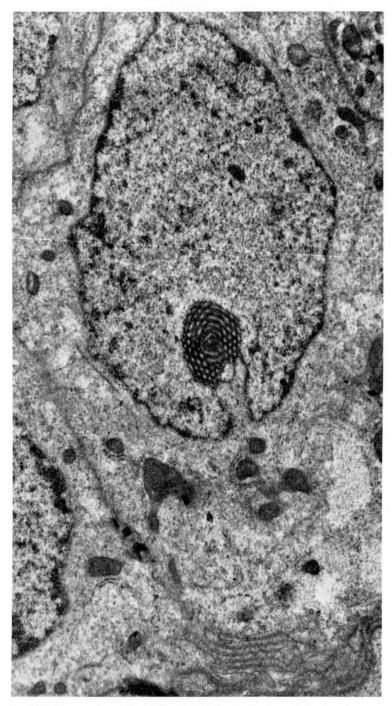

FIG. V-39. Electron micrograph of endometrium on day 19, showing nucleolar channel system.

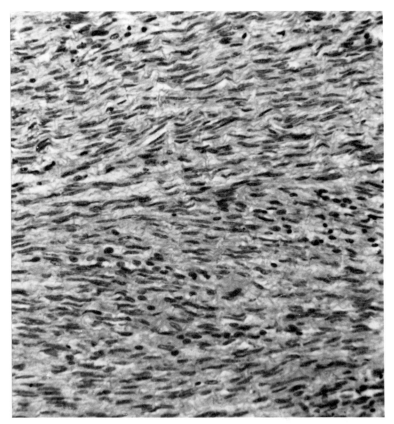

Fig. V-40. Benign cellular myoma of the uterus.

They are found most commonly in women in their thirties and forties and are larger and more common in black patients. The lesion consists of interlacing bundles of smooth muscle with only rare mitotic figures (Fig. V-40). For this reason, the tumors should be termed myomas or leiomyomas rather than fibroids. Since myomas are surrounded by a pseudocapsule of condensed uterine tissue, unlike adenomyomas or sarcomas, they may be enucleated from the normal myometrium, usually with minimal loss of blood.

The tumors range in size from microscopic lesions to huge masses filling the abdomen. They may be located within the myometrium (intramural); they may protrude from the external surface of the uterus (subserous); or they may project into the uterine cavity (submucous). The subserous and submucous varieties may be sessile or pedunculated. Tumors may grow between the leaves of the broad ligament (intraligamentous), displacing the ureters and subjecting them to danger of injury during hysterectomy. Occasionally a myoma may detach from the uterus and obtain a new blood supply from another organ (parasitic myoma).

Large myomas frequently outgrow their blood supply and undergo degeneration, including hyalinization, liquefaction, calcification (detectable radiologically), formation of bone and fat, and necrosis (occasionally characterized by pain and leukocytosis). Carneous, or red, degeneration, usually occurring during pregnancy, is one of the few changes in a myoma that is associated with pain. Sarcoma occurs in only a fraction of 1% of myomas.

Myomas appear to be under estrogenic control. They are tumors of the reproductive years and may be associated with other endocrine-dependent lesions such as endometrial hyperplasia, adenomyosis, and endometriosis. They may grow during pregnancy and with use of oral contraceptives that contain large amounts of estrogen.

Myomas do not grow after the menopause. Tumors that appear after the menopause and all cases of postmenopausal bleeding must be attributed to other causes. The most prominent sign of myomas is abnormal uterine bleeding. The bleeding typically begins as prolonged menses, which may be sufficiently severe to cause anemia. Intermenstrual bleeding may occur with extensive myomas but should suggest another lesion. The abnormal bleeding may be a result of increased surface area of the endometrium or interference by the myomas with normal uterine hemostasis.

Myomas may cause dysmenorrhea and a sensation of bearing down. Only rarely, even if large, will they obstruct the urinary tract or the bowel. A myoma protruding through the cervix may cause uterine cramps. Except when complicated by torsion, infarction, or carneous degeneration, myomas usually do not cause pain, which should therefore be attributed to another lesion, usually pelvic inflammatory disease or endometriosis.

Myomas have often been implicated in infertility, although associated lesions such as pelvic inflammatory disease or endometriosis are more often the cause. Myomas may lead to infertility by blocking the ascent of spermatozoa, occluding the oviduct, or interfering with implantation. If a pregnancy occurs, there is a greater likelihood of premature labor and delivery, abnormal presentations, dystocia, dysfunctional labor, and postpartum hemorrhage.

Diagnosis of myomas is made by history; an irregular, firm, nodular uterus on pelvic examination; and if necessary hysterosalpingography or hysteroscopy to demonstrate a filling defect (submucous myomas). Differential diagnosis includes pregnancy, ovarian tumors, and uterine anomalies. The pregnant uterus is usually softer and more symmetric, and the chorionic gonadotropin test is positive. It is impossible on physical examination to distinguish myomas from ovarian tumors with certainty after the aggregate pelvic mass has reached 12 weeks' gestational size. By that time the tumor has risen above the pelvic brim and the ovaries can no longer be palpated separately. Ultrasound may be helpful in differential diagnosis in such cases.

It is most important that the cause of bleeding in a patient with myomas be ascertained before hysterectomy. Bleeding in a patient with myomas does not necessarily stem from the myomas. It may be the result of a less serious lesion, such as an endometrial polyp, or a more serious disease such as carcinoma of the cervix or corpus. A Papanicolaou smear should therefore precede definitive therapy of myomas. If there is abnormal bleeding, a fractional curettage is also required.

Management of myomas may be conservative or may entail myomectomy or hysterectomy. No treatment is required in a woman of reproductive age if the tumors do not cause bleeding, pain, or infertility, and if they are less than 12 weeks' gestational size. In a patient near the menopause, conservative therapy may be employed after a curettage has ruled out a malignant lesion. Postmenopausal bleeding requires immediate diagnosis and treatment.

The usual treatment of symptomatic myomas is hysterectomy. Myomectomy is logically performed only in a woman of reproductive age who desires children and in whom there is no other factor preventing pregnancy. Laparotomy is indicated for any mass greater than 12 weeks' size to rule out an ovarian tumor. A smaller myoma in a patient near the menopause may be managed conservatively if asymptomatic. Rapid growth in the absence of pregnancy or oral contraceptives requires investigation. Hormonal manipulation to reduce the size of myomas offers promise.

A small uterus may be removed by the vaginal route, but large myomas are best removed by total abdominal hysterectomy. The decision to remove the ovaries is based on their condition and the patient's age.

Endometrial polyps are finger-like projections of the endometrium into the uterine cavity. They consist of glands and stroma and vary from microscopic size to several centimeters in length (Fig. V-41). In only a small percentage of cases does malignant change occur. Polyps are found in all age groups, but mostly in older women. They present with metrorrhagia or postmenopausal bleeding. Diagnosis is made by fractional curettage, which may

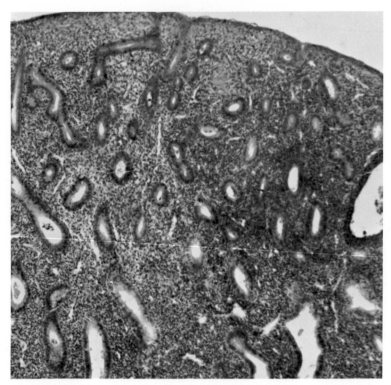

Fig. V-41. Endometrial polyp, showing numerous glands and inflammatory cells.

also be therapeutic. The differential diagnosis includes endocervical polyps, myomas, and carcinomas of the cervix and endometrium.

A placental polyp may occasionally simulate the more common endometrial polyp. It is a cause of delayed postpartum bleeding.

Hyperplasia of the endometrium is usually considered to be related to unopposed estrogen. The cystic and glandular (Swiss cheese) variety is only rarely a premalignant lesion (Fig. V-42). Adenomatous hyperplasia is more serious. Atypical adenomatous hyperplasia is often a precursor of carcinoma of the endometrium. For semantic reasons some pathologists prefer the term "adenomatoid" to "adenomatous" hyperplasia. Both diagnosis and treatment may often be achieved through curettage. High-dose progestin therapy may be used to temporize, but it will rarely cure true atypical hyperplasia. Recurrent adenomatous hyperplasia in the perimenopausal or postmenopausal patient is best treated by hysterectomy.

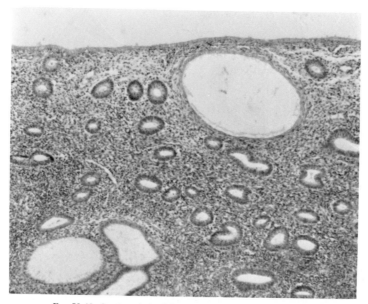

Fig. V-42. Cystic and glandular hyperplasia of the endometrium.

Carcinoma of the corpus accounts for almost half of all gynecologic cancers. In recent years it has become the most common gynecologic cancer. The estimated number of new cases for 1986 is 36,000 and the number of deaths is 2,900. Carcinoma of the corpus (endometrial cancer) affects predominantly menopausal and postmenopausal women. Its peak incidence is at age 55, or 10 years later than that of carcinoma of the cervix. In white patients of low parity and high socioeconomic status, carcinoma of the cervix is less common than carcinoma of the corpus, whereas in black patients of low socioeconomic status and high parity, the ratio of cancer of the cervix to cancer of the corpus may be as high as 10:1.

There is abundant evidence to support the relation of unopposed estrogen and anovulation to carcinoma of the corpus. The risk of carcinoma of the corpus in postmenopausal women receiving replacement therapy with estrogens is increased between threefold and eightfold (p. 332), although it can be minimized by the use of a progestin for 10 to 14 days each month. Carcinoma of the corpus is more commonly found in the obese nullipara and the patient with a late menopause and poor fertility. Hypertension, diabetes, and cardiovascular disease are often associated. Obesity appears to be the most significant risk factor in endometrial carcinoma. Adrenal androstenedione is converted to estrone in adipose tissue; the estrone, in turn, is converted to estradiol, a potent stimulator of the endometrium.

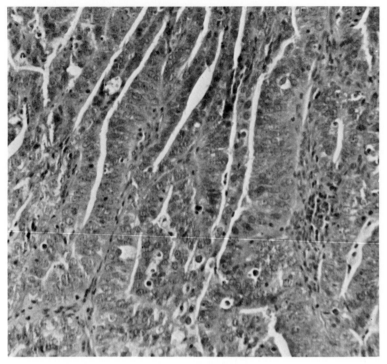

Fɪɢ. V-43. Well differentiated adenocarcinoma of the endometrium.

Cancers of the endometrium are usually adenocarcinomas (Fig. V-43). The in-situ form may be indistinguishable from severe atypical adenomatous hyperplasia. The glands are crowded back to back, with individual cells exhibiting the criteria of malignancy.

About 15% of carcinomas of the endometrium have squamous metaplasia (adenoacanthoma). This lesion does not differ significantly from ordinary adenocarcinoma with respect to therapy and prognosis. The histologic grade of the glandular component is the principal prognostic feature.

Carcinoma of the endometrium may remain localized in the uterus for a long while and then may spread widely by the vascular route. Extension may occur also along the peritoneum or by penetration of the myometrium. Pyometra is an occasional complication. About 10% metastasize early to the ovary. When spread occurs to the cervix, the behavior and treatment of the tumor resemble those of carcinoma of the cervix. Prognosis of endometrial carcinoma is adversely affected by poor differentiation of the tumor and vascular involvement. Papillary serous carcinoma of the endometrium is a particularly aggressive lesion, with early spread to distant sites.

The main sign of carcinoma of the corpus is metrorrhagia. Older women usually present with postmenopausal bleeding. In some series about one third of all cases of postmenopausal bleeding are caused by carcinoma of the corpus.

The Papanicolaou smear is less reliable for diagnosis in this disease than in carcinoma of the cervix. Results may be improved by several techniques that sample the endometrium directly, such as the aspiration curettage, but the mainstay of diagnosis is conventional curettage. A fractional curettage is required to distinguish adenocarcinoma of the corpus from that of the cervix. A hysterosalpingogram should not be performed in the presence of suspected carcinoma of the corpus. Hysteroscopy to locate the lesion precisely and describe its intrauterine extent is not yet standard practice for this purpose but it appears promising.

Stage 0 is carcinoma in situ.

Stage I carcinoma of the endometrium is confined to the corpus. In Stage I_a the length of the uterine cavity is 8 cm or less, whereas in Stage Ib the length is more than 8 cm. Stage Ia is also subdivided according to the histologic type of the adenocarcinoma. G_1 is a highly differentiated adenocarcinoma; G_2 is a differentiated adenocarcinoma with partly solid areas; and G_3 is a predominantly solid or entirely undifferentiated carcinoma. Stage II extends to the cervix. Stage III carcinoma of the corpus has spread beyond the uterus but not outside the true pelvis. In Stage IV the tumor has spread beyond the confines of the pelvis or has involved the mucosa of the bladder or rectum.

The mainstay of treatment in carcinoma of the corpus is surgical, that is, total abdominal hysterectomy and bilateral salpingo-oophorectomy. Preoperative intrauterine radium is not necessary for Stage Ia lesions that are highly differentiated, but may be beneficial in Grade 2 and Grade 3 lesions. Radium destroys superficial tumor, causes sclerosis of uterine lymphatics, and reduces the likelihood of vaginal recurrence. Although it has been standard practice to perform the hysterectomy four to six weeks after intrauterine radium, many gynecologists are now performing the operation immediately after completion of the radium therapy. The advantages of performing all the required treatment during one hospital stay include convenience for the patient and decrease in costs.

Most centers now treat all Stage I lesions with total abdominal hysterectomy, bilateral salpingo-oophorectomy, and sampling of common iliac and paraaortic lymph nodes, accompanied by cytologic washings from

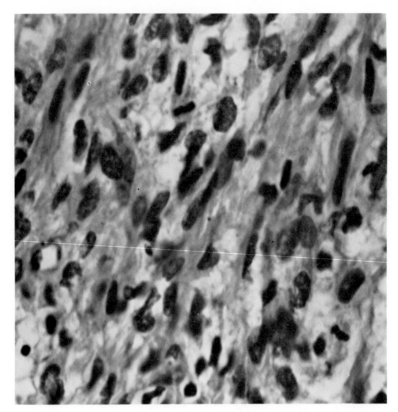

FIG. V-44. Leiomyosarcoma of the uterus, showing numerous malignant cells with bizarre nuclei.

both paracolic gutters and the pelvic peritoneal cavity. Further treatment (radiation or chemotherapy) is based on the depth of penetration of the tumor into the uterus, the histologic grade, the presence of cancer in the lymph nodes, and positive cytologic washings.

One option for treatment of Stage II lesions includes irradiation of the whole pelvis followed by intrauterine and vaginal radium and total hysterectomy with bilateral salpingo-oophorectomy; another option is radical hysterectomy with dissection of pelvic nodes. In Stages III and IV the results of both radiation and surgical treatment are poor. High doses of progestins have been used for palliation and temporary control of recurrent or metastatic lesions. Progestins are more often effective when the tumor is well differentiated.

The prognosis for disease-free survival of patients with well-differentiated Stage I lesions should be close to 100%; the prognosis for all Stage I lesions is close to 80%. In Stage II the cure rate drops to about 60%. In Stage III it is about 30%, and in Stage IV it is less than 10%. The total five-year survival in carcinoma of the corpus is between 60 and 70%.

Sarcoma of the corpus is much less common than carcinoma of the endometrium in this country. Leiomyosarcoma is the commonest of the pure homologous sarcomas (Fig. V-44). It may arise from the normal myo-

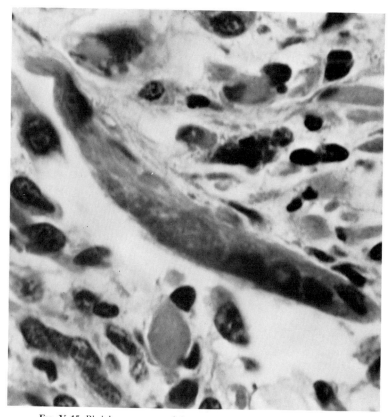

Fɪɢ. V-45. Rhabdomyosarcoma of the uterus, showing malignant "strap" cell.

metrium or from a myoma. It presents with bleeding and vaginal discharge and may be suspected when an apparent myoma grows rapidly. The treatment is total abdominal hysterectomy and bilateral salpingo-oophorectomy. The additional benefit of radiation is questionable.

Sarcomas may also arise from the endometrial stroma or from heterologous elements (Fig. V-45). These tumors, as well as mixed mesodermal malignant lesions (Fig. V-46), which are currently being reported in greater numbers, are treated by total abdominal hysterectomy and bilateral salpingo-oophorectomy. The effect of radiation is small and the prognosis is generally poor. Adjunctive chemotherapy with Adriamycin has proved helpful in patients with Stage I and Stage II sarcomas. In parts of Africa mixed mesodermal malignant tumors are much more common than they are in the United States.

Fallopian tube

Benign neoplasms of the fallopian tube include myomas, hemangiomas, and fibromas, all very uncommon lesions. The more common parovarian cysts (Fig. V-47), such as the hydatid of Morgagni, are of little

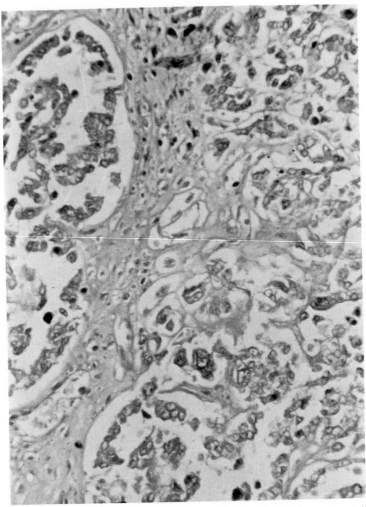

Fig. V-46. Mixed mesodermal tumor of the uterus, showing malignant stromal and epithelial components.

clinical significance. Many of these structures, formerly considered to be of mesonephric origin, are now believed to be paramesonephric. Walthard rests, which may be found in the perisalpinx and elsewhere in the female genital tract, consist of the same epithelioid cells (Fig. V-48) that are found in the Brenner tumor of the ovary (p. 286).

The fallopian tube is the least common site of carcinoma of the female genitalia. On physical examination tubal neoplasms are commonly confused with ovarian masses. Histologically, cancer of the oviduct is usually an adenocarcinoma (Fig. V-49), which spreads locally and by lymphatics. The lesion may present with vaginal bleeding, lower abdominal pain, and watery vaginal discharge (hydrorrhea). It should be suspected when

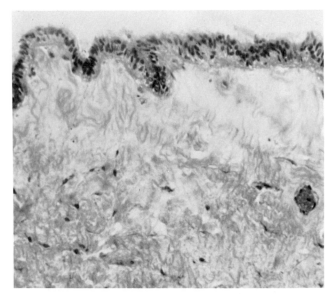

Fig. V-47. Parovarian cyst with cuboidal epithelial lining.

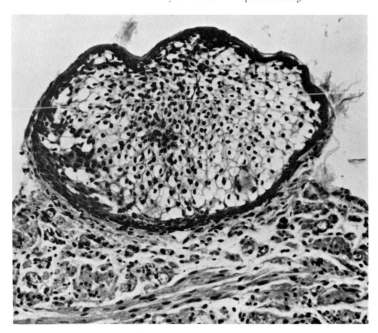

Fig. V-48. Walthard rest of epithelioid cells in the perisalpinx.

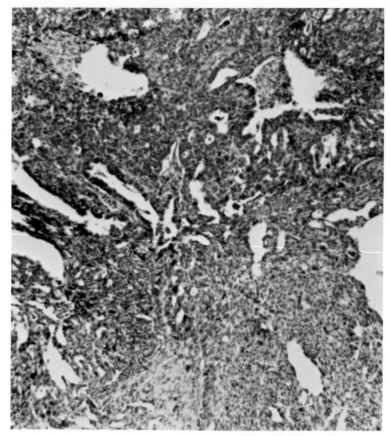

FIG. V-49. Adenocarcinoma of the fallopian tube.

curettings are negative in women with postmenopausal bleeding, particularly if there is an adnexal mass. The lesion is often found accidentally at laparotomy. Treatment is total abdominal hysterectomy and bilateral salpingo-oophorectomy, followed by chemotherapy with several agents (e.g., Cytoxan, Adriamycin, and cisplatinum) according to the pattern of spread. Carcinoma in the fallopian tube is more often metastatic, usually from the ovary or corpus.

Ovary

The gross anatomy of the ovary is discussed on page 35. The mesovarium is covered by squamous mesothelium. At the point where it attaches to the ovary, the epithelium becomes cuboidal, the so-called germinal epithelium. On section the ovary consists of an outer cortex and an inner medulla. The cortex comprises dense cellular connective tissue and many follicles and corpora lutea in

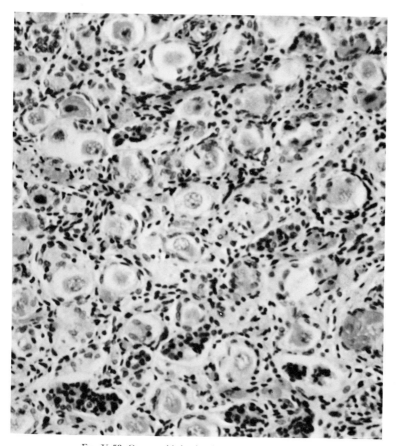

Fig. V-50. Ovary at birth, showing numerous germ cells.

various stages of maturity or degeneration. The medulla comprises loose connective tissue, large blood vessels, and degenerated corpora lutea (corpora albicantia).

The ovary at birth contains huge numbers of germ cells (Fig. V-50). Immature ovarian follicles consist of an ovocyte I (primary ovocyte, or primary oocyte) surrounded by a layer of follicular cells. As it matures, the ovocyte I develops a thick membrane, the zona pellucida. As development continues, a cellular and highly vascular theca interna forms around the zona pellucida. The fibrous layer separating the theca interna from the surrounding stroma of the ovary is the theca externa.

After each menstrual period, 15 to 20 immature follicles begin to develop under the influence of FSH from the anterior lobe of the pituitary. Development is arrested in most of these follicles at various stages, and each collapses and degenerates into a corpus

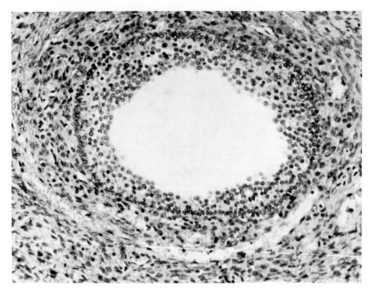

FIG. V-51. Adult ovary, showing graafian follicle lined by granulosa cells.

atreticum surrounded by a characteristic glassy membrane. Each month, however, one of the follicles continues to grow The follicular cells multiply and small intercellular spaces appear. Coalescence of these spaces forms an antral cavity, which is lined with follicular cells (the stratum granulosum) and filled with liquor folliculi. The ovocyte I surrounded by the zona pellucida is coated by one or more layers of follicular cells, the corona radiata (Fig. V-51). This complex is embedded in follicular cells on one side of the antral cavity, the cumulus oophorus. As liquor folliculi accumulates, the follicle enlarges to such an extent that it produces a bulge on the surface of the ovary. The theca interna surrounding the follicle produces estrogen.

At about midcycle, there is a surge in FSH and LH from the hypophysis. The first meiotic division occurs at this time, producing the ovocyte II (secondary ovocyte) and the reduced body I (polocyte I, or first polar body). Shortly thereafter the follicle ruptures at the stigma, and the ovocyte II inside its zona pellucida and surrounded by the corona radiata is shed into the peritoneal cavity or extruded directly into the fimbriated end of the oviduct, where it begins its journey towards the uterus. At the time of ovulation the ovocyte II begins its second meiotic division, but this process is arrested at metaphase. The reduced body II and the ovum are not produced unless fertilization, which usually takes place in the ampulla of the oviduct, occurs.

Rupture of the ovarian follicle is accompanied by some bleeding. The resulting blood clot and remaining follicular cells are organized into a corpus hemorrhagicum, which in turn gives rise to the corpus luteum. The follicular cells of the stratum granulosum develop into an inner cell mass of large vacuolated cells, the granulosa lutein cells, which produce progesterone. The cells of the theca interna continue to produce estrogen. If fertilization occurs, the corpus luteum enlarges and helps maintain pregnancy during the first trimester. If fertilization does not occur, the corpus luteum degenerates into a fibrous corpus albicans.

All adnexal masses must be considered potential ovarian neoplasms until proved otherwise. Of all ovarian tumors about 30 to 40% are malignant. As the detection and treatment of early carcinomas of the cervix and corpus improve, carcinoma of the ovary becomes increasingly important. In some series, the ovary is the most common site of gynecologic cancer, but in general ovarian carcinoma accounts for about 25% of all female genital cancers although it may be the leading cause of death from gynecologic cancer. The estimated number of new cases of cancer of the ovary for 1986 is 19,000 and the number of deaths is 11,600. Ovarian cancer affects all age groups, with the greatest frequency in the 50- to 60-year group.

The ovary is unusual in that it is a common site of both primary and metastatic lesions. The poor prognosis is related to several factors: there is no detectable in-situ form of ovarian cancer; spread occurs rapidly by peritoneal implantation as well as vascular and lymphatic channels; and there are no early signs and symptoms. Routine vaginal cytology has not been effective in detecting preclinical ovarian carcinoma.

The clinical manifestations of ovarian cancer suggest an advanced lesion. They include abdominal pain, increase in abdominal girth, palpable abdominal and pelvic masses, gastrointestinal and urinary tract complaints, ascites, and thrombophlebitis. Nonspecific lower abdominal complaints and dysmenorrhea are more common than irregular vaginal bleeding. Anorexia and cachexia occur still later. Any ovarian tumor may cause an acute surgical emergency through accidents such as rupture, torsion, hemorrhage, infection, infarction, and incarceration.

Differential diagnosis includes carcinoma of the rectum or sigmoid, diverticulosis, retroperitoneal tumors, ectopic pregnancy, pelvic kidney, endometriosis, pelvic inflammatory disease, and pregnancy. The lesion with which a solid tumor of the ovary is most commonly confused is a uterine myoma. An enlarging pelvic mass of gynecologic origin in the postmenopausal patient must be assumed to be an ovarian cancer, because myomas do not grow after the menopause (p. 262). An ovarian cyst may be differentiated from ascites by physical findings (p. 50).

Detection of an ovarian tumor is followed by laparotomy without delay except in special circumstances: in a woman in the reproductive years, a cystic unilateral mass less than 5 cm in diameter may be managed conservatively because it may well be a functional cyst of the ovary. Proper management in such cases involves reexamination of the patient in about 6 weeks. Ovulation should be suppressed by oral contraceptives during the period of observation to avoid confusion resulting from the formation of a new functional cyst. If the mass has regressed, no further treatment is required. If it has remained stationary or enlarged, laparotomy is indicated. In all other cases immediate laparotomy is required for ovarian tumors, including all solid or bilateral masses and all tumors greater than 5 to 6 cm in diameter. A palpable ovary of normal size or larger in a postmenopausal woman should be regarded as a possible malignant tumor.

Diagnostic measures before laparotomy often include computerized tomography with contrast, sonography, proctoscopy, and upper or lower gastrointestinal roentgenograms, depending on the symptoms and signs. A scout film of the abdomen may identify the opacity characteristic of a benign cystic teratoma or may visualize a tooth or piece of bone.

Staging of ovarian carcinoma is done at the time of laparotomy. Because of the enormous variety of histologic types and the individualization of management required, operations on patients with suspected carcinoma of the ovary should be performed only by the gynecologist who is thoroughly familiar with the surgical pathology. The laparotomy should include inspection and biopsy of the undersurface of the diaphragm and the retroperitoneal lymph nodes, with biopsy of other suspicious lesions, cytologic examination of peritoneal washings, omentectomy, and aggressive removal of all grossly visible tumor. A vertical incision should be used.

Staging of ovarian carcinoma is based on findings at clinical examination and surgical exploration. The histologic features of the tumor and the cytologic findings in the effusions require consideration in the staging. Biopsies of suspicious areas outside the pelvis are desirable.

Stage I lesions are limited to the ovaries. Stage Ia refers to a growth limited to one ovary, with no ascites, no tumor on the external surface, and an intact capsule. Stage Ib refers to a growth limited to both ovaries, with no ascites, no tumor on the external surface, and intact capsules.

Stage Ic refers to a tumor in either Stage Ia or Ib but with tumor on the surface of one or both ovaries, or with one or both capsules ruptured, or with ascites containing malignant cells, or with positive peritoneal washings.

Stage II growths involve one or both ovaries with pelvic extension. Stage IIa refers to extension, metastases, or both to the uterus, tubes, or both. Stage IIb refers to extension to other pelvic tissues. Stage IIc refers to a tumor in Stage IIa or IIb but with tumor on the surface of one or both ovaries, or with one or both capsules ruptured, or with ascites containing malignant cells, or with positive peritoneal washings.

Stage III lesions are tumors that involve one or both ovaries with peritoneal implants outside the pelvis or positive retroperitoneal or inguinal nodes. Superficial hepatic metastases and histologically verified malignant extension to small bowel or omentum place a lesion in Stage III. In Stage IIIa the tumor is grossly limited to the true pelvis, with negative nodes but with histologically confirmed microscopic seeding of abdominal peritoneal surfaces. Stage IIIb refers to tumors of one or both ovaries with histologically confirmed implants on abdominal peritoneal surfaces, none exceeding 2 cm in diameter, but with negative nodes. In Stage IIIc the abdominal implants are greater than 2 cm in diameter or there are positive retroperitoneal or inguinal nodes.

Stage IV lesions involve one or both ovaries with distant metastases. The pleural effusion must be cytologically positive to place the lesion in Stage IV. Parenchymal metastases to the liver place a lesion in Stage IV.

Enucleation of the tumor or unilateral oophorectomy is acceptable treatment only for well-encapsulated benign tumors or possibly Stage Ia, grade 1 carcinomas in young women. The basic surgical treatment for malignant tumors of the ovary is total abdominal hysterectomy with bilateral salpingo-oophorectomy. Aggressive removal of masses of tumor (debulking) and the omentum (to remove microscopic metastases) is indicated and even ultraradical procedures are sometimes justified. The amount of residual cancer after definitive surgical treatment is negatively correlated with ultimate survival. Occasionally, postoperative radiation may be used to treat a technically inoperable lesion. This radiation may shrink the tumor sufficiently to allow a second, more successful, operation. Because most ovarian tumors are not highly radiosensitive, the role of radiotherapy as primary treatment for ovarian carcinoma is controversial. Its success is related to accuracy of staging, adequacy of fields of treatment, and time-dose relations.

Chemotherapy is the primary means of treating persistent or recurrent ovarian cancer. Rates of response as high as 85% and long-term survival approaching 30% even in Stage III disease have recently been reported. The effectiveness of chemotherapy depends on the volume of residual tumor after surgical resection, the

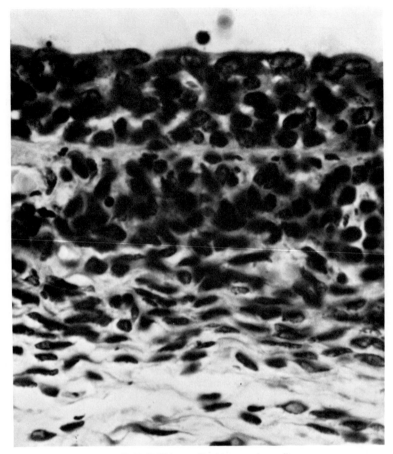

FIG. V-52. Follicle cyst lined by granulosa cells.

histologic type and grade of the tumor, and the original stage of the disease. A second laparotomy with biopsy of suspicious areas should be performed before discontinuing chemotherapy. If microscopic disease is found at the time of the "second look", intraperitoneal P^{32} may be instilled to increase salvage.

Combined chemotherapy involves use of several classes of drugs, including alkylating agents such as cytoxan, antimetabolites such as methotrexate, and antibiotics such as Adriamycin. New agents including cisplatinum and hexamethylmelamine, especially when used in combination with Adriamycin and Cytoxan, are beneficial. Although these drugs may prolong life, serious side effects may occur, including leukopenia and gastrointestinal disturbances. During chemotherapy the leukocyte and platelet counts must be carefully monitored. Intraperitoneal administration of chemotherapeutic agents is still investigational, but it shows great promise. This technique provides high local concentrations of drug with

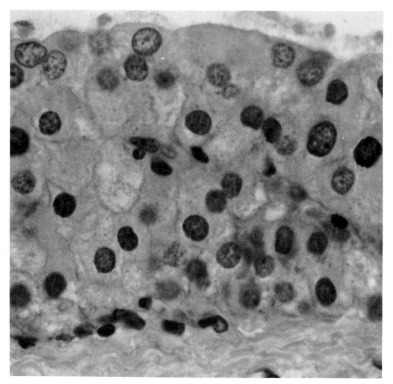

FIG. V-53. Corpus luteum cyst lined by luteinized granulosa cells.

minimal systemic toxicity. Management of incurable cancer of the ovary includes antibiotics for urinary tract infections, paracentesis for relief of ascites, and narcotics for pain in the terminal stages.

The 5-year cure rate in ovarian cancer is still only about 20 to 30% because 50 to 80% of the tumors have spread beyond the ovary at the time of laparotomy. The survival drops from about 70% in Stage I to less than 60% in Stage II, and only about 20% in Stages III and IV. The histologic type is an important determinant of the prognosis. In general, the more poorly differentiated the lesion, the worse is the prognosis. Mucinous and endometrioid carcinomas, for example, have a generally better prognosis than do serous carcinomas.

Although it is virtually impossible to construct a classification of ovarian tumors that satisfies all gynecologists and pathologists, the scheme shown in Table 12, which lists only the most common tumors, has the advantage of simplicity. A more detailed classification appears on pages 284-286.

Follicle cysts of the ovary signify failure of ovulation and may be a cause of dysfunctional uterine bleeding (Fig. V-52). They rarely exceed 6 cm in diameter and they regress in 1 or 2 months.

Table 12. Simplified Classification of Common Ovarian Tumors

I. Nonneoplastic (functional, physiologic) Ovarian Cysts
   A. Follicle cyst
   B. Corpus luteum and theca lutein cysts
   C. Endometrial cysts
II. True Neoplasms
   A. Benign
      1. Cystic
         a. Serous
         b. Mucinous
         c. Teratoma (dermoid cyst)
      2. Solid
         a. Fibroma
         b. Brenner tumor
      3. Hormonally active[*]
         a. Granulosa-theca tumors (estrogen-producing)
         b. Arrhenoblastoma (androgen-producing)
   B. Malignant
      1. Primary
         a. Adenocarcinoma
         b. Serous cystadenocarcinoma
         c. Mucinous cystadenocarcinoma
         d. Endometrial adenocarcinoma
         e. Solid teratoma
         f. Dysgerminoma†
      2. Metastatic

[*]These tumors are often considered to be of low-grade malignancy.
†This tumor is often of low-grade malignancy.

The polycystic ovary associated with the Stein-Leventhal syndrome is discussed on page 326.

A corpus luteum cyst is lined by luteinized granulosa cells, which secrete progesterone (Fig. V-53). Since the associated clinical features include delay of menses and a unilateral adnexal mass, the lesion is often confused with ectopic pregnancy (p. 125).

Theca lutein cysts form in response to high levels of chorionic gonadotropin. They are commonly associated with trophoblastic growths (p. 129), but are occasionally found with normal pregnancy. They regress after the gonadotropic stimulus is removed and should not be excised surgically. Endometrial cysts, a manifestation of endometriosis (p. 227), are also classified as nonneoplastic cysts. Because they often contain old blood they are a common variety of "chocolate cyst."

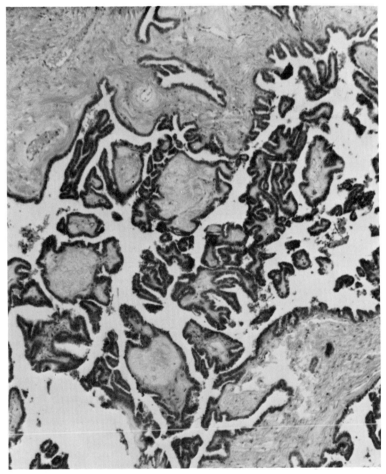

Fig. V-54. Serous cystadenoma of the ovary.

Parovarian cysts rarely reach large size. When palpable, they are often misdiagnosed as ovarian cysts.

The recent World Health Organization classification of ovarian tumors is shown in Table 13.

Serous cystadenoma is the most common true neoplasm of the ovary, accounting for 20 to 25% of all ovarian tumors (Fig. V-54). It is commonly multicystic and is bilateral in 20% or more of cases. It occurs in the reproductive and postmenopausal age groups. Histologically the epithelial lining resembles that of the fallopian tube, and calcareous concretions called psammoma bodies may be found. As may all pedunculated tumors, the serous cystadenoma may undergo torsion. The papillary variety is more likely to un-

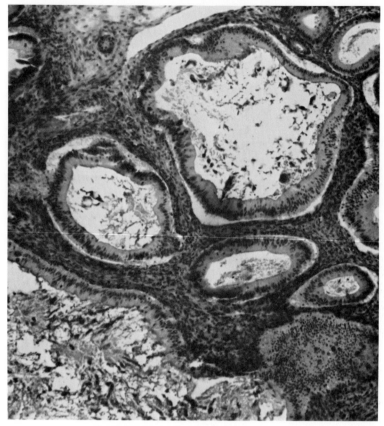

FIG. V-55. Mucinous cystadenoma of the ovary.

dergo malignant change. About 25% of the papillary serous cystadenomas are potentially or actually malignant. Bilateral tumors and those in which the capsule has been penetrated are more likely to be malignant.

The mucinous cystadenoma accounts for about 10% of all ovarian tumors (Fig. V-55). It is often multilocular, and about 5% are bilateral. The likelihood of malignant change is about 5 to 10%. The epithelial lining of the cyst resembles that of the endocervix or the small intestine. These tumors may attain very large size. Rupture of the cyst may produce the condition known as pseudomyxoma peritonei, which may be fatal.

Mesonephroid tumors of the ovary may be benign, borderline, or malignant (Fig. V-56).

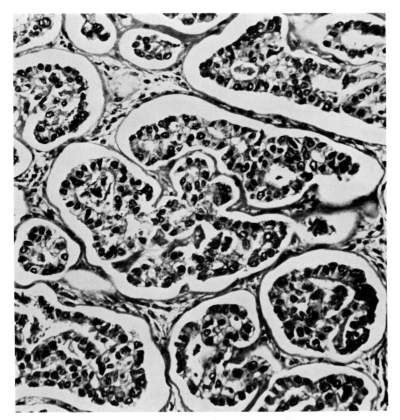

FIG. V-56. Mesonephroid tumor of the ovary.

The benign cystic teratoma (dermoid cyst) is the second most common benign ovarian tumor, accounting for about 15% of all ovarian tumors. It contains derivatives of all three germ layers, although skin and its appendages predominate (Fig. V-57). The tissues found in the benign teratoma are mature and well differentiated. They commonly occur in the third decade of life. About 25% of dermoid cysts are bilateral. Rupture of this tumor may produce a severe chemical peritonitis. Diagnosis of a dermoid cyst may occasionally be made preoperatively by roentgenologic demonstration of teeth or bone.

A special variety of dermoid, in which thyroid tissue predominates, is the struma ovarii (Fig. V-58). This tumor may produce hyperthyroidism, which regresses after removal of the neoplasm. The risk of malignant change in a benign cystic teratoma is only about 1%. The most commonly associated cancer is squamous cell carcinoma.

Table 13. W. H. O. Classification of Ovarian Tumors

I. Common Epithelial Tumors
  A. Serous tumors
    1. Benign
      a. cystadenoma and papillary cystadenoma
      b. surface papilloma
      c. adenofibroma and cystadenofibroma
    2. Borderline malignancy (carcinomas of low malignant potential)
      a. cystadenoma and papillary cystadenoma
      b. surface papilloma
      c. adenofibroma and cystadenofibroma
    3. Malignant
      a. adenocarcinoma, papillary adenocarcinoma, and papillary cystadenocarcinoma
      b. surface papillary carcinoma
      c. malignant adenofibroma and cystadenofibroma
  B. Mucinous tumors
    1. Benign
      a. cystadenoma
      b. adenofibroma and cystadenofibroma
    2. Borderline malignancy (carcinomas of low malignant potential)
      a. cystadenoma
      b. adenofibroma and cystadenofibroma
    3. Malignant
      a. adenocarcinoma and cystadenocarcinoma
      b. malignant adenofibroma and cystadenofibroma
  C. Endometrioid tumors
    1. Benign
      a. adenoma and cystadenoma
      b. adenofibroma and cystadenofibroma
    2. Borderline malignancy (carcinomas of low malignant potential
      a. adenoma and cystadenoma
      b. adenofibroma and cystadenofibroma
    3. Malignant
      a. carcinoma
        i. adenocarcinoma
        ii. adenoacanthoma
        iii. malignant adenofibroma and cystadenofibroma
      b. endometrioid stromal sarcomas
      c. mesodermal (müllerian) mixed tumors, homologous and heterologous

Table 13. Continued

D. Clear cell (mesonephroid) tumors
   1. Benign: adenofibroma
   2. Borderline malignancy (carcinomas of low malignant potential)
   3. Malignant: carcinoma and adenocarcinoma
E. Brenner tumors
   1. Benign
   2. Borderline malignancy (proliferating)
   3. Malignant
F. Mixed epithelial tumors
   1. Benign
   2. Borderline malignancy
   3. Malignant
G. Unclassified carcinoma
H. Unclassified epithelial tumors
II. Sex Cord Stromal Tumors
  A. Granulosa-stromal cell tumors
     1. Granulosa cell tumor
     2. Tumors in the thecoma-fibroma group
        a. thecoma
        b. fibroma
        c. unclassified
  B. Androblastomas; Sertoli-Leydig cell tumors
     1. Well differentiated
        a. tubular androblastoma; Sertoli cell tumor (tubular adenoma of Pick)
        b. tubular androblastoma with lipid storage; Sertoli cell tumor with lipid storage (folliculome lipidique)
        c. Sertoli-Leydig cell tumor (tubular adenoma with Leydig cells)
        d. Leydig cell tumor; hilus cell tumor
     2. Intermediate differentiation
     3. Poorly differentiated (sarcomatoid)
     4. With heterologous elements
  C. Gynandroblastoma
  D. Unclassified
III. Lipid (Lipoid) Cell Tumors
IV. Germ Cell Tumors
  A. Dysgerminoma
  B. Endodermal sinus tumor
  C. Embryonal carcinoma
  D. Polyembryoma
  E. Choriocarcinoma
  F. Teratomas
     1. Immature

Table 13. Continued

```
          2. Mature
             a. solid
             b. cystic
                i. dermoid cyst (mature cystic teratoma)
                ii. dermoid cyst with malignant transformation
          3. Monodermal and highly specialized
             a. struma ovarii
             b. carcinoid
             c. struma ovarii and carcinoid
             d. others
       G. Mixed forms
    V. Gonadoblastoma
       A. Pure
       B. Mixed with dysgerminoma or other form of germ cell tumor
   VI. Soft Tissue Tumors Not Specific to Ovary
  VII. Unclassified Tumors
 VIII. Secondary (Metastatic) Tumors
   IX. Tumor-like Conditions
       A. Pregnancy luteoma
       B. Hyperplasia of ovarian stroma and hyperthecosis
       C. Massive edema
       D. Solitary follicle cyst and corpus luteum cyst
       E. Multiple follicle cysts (polycystic ovaries)
       F. Multiple luteinized follicle cysts, corpora lutea, or both
       G. Endometriosis
       H. Surface-epithelial inclusion cysts (germinal inclusion cysts)
       I. Simple cysts
       J. Inflammatory lesions
       K. Parovarian cysts
```

The most common benign solid tumor of the ovary is the fibroma (Fig. V-59). This neoplasm accounts for about 5% of all ovarian tumors. About 90% are unilateral, and they occur more commonly after the menopause. There is less than a 1% likelihood of malignant transformation. In about 25% of cases the tumor is complicated by ascites and hydrothorax (Meigs' syndrome). The effusions regress after removal of the tumor. The cause of the hydrothorax and ascites is not clear.

The Brenner tumor (Fig. V-60), which is usually unilateral, accounts for about 1 to 2% of all ovarian tumors. It is a solid benign neoplasm with a very small likelihood of malignant change and is usually found in women above the age of 40. Histologically it consists of a fibrous stroma surrounding epithelioid cells with longitudinally grooved nuclei.

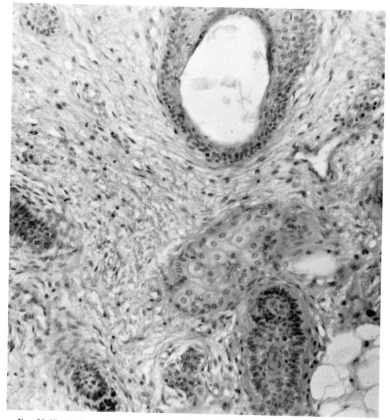

FIG. V-57. Benign cystic teratoma of the ovary, showing skin and epidermal appendages.

Endocrinologically active tumors of the ovary are difficult to classify. They are generally of a low degree of malignancy and are therefore often considered with both the benign and the malignant tumors. They may be classified according to histologic type or endocrine effects. The interconvertibility of the steroid hormones adds to the difficulty in classification. These tumors as a group are often described as gonadal stromal tumors or mesenchymomas. In the granulosa-theca cell tumors, one or the other element may predominate or occur exclusively. In general, these are estrogen-producing lesions, which account for about 10% of all solid ovarian tumors.

The granulosa cell tumor accounts for between 1 and 3% of all ovarian tumors (Fig. V-61). About 95% are unilateral, and all are generally small. Histologically the granulosa cells form a columnar or folliculoid pattern. The poorly differentiated tumors may appear

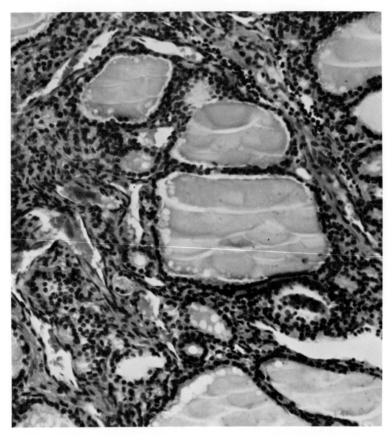

Fig. V-58. Benign cystic teratoma with preponderance of colloid-containing thyroid tissue (struma ovarii).

sarcomatoid. Granulosa cell tumors may cause precocious puberty in the child or postmenopausal bleeding in the older patient; furthermore, they may stimulate the development of endometrial cancer. In a woman in the reproductive years they are likely to cause abnormal uterine bleeding or endometrial hyperplasia. About 10 to 30% undergo malignant change. In the young patient, unilateral oophorectomy may be attempted, but in the older patient the treatment of choice is total abdominal hysterectomy with bilateral salpingo-oophorectomy.

Thecomas are also estrogen-producing tumors of the ovary (Fig. V-62). They too account for a small percentage of all ovarian tumors. In general, they are small and unilateral. Not more than 1% of these tumors have malignant potential. The tumors histologically resemble fibromas, from which they may be distinguished by appropriate lipid stains. Luteinization of an estrogen-producing

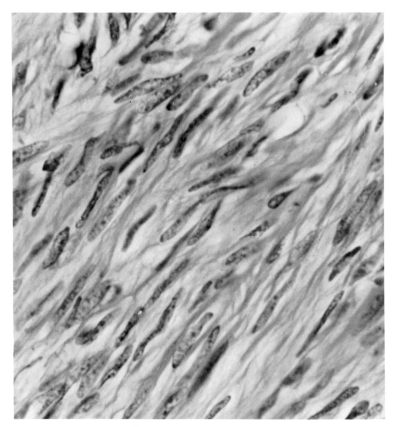

FIG. V-59. Fibroma of the ovary.

tumor may be associated with a progestational endometrium. According to some investigators, there is an increased risk of endometrial carcinoma in patients with these tumors. Treatment of thecomas is based on the same principles as that of granulosa cell tumors.

A typical masculinizing tumor of the ovary is the arrhenoblastoma. About 95% of these uncommon tumors are unilateral, and the majority occur in women under the age of 35. The malignant potential is about 20 to 25%. A well-differentiated form of the tumor is the Pick, or testicular, adenoma (Fig. V-63). The Leydig cells, which are the source of androgen, are not prominent in the highly differentiated testicular adenoma. Treatment is usually total abdominal hysterectomy and bilateral salpingo-oophorectomy. Defeminization is followed by masculinization, or virilization. The usual sequence is amenorrhea, involution of the breasts and uterus, and infertility, followed by hirsutism, acne, deepening of the voice, and hypertrophy of the clitoris.

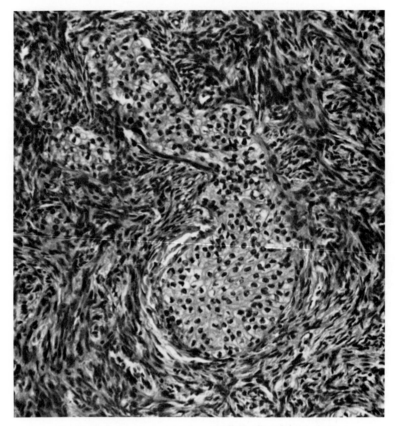

FIG. V-60. Brenner tumor, showing epithelioid cells and dense stroma.

Still less common masculinizing tumors of the ovary are the hilus cell and the adrenal rest tumors. The hilus cell tumor has about a 1% malignant potential. Microscopically, the hilus cells resemble Leydig cells and may contain crystalloids of Reinke.

Primary adenocarcinoma of the ovary is basically a solid tumor, which may contain cystic or necrotic areas. It is relatively undifferentiated, commonly bilateral, and highly malignant. Since the tumor spreads rapidly by seeding of the peritoneum and omentum, the patient with this lesion often presents with ascites.

Serous cystadenocarcinoma is the most common cancer of the ovary, accounting for about half of all ovarian carcinomas (Fig. V-64). In more than 50% of cases, it presents as bilateral cystic or loculated ovarian masses with ascites. The papillary projections may detach and implant widely in the peritoneal cavity. Several authors believe that carcinoma of this histologic variety is a mani-

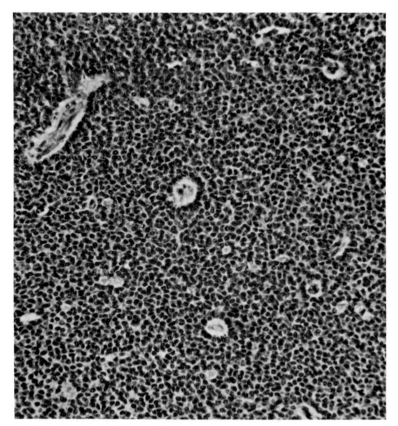

Fig. V-61. Granulosa cell tumor (folliculoid type), forming rosettes with Call-Exner bodies.

festation of generalized abdominal carcinomatosis rather than primary ovarian disease.

Mucinous cystadenocarcinoma accounts for about 10 to 15% of all ovarian cancers. The tumors are often large and multilocular, with numerous areas of hemorrhage. About 25% are bilateral.

The cure rate of endometrioid (endometrial) adenocarcinoma of the ovary is better than that of the other cystic ovarian cancers.

Solid teratomas of the ovary usually contain poorly differentiated derivatives of all three germ layers. They are found more commonly in the young patient. The degree of malignancy is high and the prognosis is poor.

The dysgerminoma arises from the undifferentiated germ cell and is histologically identical with the seminoma of the testis (Fig. V-65). The tumor is found in young adults, about 75% occurring before the age of 26. The dysgerminoma is bilateral in 10 to 20% of cases. Microscopically, it consists of large ovoid cells separated by

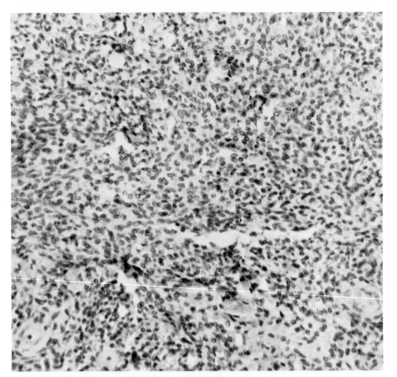

Fig. V-62. Thecoma of the ovary, composed of benign neoplastic fibrocytes.

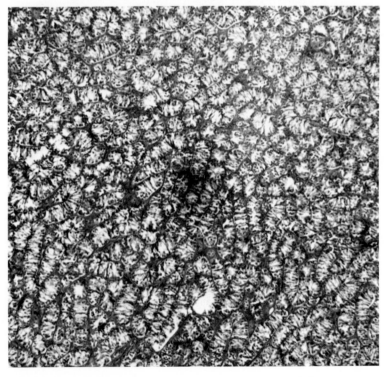

Fig. V-63. Well differentiated arrhenoblastoma (Pick's adenoma), composed of structures resembling testicular tubules.

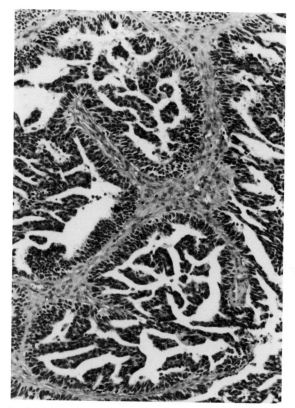

FIG. V-64. Invasive papillary serous cystadenocarcinoma of the ovary.

delicate septa of connective tissue with a sprinkling of lymphocytes. The degree of malignancy is variable. Bilateral tumors and those in which the capsule has been broken have a poorer prognosis. The tumor occasionally produces chorionic gonadotropin (with or without associated teratoid trophoblast) and is sometimes found in intersexes. The usual treatment in the patient who has completed her family is total abdominal hysterectomy and bilateral salpingo-oophorectomy. Occasionally in the young patient, a well-encapsulated unilateral tumor may be treated by unilateral oophorectomy. This tumor, unlike most ovarian neoplasms, is highly radiosensitive.

The endodermal sinus (yolk sac) tumor is a highly aggressive extra-embryonal teratoma (Fig. V-66). Alpha-fetoprotein is a useful marker for this neoplasm. New regimens of chemotherapy (e.g., Vincristine, Bleomycin, and cisplatinum) have produced high rates of cure, with frequent preservation of fertility.

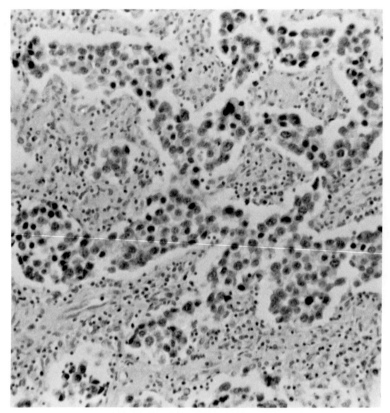

Fɪɢ. V-65. Dysgerminoma (germinoma, or seminoma), showing clusters of germ cells separated by septa containing lymphocytes.

About 20 to 25% of all ovarian tumors are metastatic. Common primary sites are the endometrium, the gastrointestinal tract, and the breast. A Krukenberg tumor is usually metastatic from the gastrointestinal tract (Fig. V-67). Microscopically, it consists of signet-ring (fat-containing) cells in a dense fibrous stroma.

Diseases of the Breast

The American Cancer Society predicted that there would be about 123,000 new cases of mammary carcinoma in the United States in 1986 and that they would result in 39,900 deaths. The respective numbers for all female genital cancers combined are 73,400 new cases and 22,400 deaths. One in 11 newborn girls is destined to have mammary carcinoma, which accounts for 27% of the estimated incidence of cancer in women and 19% of the estimated deaths from cancer. Every 15 minutes three new cases of the

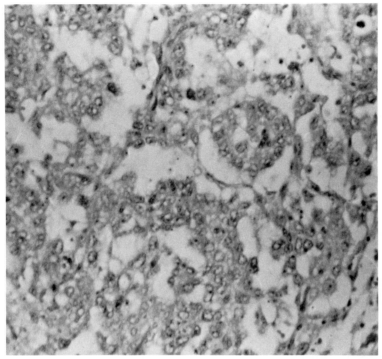

FIG. V-66. Endodermal sinus (yolk sac) tumor of the ovary, an extraembryonal teratoma, showing small cystic spaces (sinuses) lined by irregular layers of flattened endothelium into which project glomeruloid tufts with central vascular cores.

disease are diagnosed and one woman dies of it in the United States.

The obstetrician-gynecologist is well qualified to supervise the diagnosis and to some extent the management of diseases of the breast. A careful and complete examination of the breasts should precede each pelvic examination (p. 49). It is especially important in the evaluation of the pregnant patient (p. 63).

At birth the breasts consist almost entirely of ducts. With the rise in the level of estrogen at puberty, growth of the breasts occurs along with pigmentation of the areolae and enlargement of the ductal system. After the onset of ovulation and increased production of progesterone, the alveolar components appear. The alveolae, which are small sacs that lead into lactiferous ducts, are quite small and inconspicuous in the nonpregnant, nonlactating breast. The ducts, which are much larger, are embedded in a matrix of fibrous tissue and fat. Ten to 100 alveolae form a single lobule in the lactating gland. The collection of many lobules forms one lobe, which is drained by a single lactiferous duct. Each breast comprises approximately 15 to 20 lactiferous ducts and therefore 15 to 20 lobes. Each duct

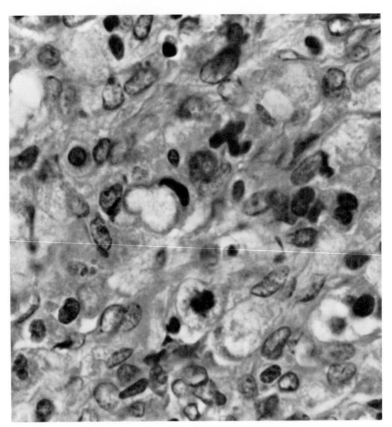

FIG. V-67. Krukenberg tumor of the ovary (metastatic from the bowel), showing typical "signet ring" cells.

terminates in a sinus as it reaches the nipple. The lobes are surrounded by fat containing blood vessels, nerves, and lymphatics.

The breast contains multiple lymphatic pathways that drain radially as well as deeply into the underlying lymphatics. Level 1 nodes are the anterior axillary chain, which includes nodes lateral to the border of the pectoralis minor muscle. Level 2 nodes comprise those beneath the pectoralis minor muscle, and level 3 those superior to the muscle. The nodes between the pectoralis minor and major muscles are known as interpectoral, or Rotter's, nodes. The internal mammary chain of nodes is particularly important in lesions that lie in the medial portion of the breast. These nodes drain from and toward the upper anterior surface of the diaphragm, the superior portion of the liver through the falciform ligament, and the upper portion of the rectus abdominis muscle and lower or inferior medial quadrant of the mammary gland.

During pregnancy, increasing amounts of estrogen, progesterone, and placental lactogen stimulate growth of functional mammary tissue (p. 116). Plasma prolactin increases from the nonpregnant level of 10 ng/ml to

200 ng/ml at term. The parallel increase in estradiol and prolactin suggests that estradiol may be related to the increase in prolactin. Although estrogen may initiate secretion of prolactin, high levels of the steroid apparently block its physiologic effect. Secretion of prolactin is controlled also by the prolactin inhibiting factor (PIF). A decrease in the level of estrogen after delivery suppresses the prolactin inhibiting factor. Suckling markedly increases the level of prolactin and leads to lactation. Engorgement of the breast occurs approximately three days after delivery, when levels of estrogen and progesterone fall markedly. Suckling stimulates release of prolactin and oxytocin. Myoepithelial cells contract in response to oxytocin and empty the alveolar lumina. Levels of prolactin return to nonpregnant values about 4 weeks after delivery but increase 10 to 20 times during suckling. By 4 months post partum the response of prolactin to suckling is lost; thereafter suckling remains the only stimulus required for lactation. Cessation of suckling terminates lactation and the release of oxytocin. Formation of milk is depressed by the effect of local pressure. Termination of suckling initiates release of prolactin inhibiting factor and a decrease in the level of prolactin.

The breasts secrete antibodies that are taken up and may be concentrated selectively from the serum. Certain antibodies are probably formed within the breast. In some species ingestion of colostral antibodies from mothers sensitized to fetal isoantigens may be deleterious to the newborn. Colostrum contains distinctive ingredients that are potentially autoantigenic for both the secretor and the recipient. Both colostrum and milk contain large numbers of living leukocytes, which may confer immunologic benefits upon the fetus. IgA, the predominant immunoglobulin in milk, probably serves an important protective function in the gastrointestinal tract of the infant. Breast milk contains IgA antibodies against *E. coli*. This finding is consistent with the clinical evidence that breast-fed babies are less susceptible to enteric infection than are bottle-fed babies. The superiority of human milk over cow's milk in protecting the newborn against infection is related to the higher content of IgA antibodies against bacteria that are pathogenic in man.

Indications of mammary disease include a dominant mass, marked increase in size or firmness of one breast, retraction of the skin, erythema or edema of the skin, spontaneous discharge from the nipple, changes in the epithelium of the nipple, and mammographic evidence of abnormalities (p. 49).

A careful history must include the date of consultation and the reason for the consultation. The duration of the signs and symptoms should be carefully recorded. The menstrual history must include the dates of menarche, last menstrual period, and menopause. The familial history must elicit information about mammary cancer or other disease in maternal and paternal relatives. The history in first-degree relatives is most important in ascertaining risk, particularly if the disease occurred in the mother or sisters premenopausally; thus, the date of onset of cancer of the breast in any family member is important. The history of intake of drugs is essential, including the use of oral contraceptives, estrogen replacement therapy, tranquilizers, and antihypertensive medications.

Mammary cancer is neither painful nor tender; nor does it undergo changes with the menstrual cycle. Benign lesions are more often painful and tender and likely to undergo cyclic changes. Bloody or serosanguineous discharge suggests cancer, whereas clear or greenish fluid is more often associated with benign lesions. A history of trauma and the finding of a firm tender area suggest fat necrosis, which may be confused with carcinoma.

A satisfactory examination of the breast requires at least five minutes if self-examination is included (p. 49). The axilla is palpated with care to support the arm with the opposite hand. This examination even if well performed is inaccurate. Approximately 40% of patients carefully examined and thought to have a disease-free axilla will at the time of axillary dissection have nodes containing tumor. It is important, however, to detect clinically evident metastatic disease before recommending treatment.

A single hard mass suggests cancer, whereas multiple indistinct nodules are more often associated with benign disease. Venous engorgement, particularly in the young patient, suggests cystosarcoma phyllodes. Bilateral venous engorgement, deviation of the nipples, and areolar excoriation are usually associated with benign lesions, whereas the corresponding unilateral alterations suggest cancer. Dimpling of the skin connotes cancer although superficial thrombophlebitis (Mondor's disease) may produce a similar change. Fixation of the lesion to the chest wall and gross involvement of regional nodes are characteristic of cancer.

Physical examination is best recorded using a diagram that indicates the location, size, and mobility of the lesion as well as nodal involvement and cutaneous changes. Diagnostic recommendations such as biopsy and mammography should be recorded with an indication that the patient will be notified of the results. The final therapeutic plan must be recorded as well.

The patient should be taught the technique of self-examination of the breast before she leaves the examining room. The value of self-examination has recently been questioned as has the assumption that it is easily learned. Lesions are still often discovered accidentally during the interval between examinations. Nevertheless, women who perform monthly self-examination of the breast usually present with earlier stages of mammary disease than do those who do not perform these examinations.

Use of a model of the breast with simulated lesions is a good technique for teaching and learning mammary examination. Gynecologists should not only teach the technique of self-examination of the breast to all their patients but should ascertain that these women are performing the examination satisfactorily.

Benign lesions include abnormalities of development, physiologic alterations, inflammations and infections, and nonmalignant neoplasms.

Abnormalities of development include accessory mammary tissue and supernumerary nipples. Because the milk ridge that forms in the embryo extends from the axilla to the groin, accessory mammary tissue (including ducts, alveolae, and nipples) may develop anywhere along this line. Macromastia, micromastia, and amastia (absence of the mammary gland) have been reported.

Physiologic alterations such as inappropriate lactation, or galactorrhea, with or without amenorrhea may result from decreases in luteinizing hormone releasing hormone (LHRH) and prolactin inhibiting factor (PIF), with an excess of prolactin (p. 116). The patient should be questioned carefully about stimulation of the breast and ingestion of medicines. Levels of gonadotropins and serum prolactin should be measured. The higher the prolactin level, the more likely is a pituitary tumor to be the cause (p. 325).

Discharge from the nipple may be related to tranquilizers (particularly the phenothiazines), oral contraceptives, and manual stimulation. The discharge should be described as unilateral or bilateral, and spontaneous or provoked. Clear or milky discharge is usually associated with physiologic alterations or manual stimulation. Serosanguineous or bloody discharge more often indicates a benign intraductal papilloma although it may rarely be associated with a malignant lesion; bilateral clear or milky discharge with or without amenorrhea may be associated with a pituitary lesion. The fluid from patients with unilateral serosanguineous or bloody discharge should be examined by means of a Papanicolaou smear. In cases of grossly bloody discharge, a mammogram is indicated. Usually the quadrant involved can be identified by careful palpation. Exploration of the ductal system is recommended.

Mastodynia, or significant pain, in the breast, particularly when it occurs premenstrually, is a common complaint among women of childbearing age although it may be found in the perimenopausal years as well. In the absence of a palpable lesion, the condition is best treated with reassurance, analgesics, and the use of a properly fitted brassiere. Diuretics, hormones including androgens, and restriction of salt are seldom effective. Recently danazol, 100 to 400 mg/day, has been used for this complaint, but long-term effects of this expensive drug have not yet been evaluated. Patients with excessive intakes of methylxanthines, as are found in coffee, tea, cola, chocolate, and certain medications, may be more likely to have symptomatic fibrocystic changes.

Almost all women have minor degrees of fibrocystic change. These lesions are usually bilateral and multiple. The pain and tenderness associated with them increase premenstrually. Early changes may be found in girls and women in their teens and twenties; they include tender tissue particularly in the axillary tail. In later stages the breast becomes multinodular, occasionally with a dominant mass. In the final stages, cysts, which may rapidly increase in size, are circumscribed, generally tender and mobile, and clear on transillumination. The fluid aspirated is usually clear or yellow. In cysts of longer duration the fluid may be dark brown or black. The prevalence of these cysts is greatest between the ages of 30 and 50 and may result from unopposed stimulation by estrogen.

The diagnosis of fibrocystic disease should not be made solely on the basis of the physical examination but should be confirmed by aspiration or biopsy. The risk of mammary carcinoma is increased in patients with dysplastic fibrocystic changes but not in those with solitary or multiple cysts without dysplasia.

Mondor's disease is probably a superficial thrombophlebitis. On physical examination the skin is dimpled and a tender cord is felt. If there is any question about the possibility of carcinoma, appropriate diagnostic studies including mammography should be performed. This self-limited disease requires no treatment. The tenderness usually diminishes over a period of 3 to 4 weeks.

Ductal ectasia or plasma cell mastitis may be manifested by discharge from the nipple. The fluid, which is usually multicolored and sticky, arises from multiple ducts in both breasts. Palpable swellings are noted under the areolae. Chronic inflammation produces a fibrosis that causes thickening of the walls of the ducts and occasionally retraction of the nipple. At this stage a hard retroareolar mass may be found. It may be necessary to excise the entire ductal system to achieve cure and exclude carcinoma.

Postpartum mastitis (p. 192) causes tenderness and induration. Occasionally there is a slight elevation in temperature. Management includes effective periodic emptying of milk from the breast and occasionally the use of antibiotics. The inflammation may progress to the formation of an abscess, which requires drainage and antibiotics.

Fat necrosis is a lesion that may obscure the diagnosis of carcinoma. Most patients give a history of trauma and complain of pain or tenderness. In about 25% of cases there is ecchymosis and ery-

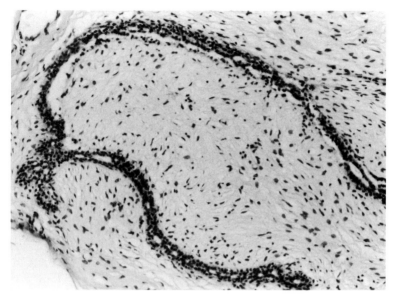

FIG. V-68. Fibroadenoma of the breast.

thema of the skin; in almost all cases a mass can be palpated. Retraction and axillary adenopathy are occasionally associated. The treatment is local excision.

Sebaceous cysts are common in the skin over the breasts. They are superficial and circumscribed. These cysts, when infected, may be associated with induration, inflammation, and formation of abscesses, and thus may be confused with carcinoma. The treatment is local excision.

Fibroadenoma (Fig. V-68) is a common benign neoplasm of the breast. It appears predominantly in young women and presents as a firm, painless, mobile mass. It may occasionally attain large size, especially in adolescents. These lesions tend to be multiple but are bilateral in only 10 to 20% of cases. The majority are discovered accidentally and, unlike fibrocystic lesions, they do not change during the menstrual cycle. They may grow rapidly during adolescence, pregnancy, and other times of endocrine upheaval. If a neoplasm increases rapidly in size, cystosarcoma phyllodes must be considered.

The predominant sign of a solitary intraductal papilloma (Fig. V-69) is discharge from the nipple. Patients with intraductal papillomas tend to be older than patients with other benign neoplasms. Most of the patients present with spontaneous, often bloody, discharge from the nipple. Surgical exploration is required. Simple excision is adequate therapy.

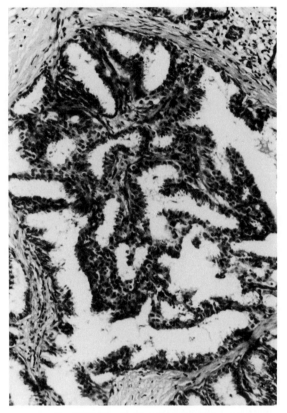

FIG. V-69. Intraductal papilloma of the breast.

Physical examination may reveal a dominant mass that is either cystic or solid, and benign or malignant. If the lesion feels
solid and the patient is under 25 years of age, observation, aspiration (needle) biopsy, or excisional biopsy, depending on the size, is
recommended. If the patient is over 25 years of age, mammography and either needle or excisional biopsy are recommended. If the
mass is cystic, an attempt should be made first to aspirate the fluid
with a 20-gauge needle. If no residual mass is palpated immediately after aspiration, reexamination in 1 month and monthly self-
examinations of the breast are recommended. If the mass persists
after aspiration or if the fluid is bloody, the patient should have a
mammogram and biopsy. If there is a residual mass on the first
reexamination, mammography and biopsy are mandatory.

Outpatient biopsy (needle or excisional) is uncomplicated and cost-effective. Occult lesions noted only on mammogram are difficult to identify by biopsy under local anesthesia. In such cases the operation is best performed in a standard operating room. A circumareolar incision is preferred. An inframammary incision is rarely necessary and a radial incision is not employed.

Outpatient biopsy for definitive diagnosis is becoming an acceptable procedure even with lesions that appear clinically malignant. Delay of definitive treatment for 1 or 2 weeks does not appear to influence survival adversely, but the operation must be performed with minimal manipulation of the mammary tissue, meticulous hemostasis, and asepsis. When the lesion is excised, a sample (preferably at least 500 mg of tissue) should be submitted fresh for estrogen-binding studies.

Carcinoma of the Breast

Systematic controlled screening for mammary carcinoma began in 1963. It utilized mammography and clinical examination. This technique of screening was shown to be of unequivocal value only in women between the ages of 50 and 59. The value of the screening was less impressive in women in other age groups.

Despite increasing enthusiasm for screening programs, many scientists and clinicians have expressed concern about the risk of radiation from mammography. The current recommendation is that mammography be continued as a screening procedure for women 50 years of age or older but that younger women be screened only in certain circumstances (p. 231). The risks associated with screening include anxiety, unnecessary operations, false security, and carcinogenesis.

The theoretic risk of developing mammary cancer is 6 cancers per 10 million person-years per rad after a 10-year latent period. It is now possible to perform acceptable mammography with an absorbed dose to the midplane of the breast that is considerably less than 0.5 rad.

In patients treated for cancer of one breast, mammography of the opposite side should be performed annually. Many physicians are recommending a baseline mammogram when the woman reaches 35 years of age and subsequent mammograms at intervals that depend upon risk factors and physical findings. In the presence of a lesion that looks or feel malignant, biopsy is indicated even when mammography suggests a normal breast or a benign tumor, for as many as 20% of palpable cancers may not be detected by mammography.

Thermography measures infrared radiation emitted by the skin and converted directly into temperatures. Although this technique is innocuous, its specificity is low.

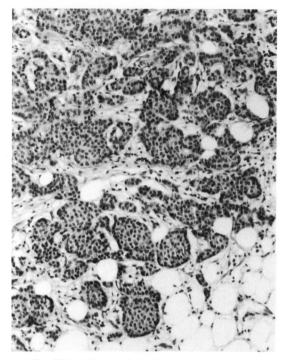

Fig. V-70. Infiltrating duct cell carcinoma of the breast.

Ultrasound is useful in delineation of mammary parenchyma in young patients and distinguishes solid from cystic lesions.

Carcinoma of the breast (Fig. V-70) is slightly more prevalent in white women and usually occurs after the age of 35. Most of these cancers begin after the age of 50 and only 1.5% under the age of 30.

The 5-year survival for mammary cancer that is diagnosed in the early localized stages has risen from 78% in 1943 to over 85% at present. When the disease is confined to the breast in its noninvasive form, rates of cure of 100% can be achieved. When the cancer is invasive but confined to the breast, the 5-year survival is 85%. When nodes are involved, the survival drops sharply to 45%. The prognosis for young women with carcinoma of the breast remains poor. More than 80% of these patients who do not die of other causes are found to die of or with their mammary cancer when they are followed for 25 years.

Major factors that determine risk of mammary carcinoma are prior cancer of one breast, age, age at menarche, age at first term pregnancy, age at menopause, and weight.

The woman with prior cancer of one breast is at risk for cancer in the opposite breast. The risk is about 1% per year. Most women who manifest cancer of the breast in the late postmenopausal years do not live long enough to develop another cancer in the opposite breast.

Women with an earlier menarche are at greater risk for mammary carcinoma. Parity is associated with a decreased risk particularly if the mother is young at the time of her first delivery. Women whose natural menopause occurs before the age of 45 have only half the likelihood of subsequent carcinoma of the breast when compared with those whose menopause occurs after the age of 55. Artificial menopause similarly reduces the risk of mammary cancer. Women who have had their ovaries removed before the age of 35 have a 70% reduction in the occurrence of carcinoma of the breast.

The relation between weight and mammary cancer, particularly in the postmenopausal woman, is strong. For women under the age of 50 there is little or no increased risk, but in those between the ages of 60 and 69 an increase in weight from 60 to 70 kilograms or more increases the risk by about 80%.

Genetic, viral, and endocrine factors have been implicated in the pathogenesis of carcinoma of the breast. Relatives of women who had mammary cancer, particularly if bilateral, in the premenopausal years are at particular risk. The pattern of inheritance in most patients, however, is not clear and environmental factors have been implicated. Viruses have been suspected, but there is no proof that they are etiologic in mammary carcinoma. The most popular hypothesis relates to increased estrogens, either exogenous or endogenous, which usually arise from increase in peripheral conversion of androgens. Estrone is the most important estrogen after the menopause. Recent evidence suggests that although estrone binds to the receptor with less affinity than does estradiol, both induce specific estrogenic effects. The primary site of the peripheral conversion of androgens to estrone is fat. The major factor related to increase in susceptibility to carcinoma of the breast over which control can be exerted is therefore obesity.

Because many patients with cancer of the breast present with metastatic disease, previously held concepts of therapy must be reassessed in the light that this carcinoma may be a systemic disease. Evaluation of the patient with mammary cancer includes a complete physical examination, roentgenogram of the chest, tests of hepatic function, and mammography. Isotopic scanning and films for metastatic disease are obtained when indicated by signs and symptoms and in the presence of lesions greater than 2 cm in diameter. Bone scans are often obtained, particularly if adjuvant chemotherapy is planned.

The TNM system provides for the preoperative and postoperative staging of the primary lesion. T refers to the primary tumor, N to the regional nodes, and M to distant metastases. TO means no evidence of primary disease; TIS is carcinoma in situ; and T1, T2, T3, and T4 refer to progressive increases in size of the tumor.

For most patients a two-step plan of diagnosis and therapy is recommended. A frozen section of the specimen obtained by biopsy, on an outpatient or inpatient basis, is examined to ascertain whether cancer is present. If cancer is found, appropriate estrogen and progesterone binding studies are performed. After permanent sections are reviewed, the options for treatment are discussed with the patient. There is no evidence that a delay of 1 or 2 weeks between diagnosis and definitive treatment adversely affects prognosis.

In the 1970s radical mastectomy was the most widely performed operation in the United States for the primary treatment of mammary cancer. It is still the standard against which the results of all other procedures must be judged. With radical mastectomy, the pectoral muscles are removed and a complete axillary dissection performed. In about 20% of the cases significant morbidity or functional impairment follows this operation.

Total mastectomy with axillary dissection (modified radical mastectomy) has largely supplanted the radical operation and is the operation of choice of most surgeons for Stages T1 and T2 curable carcinoma of the breast.

Total removal of the breast with axillary dissection is common to both radical and modified radical procedures, although complete axillary dissection is technically more difficult when the muscles of the chest wall are not removed. When both pectorales (major and minor) are preserved, complete dissection of level 1 and level 2 nodes is difficult. When the pectoralis minor is removed, access to the axilla is facilitated. Preservation of the bulk of the pectoralis major decreases edema and deformity of the chest wall and leads to greater strength and mobility of the arm. Furthermore, preservation of the musculature of the chest wall permits more effective reconstructive procedures. The modified radical mastectomy is probably as effective as the classical radical operation in the surgical treatment of curable mammary cancer.

Radiation compared with surgery achieves better functional and cosmetic results with equal or decreased morbidity. Complete excision of the tumor is important for adequate local control and cosmetic appearance with radiation therapy. The high doses of radiation that are necessary for control of a bulky tumor occasionally produce unacceptable cosmetic and functional results.

After removal of macroscopic masses of tumor, 5000 rads may be adequate to control microscopic disease. Additional therapy (a "boost") to the area of excision can be provided with a variety of techniques. Primary radiotherapy should be reserved for patients whose lesions are small in comparison with the size of the breast. In premenopausal patients with Stage T1 or T2 lesions, sampling of axillary nodes is important to ascertain which women may benefit from adjuvant chemotherapy.

With optimal combinations of surgical therapy and radiation fewer than 5% of patients with mammary cancer will have a local recurrence. More than 70% of all patients with carcinoma of the breast, however, will die of or with active mammary cancer in the 30-year period after initial diagnosis (before metastasis) and treatment of microscopic metastases immediately after local therapy.

Adjuvant chemotherapy is most effective in premenopausal patients with significant axillary involvement. No single agent, however, can yet be considered the standard drug of choice. Patients with Stages T1 and T2 lesions with no histologic evidence of nodal involvement do not require treatment.

Tumors positive for estrogen receptors respond to hormonal therapy with a prolonged interval between diagnosis of cancer and recurrence. If the estrogen receptor (ER) analysis is positive (greater than 10 femtomoles/mg protein), the likelihood of response is greater than 50%. If the ER is negative (less than 10 femtomoles/mg protein), the rate of response is less than 8%. A high content of receptor (greater than 100 femtomoles/mg protein) is associated with a rate of response greater than 80%. The estrogen receptor assay should be used in conjunction with other clinical factors that predict response to hormonal therapy. These factors include a tumor-free interval of greater than 2 years, postmenopausal status, prior response to hormonal therapy, and metastatic or recurrent disease predominantly in skin or lymph nodes. The relation of the estrogen receptor assay to clinical response to cytotoxic chemotherapy remains controversial.

Treatment of recurrent or metastatic mammary cancer comprises hormonal manipulation that is based on analysis of endocrine receptors, the menopausal or postmenopausal status of the patient, and the location of the metastatic disease. Oophorectomy, possibly followed by adrenalectomy or hypophysectomy, may be indicated in the premenopausal patient with estrogen receptors. If the analysis of estrogen receptors is negative or if there is rapidly advancing visceral disease, chemotherapy should be started at once. If there is no response to oophorectomy or other hormonal manipulations, chemotherapy should be instituted. For the post-menopausal patient with estrogen receptors, estrogens or tamoxifen followed by adrenalectomy may be employed. If endocrine therapy fails, the patient should receive chemotherapy. Combined chemotherapy given either weekly or cyclically seems to achieve the highest rate of response, the greatest complete response, the longest duration of remission, and the greatest increase in survival. Single drugs appear to be less effective. Tamoxifen is probably the best drug for patients with metastatic mammary cancer in whom conventional endocrine therapy and combined chemotherapy have failed. A panel at the National Institutes of Health recently concluded that treatment with tamoxifen should be the standard for follow-up in women over 50 whose mammary cancers involve lymph nodes and whose tumors are positive for hormone receptors.

About 2% of all mammary carcinomas occur in pregnancy. Discovery of the lesion in its early stages in the pregnant patient leads to a rate of survival, after proper treatment, similar to that in the nonpregnant patient.

For certain patients a reconstructive procedure after mastectomy is an important part of their rehabilitation. Although anatomic results are imperfect, the psychologic benefits are significant. As a result, more women are likely to perform self-examination of the breast and to consult their physicians earlier.

The diagnosis and treatment of mammary cancer often require the talents of the surgeon or gynecologist, diagnostic radiologist, medical oncologist, radiotherapist, and plastic surgeon, in addition to the psychologic support that can be provided by professionals in the fields of psychiatry, nursing, and social work.

VI

Gynecologic Endocrinology and Related Topics

Endocrine Syndromes

Basic understanding of gynecologic endocrinology requires knowledge of general endocrinology, for lesions of the central nervous system, hypothalamus, pituitary and other endocrine glands directly affect the function of the ovary and uterus. Furthermore, reproductive endocrine function is affected by metabolic disorders, systemic diseases, and psychogenic factors. The information in this unit is helpful in understanding further the physiologic changes in pregnancy (p. 61) and the mode of action and side effects of steroidal contraceptives (p. 348).

The most common endocrine problems are menopause; a delay in menarche or puberty; amenorrhea; defeminization, virilization, and hirsutism; and ambiguous genitalia, or intersexuality. In addition, management of infertility often includes endocrinologic diagnosis and therapy.

Abnormal uterine bleeding frequently results from endocrine dysfunction, but it is mandatory to rule out all other causes, especially neoplasms, before instituting hormonal therapy.

Dysmenorrhea and premenstrual tension are common problems that may have an endocrine component.

Patients with complicated problems should be referred to a specialist in gynecologic endocrinology for diagnosis and therapy.

Finally, a knowledge of normal endocrine function is requisite to a rational discussion of human sexuality (Unit VIII).

Action of Hormones

The hypothalamus is controlled by neurohumoral secretions (neurotransmitters) from higher areas in the central nervous system. Several that play a role in reproduction are dopamine, norepinephrine, and serotonin, which originate in the nerves of the limbic system. These substances cause the hypothalamus to produce releasing hormones, which inhibit or stimulate the release of tropic hormones from the adenohypophysis (anterior lobe of the pituitary gland).

The neurotransmitters stimulate the cells of the anterior hypothalamic area; the preoptic, arcuate, and ventromedial nuclei; and the prechiasmatic area and median eminence. The gonadotropin-releasing hormone (GnRH), a decapeptide, originates in the preoptic, prechiasmatic, and anterior hypothalamic areas. It stimulates synthesis and release of LH and FSH from the gonadotropic cells of the pituitary.

FSH and LH attach themselves to specific portions of the membranes (receptor sites) of the target cells. After the hormone is bound to the receptor, the resulting complex is brought into the cell membrane. The internalized hormone-receptor complex then activates the adenylate cyclase system and generates cyclic AMP, which acts as a second messenger to initiate the biochemical processes that culminate in synthesis of protein. Ovarian follicles and seminiferous tubules may produce a polypeptide hormone (inhibin) that exerts negative feedback on secretion of gonadotropin, primarily FSH.

The lipid-soluble, free steroid hormones of the end organs diffuse across the plasma membrane of the target cell into the cytoplasm. Free estradiol (E_2), for example, binds to its receptor in the endometrial cell. The hormone-receptor complex (E_2-R) is then translocated into the nucleus, where it binds to DNA. The resulting complex activates the genome, causing "transcription," or production of messenger RNA, which enters the cytoplasm and binds to the ribosome, where synthesis of protein is "translated." The effects include mitosis and synthesis of enzymes and proteins, among which are receptors for estrogen and progesterone, which provide additional capacity for binding. The complex dissociates in the nucleus after activating DNA. Free hormones are metabolized or excreted from the cell and the receptor is recycled back into the cytoplasm. Progesterone reduces the replenishment of new cytoplasmic estrogen or progesterone receptors, thus exerting an antiestrogenic action.

The secretion of pituitary gonadotropins is modulated by hormonal signals originating in the target organs, the pituitary, and the hypothalamus itself through feedback mechanisms. In the case of positive feedback, increased secretion of a hormone stimulates secretion by the pituitary; with negative feedback, the secretion of a hormone inhibits the output of the pituitary.

Through the long feedback loop, estrogens may exert negative feedback on secretion of both FSH and LH, as well as positive feedback on secretion of LH (as with the preovulatory surge, which precedes the LH peak at midcycle). LH itself may exert negative feedback on the hypothalamus, resulting in decrease in GnRH and subsequent lowering of LH through a short feedback loop. It is also possible that LH may exert positive feedback with respect to its own secretion. In the ultrashort feedback loop, the synthesis, storage, and release of the hypothalamic releasing hormones are influenced by changes in their own titers. A negative ultrashort feedback has been demonstrated to affect GnRH.

Masculinization of the hypothalamus and perhaps other parts of the central nervous system during fetal life causes the male, or tonic, pattern of secretion of FSH or LH. In the male, only negative feedback of sex steroids occurs, which results in rather constant secretion of FSH and LH. If the fetus is not exposed to an-

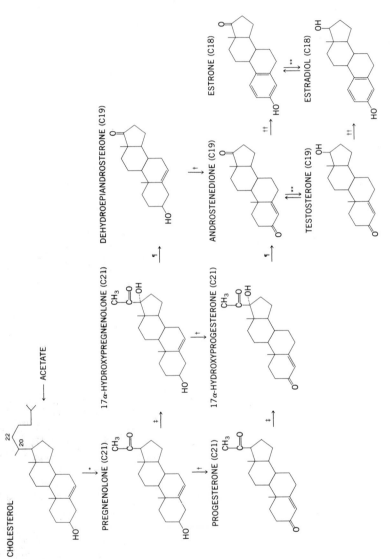

Fig. VI-I. Biosynthetic pathways of gonadal steroids. Enzymes involved are as follows:

* = 20-hydroxylase, 22-hydroxylase, and 20,22-desmolase   ¶ = 17,20-desmolase
† = 3β-ol-dehydrogenase and $\Delta^4 - \Delta^5$ isomerase   ** = 17β-ol-dehydrogenase
‡ = 17α-hydroxylase   †† = aromatizing enzyme system

drogens, it develops a female, or clonic, pattern of secretion of gonadotropins, in which both negative and positive feedback occur.

The sex steroids produced by the gonads are classifiable physiologically into three groups: progestins, estrogens, and androgens. Progestins have 21 carbon atoms (C21), androgens have 19 (C19), and estrogens have 18 (C18). In estrogens, furthermore, the A ring of the steroid nucleus is aromatized. The biosynthetic pathways leading to formation of the principal gonadal hormones are diagrammed in Figure VI-I.

Puberty

Puberty is the period when a person becomes sexually mature, the reproductive organs become functional, and the secondary sexual characteristics become developed. Its onset varies somewhat with racial, hereditary, social, and nutritional factors. Menarche, or the onset of menses, occurs about two years after the onset of puberty, which normally lasts between four and eight years. Puberty begins about two years earlier in girls than in boys. Menarche normally occurs between 10 and 16 years of age, with an average of 12.5 years in North America. The age of menarche appears to have fallen gradually during the last few decades. Since the first few cycles are usually anovulatory, fertility is ordinarily not established until about two years after menarche. The changes accompanying puberty normally occur in a well-defined sequence: development of the breasts (thelarche), growth of pubic hair (adrenarche), growth of axillary hair, and finally menses.

The first sign of puberty is usually the appearance of downy pubic hair. A small growth spurt in height and weight is then followed by elevation of the nipples and the growth of coarse and curly pubic hair. Budding of the breasts and enlargement of the areolae precede the marked growth spurt. Enlargement of the labia, further growth of pubic hair, and filling out of the breasts accompany the development of axillary hair. Menarche then occurs, followed by further growth of the labia and a decrease in the rate of general growth. The distribution of pubic hair is now of the adult type. Axillary hair is more abundant and the breasts approach the adult configuration. Labia are now of the adult type, annual growth decreases, and menstruation is well established.

The growth spurt in puberal girls reaches a peak about two months before menarche, or at 12.3 years of age. The growth rate then declines and ceases about 2.5 years after menarche. The epiphyses close at 16 to 17 years of age.

Precocious puberty is defined as puberty before the age of 8 in girls (or 10 in boys). It is more common in girls. Another definition is menarche before the age of 10 and adrenarche before the age of 9 in girls.

True precocious puberty, the premature initiation of the usual events of puberty, proceeds in an orderly manner and results from malfunction of the hypothalamus. It is always isosexual; in girls it culminates in ovulation. Its cause is usually unknown (idiopathic, or constitutional), but it may result from a variety of rare diseases of the central nervous system or from polyostotic fibrous dysplasia (Albright's syndrome).

Precocious pseudopuberty (pseudopuberal precocity) implies the premature appearance of one or more secondary sexual characteristics without the development of normal reproductive capabilities. It may result from abnormal hormonal (steroidal) stimulation or abnormal sensitivity of the end organs to normal levels of steroidal hormones. In the isosexual variety, estrogenic effects are evident in the female, and androgenic effects in the male; in the heterosexual variety, estrogenic effects are evident in the male, and androgenic effects in the female.

In all forms of sexual precocity the patients initially will be tall for their age but because their epiphyses close prematurely, they will ultimately be shorter than average for their age. Diagnosis requires expert evaluation. Gonadotropins and gonadal steroidal hormones should be measured to distinguish true precocity from pseudoprecocity. In true precocity, all hormonal levels are within normal adult limits. In pseudoprecocity, the levels of serum estrogens or androgens are elevated or, if the end organs are abnormally sensitive, within the normal range for children. The requirement for additional tests depends upon the preliminary diagnosis.

Investigation of true precocity requires evaluation of the central nervous system with neurologic examination and radiologic techniques such as computerized tomography (CT scan) and cerebral angiography. Investigation of pseudoprecocity requires techniques to localize the site of origin of the steroids. An estrogen-producing neoplasm in the young girl should be easily palpable on physical examination.

Treatment of precocious puberty depends on the cause. True precocity without an organic lesion requires no direct treatment, but pregnancy must be prevented if the patient is ovulating. Counseling is helpful to aid the girl in her psychosexual adjustment. In the pseudosyndrome, treatment may be directed toward removing the tumor or suppressing the hyperplastic adrenal cortex. (p. 324).

The onset of puberty occurs when the hypothalamus begins to secrete luteinizing hormone releasing hormone in periodic bursts, which stimulate the pituitary gland to produce gonadotropins. These hormones, in turn, stimulate the gonads to produce the sex steroids, which induce the changes that characterize puberty. Unless the releasing hormone is secreted intermittently, the pituitary will not release enough gonadotropin to stimulate production of sex steroids. If it is secreted continuously, the pituitary becomes desensitized and ceases to release gonadotropin. With the use of a synthetic analog of luteinizing hormone releasing hormone that is more potent and longer acting than the natural hormone, the pituitary may be desensitized. This promising technique may be the most effective method of arresting precocious puberty.

Retarded puberty may be associated with low or elevated gonadotropins and arise from dysfunction of the ovary, pituitary, or central nervous system or from genetic causes. It should be evaluated by the age of 15. Gonadal dysgenesis, testicular feminization, and diencephalic lesions must be excluded. Any associated emaciation or obesity should be corrected.

Causes associated with low gonadotropins include: constitutional delay, tumors and malformations of the central nervous system, gonadotropin deficiencies, and miscellaneous syndromes such as Prader-Willi and Laurence-Moon-Biedl.

Causes associated with elevated gonadotropins include: gonadal dysgenesis, cytotoxic drugs and radiation, galactose intolerance, gonadotropin resistance, and deficiencies of steroidal enzymes such as cholesterol desmolase, 17α-hydroxylase, and 17-20 lyase.

Amenorrhea

Of all the stigmata of endocrine disorders, amenorrhea results from the greatest diversity of causes. It figures prominently in the differential diagnosis of defeminization, intersexuality, and infertility. An entirely satisfactory simple classification of the amenorrheas is therefore almost impossible to construct since the various etiologic subgroups are often interrelated. Investigation and treatment of amenorrhea require basic knowledge of developmental and chromosomal abnormalities and general endocrinology.

Primary amenorrhea is lack of menarche by the age of 18. Amenorrhea should be investigated by the age of 16, and preferably earlier. Secondary amenorrhea is the cessation of menstruation for at least 6 months in a woman who has had her menarche.

The causes of amenorrhea may be considered physiologic or pathologic. Amenorrhea is normal (physiologic) in childhood, pregnancy, lactation, and the menopause. By far the commonest cause of amenorrhea in a woman in the reproductive years is

Table 14. Etiology of Amenorrhea

I. Physiologic
   A. Prepuberal state
   B. Pregnancy
   C. Postpartum lactation
   D. Menopause
II. Congenital Anatomic
   A. Imperforate hymen
   B. Developmental anomalies of vagina, cervix, or corpus
III. Chromosomal and Genetic
   A. Gonadal dysgenesis
   B. Testicular feminization
   C. True hermaphroditism
   D. Other forms of pseudohermaphroditism and intersexuality
IV. Central Nervous System-Hypothalamic-Pituitary
   A. Hypothalamic dysfunction
   B. Pituitary insufficiency
   C. Tumors and other organic lesions
V. Psychogenic
   A. Psychosis and anxiety
   B. Emotional shock
   C. Pseudocyesis
   D. Anorexia nervosa
VI. Systemic
   A. Chronic disease
   B. Nutritional disorders
   C. Drugs
VII. Other Endocrine Causes
   A. Adrenal hyperplasia, tumors, or insufficiency
   B. Hyperthyroidism or hypothyroidism
   C. Steroidal contraceptives
VIII. Ovary
   A. Insensitive ovocytes
   B. Destructive lesions
   C. Estrogen-producing and androgen-producing tumors
   D. Premature ovarian failure
IX. Uterus
   A. Endometrial destruction (Asherman's syndrome)
   B. Cervical stenosis

pregnancy. Amenorrhea may persist normally from 6 weeks to 6 months after pregnancy and may be prolonged somewhat by breastfeeding or stimulation of the nipples. Amenorrhea lasting longer than 6 months post partum may reflect a significant underlying disorder.

Pathologic amenorrhea may stem from anatomic, congenital, or chromosomal defects or may reflect dysfunction of the central nervous system, hypothalamus, pituitary, ovary, or uterus. It may also follow in the wake of systemic diseases, dysfunction of the other endocrine glands, or psychogenic factors (Table 14). Before a diagnosis of amenorrhea is undertaken, pregnancy must be excluded. When the cause of amenorrhea cannot be ascertained, the disorder is often termed idiopathic (Table 15).

Development anomalies occasionally cause primary amenorrhea. In such cases, the diagnosis is usually obvious, as with an imperforate hymen. This lesion and vaginal atresia may result in uterine bleeding that cannot escape from the body (cryptomenorrhea).

Embryology of the Genital System

Knowledge of normal development of the genitourinary system is prerequisite to understanding the numerous anatomic malformations that may cause amenorrhea or otherwise interfere with reproductive function. The urinary and reproductive systems develop from the intermediate mesoderm (p. 71). During folding, the intermediate mesoderm migrates ventrally and forms two longitudinal masses named the nephrogenic cords, which produce the urogenital ridges.

Three sets of excretory organs develop in human embryos. The first is the pronephros, which appears in human embryos as a few small cords or tubules on day 22. Its regression is complete by the beginning of the fifth week and it probably is never functional. It consists of several pairs of tubules and a pronephric duct. Caudad to the pronephros, the blind end of the pronephric duct continues to grow toward the cloaca, which it perforates on about day 30. The mesonephros appears during the fourth week, caudad to the pronephros. Clusters of cells within the nephrogenic cord differentiate into S-shaped mesonephric tubules, which become continuous with the pronephric duct, which at this stage is designated the mesonephric duct. The medial end of each tubule expands, is invaginated by capillaries, and forms a glomerulus. Although they are functional in some mammals, the tubules are not believed to function in man. Their importance is in formation of part of the male reproductive system. By the tenth week most of these tubules have degenerated. A few caudal tubules persist as genital ducts in men or as vestigial structures in women. The metanephros, or adult kidney, develops from the ureteric bud and the metanephrogenic mass. The ureteric bud, which arises during the fifth

Table 15. Diagnosis of Amenorrhea

ADMINISTRATION OF PROGESTERONE

├─ MENSES
│ Indicates:
│ Intact endometrium
│ Estrogen priming
│ Secretion of gonadotropins
│
│ Amenorrhea caused by:
│ Psychogenic factors
│ Ovulatory failure:
│ Failure of LH release or production
│ Thyroid dysfunction
│ Adrenal dysfunction
│ Ovarian dysfunction
│ Hyperprolactinemia
│
└─ NO MENSES
   ESTROGEN-PROGESTERONE CYCLIC THERAPY

   ├─ MENSES
   │ Indicates:
   │ Ovarian failure or Pituitary failure
   │ High gonadotropins   Low gonadotropins
   │ Low estrogens
   │
   └─ NO MENSES
      Indicates:
      Pregnancy
      Persistent corpus luteum
      Endometrial failure:
      Congenital
      Inflammatory
      Mechanical
      Radiational
      Idiopathic

week from the mesonephric duct just anterior to the cloaca, gives rise to the ureter, renal pelvis, calyces, and all the collecting ducts of the adult kidney. Mesenchymal cells from the metanephrogenic mass form a cap over the blind end of each newly formed collecting duct. Clusters of cells in each cap differentiate into Bowman's capsule and its associated tubules to form a nephron. Communication is then established between nephron and collecting duct. By early in the third month the fetal kidney has become functional. The mature fetus may void as much as 450 ml/day into the amnionic sac.

The cloaca, a common endodermal chamber, is divided into a dorsal rectum and a ventral region comprising bladder and urogenital sinus. The apex of the bladder tapers to form an elongate tube, the urachus, which is the proximal remnant of the allantois. After birth the urachus persists as the median umbilical ligament.

Sex cannot be ascertained in the human embryo except by chromosomal analysis until approximately the sixth to seventh week. In early development the genital systems in both sexes are similar and potentially bisexual. This indifferent stage persists until the seventh week of development.

The gonads are derived from three sources: the celomic epithelium of the urogenital ridge, the underlying mesenchyme, and the primordial germ cells. A bulge on the medial side of the mesonephros forms the gonadal ridge. The celomic epithelium gives rise to primary sex cords, which grow into the underlying mesenchyme. The primordial germ cells are first seen early in the fourth week in the wall of the yolk sac near the origin of the allantois. They migrate along the dorsal mesentery of the hindgut into the gonadal ridge. During the sixth week they are incorporated into the primary sex cords.

In embryos with a Y chromosome, the seminiferous cords form branches the ends of which anastomose to form the rete testis. Mesonephric tubules that communicate with the mesonephric (wolffian) duct give rise to the efferent ductules, whereas the mesonephric duct forms the epididymis and ductus (vas) deferens. Mesenchymal elements give rise to the interstitial cells of Leydig.

In embryos that lack a Y chromosome, gonadal development occurs slowly. The primary sex cords do not become prominent but they form a rudimentary rete ovarii. During the fourth month the definitive cortex of the ovary first appears. The germinal epithelium produces the secondary sex cords, or cortical cords, which incorporate primordial germ cells.

The paramesonephric (müllerian) duct first appears during the sixth week as a dimple or groove in the thickened epithelium on the lateral aspect of the urogenital ridge. The groove never closes at its cephalic end but remains open to the celomic cavity. Distally the edges of the groove fuse to form the paramesonephric duct, which runs parallel to the mesonephric duct. Caudally the paramesonephric ducts cross ventrad to the mesonephric ducts, fusing in the midline into a Y-shaped uterovaginal primordium. This primordium reaches the urogenital sinus during the eighth week, producing an elevation named the müllerian tubercle.

In the absence of testes, and the müllerian duct inhibitor, the paramesonephric ducts develop into the female genital tract. The cranial longitudinal segments form the oviducts, their ostia becoming the fimbriated extremities. The uterus develops from the middle transverse portion of the paramesonephric duct as a result of proliferation of cells in this region and elevation of the cranial aspect of the uterovaginal primordium. The cervix and part of the vagina develop from the caudal longitudinal segment of the paramesonephric duct. The caudal tip of the uterovaginal primordium proliferates to produce a solid vaginal cord. Paired sinovaginal bulbs grow from the urogenital sinus and fuse with the vaginal cord. This solid cord of endodermal and mesodermal cells forms the vaginal plate. The central cells of this plate subsequently break down and form the lumen of the vagina, part or all of which is lined by endodermal cells derived from the sinovaginal bulbs.

In the female, buds grow out from the urethra into the surrounding mesenchyme to form the urethral and paraurethral (Skene's) glands. Similar outgrowths from the urogenital sinus form the greater vestibular (Bartholin's) glands.

The entire mesonephric system undergoes atrophy in the female in the absence of male hormone. The cranial group of tubules persists as a functionless vestige, the epoophoron, which is located within the mesosalpinx. The caudal group of mesonephric tubules forms the small paroophoron, which usually disappears before adult life. Vestiges of the caudal portion of the mesonephric duct (Gartner's duct) may be found anywhere between the epoophoron and the hymen.

During the indifferent stage of genital development, the mesoderm surrounding the cloacal membrane undergoes proliferation (at about the fourth week), producing, cranially, the genital tubercle, and, laterally, the labioscrotal swellings and urogenital folds. The phallus develops as the genital tubercle elongates. The rectouterine septum fuses with the cloacal membrane at the end of the sixth week. Rupture of this membrane forms the anus and the urogenital opening.

The external female genitalia develop during the ninth to twelfth weeks. The phallus develops into the clitoris, with glans and prepuce. The urogenital folds, which form the labia minora, do not fuse except in front of the anus. Laterally, the labioscrotal folds, which form the labia majora, remain unfused except posteriorly, to form the posterior labial commissure, and anteriorly, to form the mons pubis.

Of the numerous malformations of the genital tract from the external genitalia to the uterus, only a few will prevent or conceal menstruation. In children, agglutination of the labia may be confused with an imperforate hymen. The simplest effective treatment is gentle digital separation of the adhesions and the local use of petroleum jelly or estrogen creams.

A true imperforate hymen at the onset of menses will result in retention of blood within the vagina (hematocolpos), uterus (hematometra), and fallopian tube (hematosalpinx), and even the peritoneal cavity. Treatment is incision of the hymen and sometimes excision of a wedge of tissue. Ultimate fertility is preserved if the tubes are not damaged by the collections of blood.

Aplasia of the vagina may be associated with absence of the uterus and anomalies of the urinary tract. If the corpus and cervix are normal, fertility may be restored after reconstruction of a vaginal canal.

A transverse septum of the vagina may be mistaken for congenital absence of the vagina. A longitudinal septum has no effect on menses or fertility in general. Aplasia of the vagina results from agenesis of the vaginal cord. Atresia results from failure of canalization (p. 320).

Most anomalies of the uterus result from aplasia, abnormalities of differentiation, regression, or fusion of the müllerian ducts. In the case of aplasia, a cord of connective tissue replaces the uterus. This malformation is usually accompanied by vaginal anomalies. Only a few of the uterine malformations are clinically significant.

A unicornuate uterus, which results from aplasia of one müllerian duct, is not clinically important. A noncommunicating rudimentary horn may collect blood to form an enlarging mass. In a septate uterus, fusion is complete but the septum persists. In a bicornuate uterus, fusion occurs only in the lower portion of the müllerian ducts, resulting in a single cervix and a single vagina. With complete duplication of the müllerian ducts (uterus didelphys), the uterus and cervix are double and the vagina is septate. The ovaries are normal, however, and there is no disturbance of menstruation.

Chromosomal and genetic causes of amenorrhea include several fairly common disorders such as gonadal dysgenesis and testicular feminization and a great variety of rare hermaphroditic and intersexual syndromes, some of which reflect specific biochemical defects.

Patients with gonadal dysgenesis typically have "streak gonads." The müllerian ducts form, but the uterus and oviducts remain prepuberal. The external genitalia are female and the children are usually reared as girls, although they fail to manifest secondary sexual characteristics.

Diagnosis is suspected on clinical grounds and confirmed by karyotype, studies of chromosomal fluorescence, and laparoscopy. The levels of FSH and LH are elevated but those of other hormones are usually normal. Differential diagnosis includes ovarian hypoplasia, delayed puberty, and pituitary dwarfism.

Gonadal Dysgenesis

The common forms of gonadal dysgenesis are Turner's syndrome and pure gonadal dysgenesis. Patients with Turner's syndrome classically are short, with low-set ears, webbed neck, shield chest, coarctation of the aorta, nevi, and edema at birth. The karyotype is classically 45,X but mosaics have been described as well as chromosomal patterns containing an iso-X or a ring chromosome. Of all fetuses with a single X chromosome, only about 20% are born alive.

Patients with pure gonadal dysgenesis are of normal stature or may even be taller than average and they have no somatic abnormalities other than the absence of secondary sexual characteristics. The karyotype is usually 46,XX but mosaics have been described in this syndrome also.

In the rare condition of gonadal agenesis, the entire gonadal anlage is missing. These patients may have an XX or an XY chromosomal pattern, but they will be amenorrheic and their gender role will be female.

Treatment of all patients with gonadal dysgenesis or agenesis comprises cyclic estrogen and progestin. Estrogen alone may be given for the first several months. Treatment should be delayed until around age 14 to prevent premature closure of the epiphyses. Patients with Turner's syndrome do not achieve normal height, and development of the breasts may be suboptimal even after treatment.

Klinefelter's syndrome is the commonest sex chromosomal anomaly. These phenotypic males have a chromosomal pattern of 47,XXY, atrophic testes, and oligospermia or azoospermia. They frequently have gynecomastia and some degree of mental retardation.

The 47, XXX "superfemale" may be a phenotypically normal woman. There is an increased incidence of mental retardation, but the patients are sometimes fertile.

Hermaphroditism

Testicular feminization is a fairly common cause of amenorrhea in phenotypic females with an XY chromosomal constitution. This disorder may be considered a form of intersexuality or pseudohermaphroditism and it tends to be familial. The patients have scanty sexual hair (pubic and axillary) but may have moderately well developed breasts. Because müllerian development is lacking, the uterus is absent or rudimentary, and oviducts are missing. Testes may be abdominal, inguinal, or vulvar. The vagina commonly ends in a short blind pouch. Levels of serum estrogen and androgen are in the normal male range.

The main cause is probably a defect in androgen receptors or androgen receptor-effector mechanisms in the end organs. The testes should be removed because of the increased incidence of neoplasia in these ectopic gonads. Estrogen therapy should be initiated preoperatively and continued permanently. It may be necessary to construct a functional vagina when the patient indicates a desire to initiate coitus. These patients should not be told that they are genetic males, for their psychologic orientation and sex of rearing are female. Great care must be taken to give them sufficient psychologic support so that they can perceive themselves as sexually adequate women. In incomplete forms of the syndrome the external genitalia are ambiguous.

True hermaphrodites have both ovarian and testicular tissue, either in the form of one ovary and one testis or as bilateral mixed gonads containing both tissues. The hermaphrodite may have associated anomalies of the urinary tract. The most common chromosomal pattern is 46,XX and the sex chromatin is usually positive, but the phenotype depends on the predominant tissue. The external genitalia are usually ambiguous. Although these patients may menstruate, they are usually infertile.

The female pseudohermaphrodite has ovaries, but the genital ducts and external genitalia differentiate to some extent along male lines. The male pseudohermaphrodite has testes, but the genital ducts, external genitalia, or both differentiate to some extent in the female direction.

Sexual differentiation depends on genetic and environmental factors. A discrepancy among the various criteria of sexual identification results in intersexuality.

Criteria of sexuality include chromosomal pattern, sex chromatin, gonadal structure, differentiation of the genital ducts (internal genitalia), external genitalia, hormonal status, sex of rearing, and gender role (psychologic orientation). Since the sex of rearing is crucial to the psychologic development of the child and is well established after the second year of life, it is important to assign sex definitively as early as possible.

All fetuses are potentially bisexual. In the fourth week of gestation an indifferent gonad appears in both sexes. Gonadal differentiation occurs at about the sixth week. Normally a Y chromosome leads to the development of a testis, which in turn produces a male phenotype, with certain exceptions such as testicular feminization. The primordia differentiate into the internal genitalia, or genital ducts, at about the seventh week. Testes produce an androgenic steroid, which stimulates the wolffian ducts and induces the development of male external genitalia. The testes normally produce also a nonsteroid (Factor X, or müllerian inhibiting factor), which inhibits the müllerian ducts. In normal female differentiation the wolffian ducts regress and the müllerian ducts develop into uterus, oviducts, and possibly a portion of the upper vagina. Normal sexual development requires appropriate stimulation of one ductal system and repression of the other. Development of the external genitalia is hormonally determined. In brief, androgen (usually testosterone) causes development of the male external genitalia. In the absence of androgen, female genitalia develop.

The mammalian Y chromosome plays a dominant role in the initiation of fetal testicular differentiation. Testicular differentiating genes on the Y chromosome can be detected serologically as H-Y antigen. The correlation of numerical and structural abnormalities of the sex chromosomes combined with reactivity of the H-Y antigen, gonadal histology, and phenotype has led to mapping the loci of these genes on the Y chromosome.

Genes on the X chromosome may regulate the activity of testicular differentiating genes on the Y chromosome.

Clinical investigation of the child with ambiguous genitalia should occur in a systematic sequence. A history of the pregnancy with special references to drugs or hormones ingested by the mother should be obtained. Physical examination of the infant should detect associated anomalies, as in Turner's syndrome, or small testes, as in Klinefelter's syndrome. Small testes in a virilized male infant may suggest the adrenogenital syndrome. A karyotype should be performed to ascertain genetic sex and to detect aneuploidy and mosaicism. Urethroscopy or injection of contrast medium into the "vagina" or urogenital sinus may be necessary to reveal the internal genitalia.

Hormonal studies may provide diagnostic information. Urinary 17-ketosteroid and pregnanediol levels as well as serum DHEA-S and 17$\propto$-OH progesterone concentrations are elevated in the congenital adrenogenital syndrome, whereas they are normal if the masculinization results from exogenous androgens transferred from the maternal circulation. In certain cases laparotomy with biopsy of the gonads may be required for definitive diagnosis. Intravenous pyelography should be performed to detect associated anomalies of the urinary tract.

In the adult, two primarily psychiatric problems should be distinguished from hermaphroditism. The transsexual patient has no discrepancies among the anatomic criteria of sex but feels "trapped in the body of the wrong sex." Such patients may request surgical change of gender. These extensive operations should be performed only after psychiatric evaluation.

A transvestite is a patient who derives pleasure from wearing the clothes of the opposite sex. These patients do not request operations to change their sex. When their behavior conflicts with the law, they require psychiatric care. Neither transvestites nor transsexuals are necessarily homosexual.

Female pseudohermaphrodites have a 46,XX karyotype but external genitalia that do not develop in the normal female direction. Female pseudohermaphroditism usually results from either congenital adrenal hyperplasia in the fetus or excessive maternal androgen arising from exogenous hormones or a masculinizing tumor of the ovary. The external genitalia are ambiguous or masculinized but the internal genitalia are normal.

Congenital adrenal hyperplasia is the most common cause of female pseudohermaphroditism. It results from a defect in enzymatic hydroxylation in the zona fasciculata of the adrenal cortex, which causes a deficiency of cortisol. Negative feedback results in an increase in ACTH, which in turn stimulates the zona reticularis to produce androgen. The most common form of the syndrome results from a block in 21-hydroxylase, although other enzymatic defects may occur.

Patients usually first come to the attention of the physician either as newborns with ambiguous external genitalia, which present a problem in gender identity, or as adolescents with amenorrhea and a somewhat masculine habitus. Because it is difficult to change a gender role from female to male in later life, in cases of doubt the children should be raised as girls.

Adolescents with congenital adrenal hyperplasia frequently demonstrate precocious growth until age 10 or 11, when they cease to grow. They manifest signs of puberty but fail to menstruate. Manifestations of excessive androgen, such as masculine habitus, hirsutism, and clitoromegaly, also may appear.

The diagnosis can be made from tests performed on urine or serum. Urinary 17-ketosteroids and pregnanediol and serum dehydroisoandrosterone and 17α-hydroxyprogesterone are all elevated. The treatment is a corticosteroid to suppress ACTH, with resulting decrease in adrenal androgen. Plastic surgical procedures may be required if the external genitalia are significantly masculinized.

Amenorrhea may be caused by a variety of abnormalities in the central nervous system, hypothalamus, or pituitary. The most common cause is hypothalamic dysfunction. If the dysfunction first appears when puberty is expected, the manifestations will be delay of puberal changes and primary amenorrhea. If it first appears after menarche, a secondary amenorrhea results. The essential common dysfunction in these patients is lack of cyclic hypothalamic stimulation of the pituitary. The levels of FSH and LH are normal or only slightly depressed but they do not undergo the periodic elevations that are characteristic of the normal female reproductive cycle. Inasmuch as stimulation of the pituitary by releasing hormones causes a normal response, the primary dysfunction cannot be attributed to the pituitary. Because of the lack of stimulation by gonadotropin, the ovaries are hypoplastic and the levels of estrogen are low or at least slightly depressed. Most patients with amenorrhea of this cause do not bleed after withdrawal of progestin.

A variety of neoplastic, inflammatory, and destructive lesions in the hypothalamus or pituitary may be associated with amenorrhea. The most common lesion is a prolactin-secreting tumor of the pituitary. Galactorrhea may or may not accompany the amenorrhea. The elevation of the level of prolactin in the serum is positively correlated with the size of the tumor. If the lesion is smaller than 1 cm in diameter, it is a microadenoma; if larger, it is a macroadenoma. Most patients with these lesions have no abnormalities other than amenorrhea, elevated levels of prolactin, and possibly galactorrhea.

Diagnosis of the lesion is made by history, elevated levels of prolactin, and radiologic identification of a sellar or suprasellar mass. The most accurate radiographic technique is computerized tomography with the newest scanners, which can identify a lesion smaller than 4 mm in diameter. Arteriography may occasionally be useful. Neurologic findings such as changes in the visual fields are uncommon because most of the tumors are small, but they can occur with larger lesions.

Possible methods of management of pituitary prolactinomas include observation alone, therapy with bromocriptine (Parlodel), and surgical removal. If the lesion is small, it can usually be removed transsphenoidally.

Pituitary insufficiency may manifest itself as an inability to produce one or more tropic hormones. Isolated or partial deficiencies are more common than complete hypopituitarism (panhypopituitarism). Although the causes are usually unknown, etiologic factors include pituitary tumors, cysts, and necrosis. Hypopituitarism may follow hemorrhage and shock. When it occurs in association with pregnancy it is called Sheehan's syndrome. Hypopituitarism unassociated with pregnancy is known as Simmond's disease. A selective deficiency of gonadotropins produces hypogonadotropic hypogonadism.

A deficiency of gonadotropins that results in anovulation and infertility is the classic indication for gonadotropin therapy. Complications of the therapeutic use of these hormones for any cause include ovarian cysts and plural gestations.

The polycystic ovary (Stein-Leventhal) syndrome characteristically includes bilateral pearly white ovaries. These patients have amenorrhea or oligomenorrhea with anovulatory irregular uterine bleeding and infertility. Some degree of hirsutism (p. 330) and moderate obesity are commonly associated. Diagnosis is made on the finding, by laparoscopy or laparotomy, of large white ovaries with numerous small cysts and a thickened capsule. FSH levels are within the normal range, but LH levels are usually elevated. Inappropriate secretion of LH results in an elevated LH : FSH ratio. Dexamethasone does not suppress the androgens significantly in the Stein-Leventhal syndrome. The differential diagnosis includes mild adrenal hyperplasia and Cushing's syndrome. Medical treatment by stimulation of ovulation with clomiphene is the method of choice. Wedge resection of the ovary is rarely used today because it may result in ovarian adhesions and subsequent infertility.

Clomiphene (Clomid) is a nonsteroidal estrogen antagonist. It is indicated in the anovulatory patient who has follicular function and adequate endogenous estrogen but lacks cyclic stimulation by pituitary gonadotropins. The dosage must be carefully regulated to minimize the likelihood of cystic ovarian enlargement and multiple ovulations with resulting plural gestations. Chorionic gonadotropin may be added to induce ovulation in refractory cases. Its long half-life makes it more effective than LH for this purpose.

In patients with deficiencies in pituitary gonadotropins (serious hypothalamic-pituitary disease), human menopausal gonadotropin (hMG) is effective in inducing ovulation. This substance, which is purified from the urine of postmenopausal women, consists of both FSH and LH, but its effect is mainly that of FSH. Overstimulation of the ovaries with hMG (Pergonal) is a serious drawback to the use of this hormone.

Clomiphene is administered in an initial dose of 50 mg/day for five days beginning early in the cycle. The dose may be increased to 100 or 150 mg/day for 5 days if necessary. Ovulatory function improves with this drug alone in about 75% of women, but rates of pregnancy are only about 35%. Some patients require addition of 100,000 units of hCG at midcycle to complement the LH surge and facilitate ovulation. If this therapy is unsuccessful, human menopausal gonadotropins (menotropins, or Pergonal) may be tried. These substances, which substitute for pituitary FSH and LH, may lead to a rate of ovulation of 90% and a rate of pregnancy of 60% in carefully selected patients.

Polycystic ovarian disease is now considered to result from primary dysfunction of the hypothalamus and pituitary rather than the ovary. Overstimulation by gonadotropins is found in association with an excess of ovarian steroids, indicating that the sex hormones do not suppress the gonadotropins, as in normal feedback mechanisms. As a result, there is an exaggerated response to gonadotropins. Like Cushing's disease, the Stein-Leventhal syndrome represents increased pituitary activity in conjunction with a paradoxical excess of the target hormone. The rationale for use of clomiphene is the blockage of the action of estrogen at the level of the hypothalamus.

The elevated level of LH may result from an increased pituitary response to estradiol (increased positive feedback). There may be in addition an increased pituitary response to luteinizing hormone releasing hormone. The histologic changes in the ovaries are related to increased levels of androgens.

Amenorrhea after discontinuing oral contraceptives is uncommon in proportion to the number of women using these drugs. If spontaneous menses do not resume within 6 to 12 months after discontinuation of the oral contraceptive, the patient should be evaluated in the manner appropriate for any patient with secondary amenorrhea.

Psychogenic causes of amenorrhea include psychosis, severe emotional shock, anxiety, pseudocyesis (false, or spurious, pregnancy), and anorexia nervosa. In anorexia nervosa, unlike Sheehan's syndrome, no organic lesion of the pituitary is found, and thyroid and adrenal functions are not depressed. The patient with anorexia nervosa is cachectic and hypotensive. The underlying emotional problem may respond to psychotherapy.

A variety of chronic diseases such as tuberculosis and nutritional deficiencies may cause oligomenorrhea or amenorrhea. Diabetes mellitus, particularly if untreated, also will adversely affect menstrual function. Hepatic or renal dysfunction may interfere sufficiently with the metabolism of hormones to prevent normal menstruation. Many drugs in addition to hormones may depress menstrual function. The commonest etiologic agents are phenothiazines and narcotics.

Dysfunction of the other endocrine organs may also interfere with menstrual function. Adrenal hyperplasia, neoplasms, or insufficiency (Addison's disease) may lead to amenorrhea.

Unlike congenital adrenal hyperplasia, Cushing's syndrome represents hyperfunction of the zona fasciculata as well as the zona reticularis. Cushing's syndrome classically includes obesity, amenorrhea, hirsutism, and hypertension. In this syndrome overreaction to ACTH occurs, corticosteroids are elevated, and the adrenal cortex cannot be suppressed with cortisone. Loss of diurnal fluctuation in the level of cortisol is found.

Hyperthyroidism as well as hypothyroidism may affect menstrual function unpredictably. Aside from pregnancy, perhaps the commonest endocrine cause of decreased menses is ingestion of oral contraceptives. The patient should always be asked whether she has used these agents before other endocrine causes of amenorrhea are considered.

The ovary itself may be the cause of amenorrhea as a result of biochemical defects, insensitivity to tropic hormones, or destructive lesions. Functioning tumors of the ovary also may produce menstrual abnormalities including amenorrhea. Androgen-producing tumors (arrhenoblastoma, hilus cell tumor, and adrenal rest tumor) and estrogen-producing varieties (granulosa cell and theca cell tumors) may all cause amenorrhea or other menstrual abnormalities.

Premature menopause, is the cessation of ovarian function before the age of 40. Ovarian failure results from premature aging of the ovaries. Finally, the uterus itself may be the cause of amenorrhea. Uterine trauma sufficient to destroy the endometrium may occur after infection or overly vigorous curettage, particularly after pregnancy (Asherman's syndrome). The intrauterine synechiae are often treated successfully by gentle curettage.

Cervical stenosis, which may also result from trauma, prevents the escape of menstrual blood. It may be treated by cervical dilatation.

Diagnosis of the cause of amenorrhea can often be made by careful history and physical examination alone. After pregnancy, chronic disease, and drug-induced amenorrhea are ruled out, consultation with a gynecologic endocrinologist is desirable.

The next tests to perform in the diagnosis of secondary amenorrhea are a progestin challenge and measurements of FSH, LH, and prolactin. Other tests that are sometimes helpful include measurement of serum TSH, T_3, T_4, and cortisol; karyotype; and radiologic evaluation of the pituitary. Laparoscopy, hysterosalpingography, endometrial curettage, and hysteroscopy may detect local lesions. Stimulation of the adrenal or pituitary glands less frequently provides diagnostic information in the initial evaluation of secondary amenorrhea.

The administration of metyrapone (metopirone) has been used as a test of pituitary function. The drug by interfering with 11-hydroxylation causes a negative feedback that stimulates a normal pituitary gland, as indicated by an increase in 17-hydroxycorticosteroids. Insulin-induced hypoglycemia normally results in increases in growth hormone and ACTH; TRH normally causes increases in TSH and prolactin; and GnRH normally results in increases in LH and FSH.

The treatment of secondary amenorrhea is determined by the etiologic factor and the reproductive desires of the patient. Diagnosis and correction of the disorder rather than the induction of menstruation are the primary goals. It is not necessary to induce ovulation except in patients who want to become pregnant.

Defeminization, Virilization, and Hirsutism

Defeminization, the relative loss of female sexual characteristics, usually precedes virilization, or masculinization. Defeminization involves diminution in mammary tissue and female distribution of fat, amenorrhea, and ovarian failure. Virilization is the development of male secondary sexual characteristics in a woman as a result of stimulation of the responsive tissues by excessive androgen. A common sequence of masculinization is deepening of

Table 16. Etiology of Hirsutism

    I. Genetic, Familial, or Racial
   II. Pituitary-Hypothalamic
       A. Acromegaly
       B. Cushing's syndrome
       C. Polycystic ovary syndrome
  III. Other Endocrine Defects
       A. Adrenogenital syndrome (congenital or acquired)
       B. Cushing's syndrome
       C. Adenoma and carcinoma of the adrenal
       D. Hypothyroidism in children
   IV. Ovarian
       A. Masculinizing tumors
       B. Menopause
    V. Systemic Physical and Emotional Illnesses
       A. Porphyria
       B. Anorexia nervosa
   VI. Local Effects
       A. Plaster casts
       B. Roentgen therapy
  VII. Drug-Induced
       A. Dilantin
       B. Androgens
       C. Corticosteroids
       D. Diazoxide

the voice, hirsutism, a male pattern of baldness, increased secretion of sebaceous glands with occasional acne, hypertrophy of the clitoris, and increased muscle mass.

Hirsutism is the excessive growth of hair on the body or face of a woman, usually involving the upper lip, chin, chest, abdomen, or legs. The major causes are listed in Table 16. Genetic, familial, and racial predispositions are the most common etiologic factors in hirsutism. Hairiness, or hypertrichosis, is more common in Mediterranean races, for example. It is therefore necessary in such people to compare the patient with other members of her family. In this idiopathic form of hirsutism the levels of serum testosterone and dehydroisoandrosterone are within normal limits.

Hirsutism of some degree is noted in many syndromes involving amenorrhea of central, constitutional, or peripheral origin, such as the polycystic ovary, Cushing, and adrenogenital syndromes. Most of the causes of hirsutism are discussed elsewhere in this unit under the appropriate syndromes. Masculinizing tumors of the ovary or adrenal almost always cause rapidly progressive results. They should be suspected when the level of serum testosterone exceeds 250 ng/dl or that of dehydroisoandrosterone exceeds 700 ng/dl. Hirsutism caused by adrenal hyperplasia can be distinguished from that resulting from adrenal neoplasms in that the androgens from adrenal tumors are not suppressed by the administration of dexamethasone. Production of adrenal androgen may be suppressed by spironolactone, an antagonist of aldosterone.

Elevated levels of dehydroisoandrosterone suggest an adrenal source of excess androgens; elevated levels of testosterone suggest an ovarian source. Precise identification of the source, however, may require catheterization of the ovarian and adrenal veins to measure the concentrations of the androgens. Testosterone-producing tumors or areas of hyperplasia of the ovary may be too small to visualize at laparoscopy or laparotomy.

Menopause

Menopause is the cessation of menstruation for a year or more. It is caused by ovarian failure and is frequently preceded by anovulatory bleeding. It occurs normally between the ages of 40 and 55 and is often accompanied by the symptoms of the climacteric, including hot flashes, excessive perspiration, and depression or agitation. Menopause is frequently followed by endocrine and metabolic changes. Secretion of estrogens by the ovary is markedly decreased, although peripheral conversion of adrenal steroids to estrone continues after the menopause. In obese women there is greater production of estrone. Production of gonadotropin, mostly FSH, is high, particularly in the early postmenopausal years. Later, atrophy of the introitus and the vagina, with occasional dyspareunia and pruritus, occur. Involution of the breasts is common. Atrophy of the epithelia of the genitourinary tract may predispose to cystitis, and in some women osteoporosis and cardiovascular degeneration may occur.

The routine use of estrogen for all postmenopausal women remains controversial. The treatment of women with climacteric symptoms, however, is indicated. Estrogen should be used in the smallest dose that is sufficient to alleviate symptoms and it should be combined with cyclic progestational therapy of at least 10 days' duration. One commonly employed regimen is estrogen on days 1 through 25 of the month and progestin on days 16 through 25.

The rationale for the replacement of estrogen in asymptomatic postmenopausal women is prevention of osteoporosis. Estrogen prevents the accelerated loss of bone in women who are estrogen-deficient; the hormone is most efficacious when it is started before loss of bone has occurred and when it is combined with increased intake of calcium and exercise. If the patient has her uterus, the estrogen should always be given with a progestin. In evaluating and treating climacteric patients, environmental stresses associated with the postmenopausal era of life must be recognized, for not all the symptoms attributed to the menopause result from decline in ovarian function. Mild discomfort may be managed with tranquilizers and mild sedation, or these drugs may be used to reduce the dose of estrogen. Symptoms of vasomotor instability and urogenital atrophy with pruritus are indications for estrogen replacement. Less vaginal atrophy has been reported in women who are sexually active than in those who are inactive. Women with less vaginal atrophy, furthermore, are reported to have higher levels of androgen and gonadotropins, particularly LH.

Low-dose estrogen given to postmenopausal women may decrease the risk of myocardial infarction and possibly cerebrovascular accidents. It is not certain whether estrogen given to postmenopausal women causes an increased incidence of mammary tumors, but it is clear that such treatment does not prevent these tumors. Baseline mammographic studies are appropriate prior to hormonal replacement. Treatment with estrogen does, however, increase the risk of endometrial carcinoma in postmenopausal women (p. 265), but the relation appears to be strongly dose-dependent.

Estrogen may be used in doses sufficient to treat climacteric symptoms without stimulating the endometrium or causing postmenopausal bleeding. The desired duration of therapy remains controversial. Although the duration of treatment of climacteric symptoms may be short, prevention of osteoporosis requires long-term therapy. A progestational agent administered cyclically for 10 to 14 days each month protects against the carcinogenic effect of estrogens on the endometrium but may produce adverse effects on serum lipids, with resulting increases in cardiovascular disease and stroke.

Medroxyprogesterone acetate can be used to treat the vasomotor flushes of women to whom the administration of estrogen is undesirable. Certain complaints can be alleviated by psychotherapy and tranquilizers; several other substances, such as naloxone, bioflavonoids, and clonidine, may be effective in relieving climacteric vasomotor instability. All postmenopausal patients receiving estrogen should have frequent measurements of blood pressure to exclude the possibility of hormone-induced hypertension. Regular manual examinations of the breast and mammography are required. Postmenopausal bleeding demands the prompt exclusion of neoplastic diseases, particularly carcinoma of the endometrium.

Infertility

Infertility is diminished fertility, unlike sterility, which is absolute inability to reproduce. Female sterility is the inability to conceive. Male sterility is the inability to fertilize an ovum. Primary infertility means diminished fertility throughout the reproductive years, whereas secondary infertility implies one or more earlier successful pregnancies. Diagnosis of infertility is not made until failure to conceive has occurred despite 12 months or longer of attempting pregnancy. A female factor may be uncovered in not more than half the cases of infertility.

Male causes include impotence, failure to ejaculate, disturbances in numbers or motility of spermatozoa, and defective seminal plasma. Female causes include anovulation, tubal disease, and abnormalities of cervical mucus.

Anovulation is evaluated by means of a daily morning temperature graph (basal body temperature, or BBT), progesterone assay or endometrial biopsy to demonstrate lack of a secretory endometrium, and inadequate cyclic changes in the cervical mucus or vaginal cytologic smear. The ovaries may be visualized directly by endoscopy.

Tubal disease (occlusion or dysfunction) may be evaluated by three means. The simplest is insufflation of CO_2 through the cervix (Rubin's test, p. 187), although this test is infrequently used today because it provides less information than do other methods. Patency of the tubes is suggested by shoulder pain (diaphragmatic irritation). The second technique, which provides much more information, is hysterosalpingography, in which contrast medium is injected into the cervix for visualization of the lumens of the uterus and tubes. The third technique is endoscopy (laparoscopy or culdoscopy), in which the tubes may be visualized directly while dye is injected through the cervix. Hysterosalpingography combined with laparoscopy may provide maximal information.

Abnormalities of cervical mucus are detected by careful examination of amount and quality throughout the cycle. The cervical mucus should exhibit a fernlike pattern in the first half of the cycle, and Spinnbarkeit (ability of the mucus to be drawn into long threads) should be maximal at ovulation. In a normal Sims-Hühner (postcoital) test, ten or more motile spermatozoa per high-power field should be seen in cervical mucus at midcycle, 2 hours after coitus. In any investigation of infertility the couple should be interviewed together early and any male factor ruled out before complicated procedures are performed on the woman. Ovulation, adequate production of sperm, patency of the fallopian tubes, and a histologically normal endometrium may be detected by relatively simple means. Further diagnosis and treatment often require referral to a specialist in infertility.

Common male factors are defects in number, motility, or proportion of morphologically normal spermatozoa. In evaluation of the semen, the total ejaculate should be obtained, preferably by masturbation. In certain cases of oligospermia, a homologous insemination may be performed with the husband's semen. The use of a split ejaculate, in which only the first portion is used for insemination, is occasionally valuable in homologous insemination for oligospermia. The first portion, containing fluid from the prostate and Cowper's glands, contains most of the viable spermatozoa and can be effectively separated from the third portion, which contains fluid from the seminal vesicles. With azoospermia, a heterologous (donor) insemination may provide an alternative to adoption. Causes of male infertility include: congenital defects of the genitalia, such as cryptorchidism, testicular hypoplasia, absence of the vasa deferentia, hypospadias, and epispadias; acquired defects, such as varicocele, local infections and trauma, and neoplasms; physical and toxic factors, such as heat, radiation, and drugs; chromosomal aberrations, such as Klinefelter's syndrome with dysgenesis of the seminiferous tubules; retrograde ejaculation, of idiopathic or diabetic origin; neuropsychiatric problems; and nutritional and endocrine factors. Improved production of sperm often follows ligation of the spermatic veins in a man with a varicocele and oligospermia or asthenospermia.

Semen for analysis should be collected after a period of abstinence of 3 to 4 days. The normal volume after 3 days of abstinence is 1 to 6 ml. Normally at least 60 to 80% of the sperm should be motile 1 hour after ejaculation. The normal sperm count varies between 40 and 125 million/ml. Counts under 20 million/ml reflect true oligospermia. In a fertile semen sample at least 60% of the cells are morphologically normal. The concentrations of fructose and citric acid in the semen are indices of function of the seminal vesicles and prostate, respectively. Complete absence of fructose in azoospermic men indicates congenital bilateral absence of the vasa deferentia, inasmuch as the seminal vesicles and the vas deferens arise from the same embryologic structures. In men with hypogonadotropic hypogonadism and lowered levels of gonadotropin, the enhancement and completion of spermatogenesis may be accomplished through the use of Pergonal (human menopausal gonadotropin) combined with hCG.

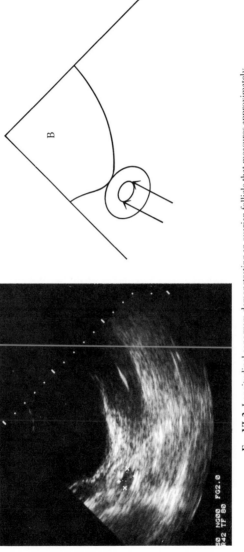

Fig. VI-2. Longitudinal sonogram demonstrating an ovarian follicle that measures approximately 12 × 13 mm, demarcated by arrows. Precovulatory follicles are usually about 20 mm in diameter. After ovulation the follicle can be shown to collapse.

Ovulation is suggested by a history of regular menses at intervals of between 23 and 33 days, associated with premenstrual molimina such as backache, fullness of the breasts, swelling of the hands and feet, bloating, acne, and irritability. A biphasic BBT curve is associated with ovulation, as are an increase in amount and a decrease in viscosity of cervical mucus at the time of ovulation, followed by the disappearance of a fern. The best evidence is provided by measurement of serum progesterone or an endometrial biopsy that shows secretory changes. Ovarian follicles may be measured accurately by sonography (Fig. VI-2).

Ovulation may be predicted clinically by "ovulation pain" or by the passage of clear, liquid mucus from the cervix. Useful laboratory methods include serial measurements of estrogen and LH and serial sonographic examinations of the ovary.

Anovulation may result from disturbances anywhere between the central nervous system and the ovary. The major causes are discussed in the section on amenorrhea (pp. 315–329). The treatment is induction of ovulation.

Abnormal cervical mucus may create an environment "hostile" to the sperm. In the postcoital test, semen is aspirated from the vaginal pool and the endocervix shortly after intercourse to assess the motility of the spermatozoa.

Less commonly, infertility may stem from lesions of the vagina (anomalies or stenosis) or cervix (trauma, inflammation, stenosis, and incompetent os). Abnormalities of the corpus that occasionally lead to infertility include congenital anomalies, submucous myomas, and traumatic scarring of the endometrium (Asherman's syndrome), which may be treated by gentle curettage.

A luteal phase defect is detectable by endometrial biopsy, or measurement of serum progesterone. In such cases either the endometrium is not responsive or the ovary produces insufficient progesterone. In this condition exogenous progesterone or hCG may be therapeutic. Inflammatory occlusions of the oviduct or adhesions may be treated surgically with moderate success, especially if the fimbriae and tubal peristalsis remain unimpaired. Tuberculosis must be ruled out during the investigation of the woman. Immunologic causes, such as antibodies to components of the semen, are difficult to treat and require referral to specialized centers.

In vitro fertilization of human ova with transfer of the embryo to the recipient's uterus (I.V.F.-E.T.) has resulted in normal pregnancies. An alternative method is gamete intrafallopian transfer (G.I.F.T.), in which an ovum and washed sperm are placed directly in the fallopian tube.

Ovum transfer involves a different principle, in which the donor of the ovum is inseminated and the resulting fertilized ovum is transferred to the uterus of the infertile recipient. The three procedures provide options for couples with previously untreatable infertility.

Psychogenic factors are said to cause spasm of the reproductive tract on occasion. In rare instances, psychiatric treatment may be helpful.

Abnormal Uterine Bleeding

Abnormal or excessive uterine bleeding may result from endocrine dysfunction, but neoplasms and other anatomic causes and complications of pregnancy must be ruled out before hormonal therapy is initiated. Dysfunctional uterine bleeding (bleeding without an obvious anatomic abnormality) is usually anovulatory and is associated with a nonsecretory endometrium. It is most common shortly after the menarche or just before the menopause, but it may occur at other times as well.

Prolonged dysfunctional bleeding may result from a persistent graafian follicle. In such cases, withdrawal of estrogen leads to delayed endometrial shedding and irregular bleeding. The bleeding is caused by estrogenic overstimulation followed by withdrawal or diminution of estrogen, unopposed by progesterone. Estrogenic stimulation results in bleeding from a proliferative or hyperplastic endometrium, or occasionally from endometrial polyps or carcinoma. A related cause is "breakthrough bleeding" during the use of oral contraceptives.

Dysfunctional bleeding may result from disorders of the central nervous system, pituitary, or ovary, or from the effects of exogenous or endogenous steroids. Etiologic factors related to systemic metabolic disorders include hyperthyroidism, hypothyroidism, hepatic dysfunction, and a variety of chronic diseases. Anovulatory bleeding requires consideration of nutritional, metabolic, and emotional factors. Polycystic ovaries may be ruled out by measurement of FSH and LH or laparoscopy.

Bleeding from a secretory endometrium, which indicates ovulation, usually implies an anatomic lesion rather than an endocrine disorder. The investigation of ovulatory bleeding should include a hysterogram and hematologic studies.

Most important, any abnormal bleeding in an adult requires a Papanicolaou smear and endometrial sampling before treatment. For greatest accuracy of diagnosis, curettage is best performed just before menses. In an adolescent patient presumptive dysfunctional bleeding may be treated without curettage.

Ovulatory bleeding may occasionally produce minimal midcyclic bleeding in the absence of an organic lesion. Abnormal uterine bleeding may result from organic lesions of the ovary, oviduct, corpus, cervix, or vagina. Complications of pregnancy include ectopic gestation, abortion, bleeding corpus luteum, hydatidiform mole, and choriocarcinoma.

Genital causes unassociated with pregnancy include myomas, and carcinoma, polyps, or hyperplasia of the endometrium; chronic cervicitis; polyps and carcinomas of the cervix; carcinoma of the vagina; functional ovarian cysts; and functioning ovarian neoplasms.

Extragenital causes include blood dyscrasias, thrombocytopenia, deficient clotting factors, endocrinopathies, and, uncommonly, hypertension. In addition, bleeding from the urinary tract and rectum must be excluded.

Treatment of uterine bleeding depends on the cause. In adolescents, cyclic progestin or estrogen-progestin therapy may be instituted after a Papanicolaou smear without a preliminary curettage. If irregular bleeding persists after cyclic estrogen-progesterone therapy (medical curettage), a complete diagnostic investigation including formal curettage is required. In cases of recurrent apparently dysfunctional bleeding in younger patients, progesterone may be used while the investigation continues.

Attempts to induce ovulation are justified only when fertility is part of the goal of therapy. In premenopausal patients medroxyprogesterone acetate administered cyclically may induce regular withdrawal bleeding and preclude the need for further therapy. In patients who have completed their families, recurrent irregular uterine bleeding that is unresponsive to progestin therapy may be treated by hysterectomy.

Dysmenorrhea

Dysmenorrhea, or painful menstruation, is a symptom and not a disease. Dysmenorrhea may be the commonest gynecologic symptom. It is the direct cause of the loss of countless woman-hours of work.

Primary dysmenorrhea occurs in the absence of a significant pelvic lesion. It is essential, or functional, dysmenorrhea and is caused by factors intrinsic to the uterus. Primary dysmenorrhea is the more common form of the symptom. Its onset is usually in adolescence, within two years of the menarche. It is generally associated with ovulatory cycles and appears to be caused by an excessive production of endometrial prostaglandins, which stimulate painful uterine contractions.

In secondary dysmenorrhea, pelvic disease can be demonstrated, for example, endometriosis, adenomyosis, and chronic pelvic inflammatory disease. Even if palpable findings are absent on pelvic examination, endometriosis may still be the cause of the dysmenorrhea. It should therefore be ruled out by laparoscopy. The secondary form begins in adult life, affecting a previously symptom-free woman.

The principal treatment of primary dysmenorrhea is administration of inhibitors or antagonists of prostaglandin. In more severe cases, ovulation may be inhibited by oral contraceptive drugs.

Psychotherapy and surgical procedures play small roles today in the management of primary dysmenorrhea. The principal drugs currently employed are nonsteroidal, anti-inflammatory agents that inhibit synthesis or activity of prostaglandins. Many are indoles, indole-like compounds, or arylpropionic acids. Effective compounds include indomethacin, various fenamates such as flufenamic acid and mefenamic acid, ibuprofen, and naproxen sodium. The fenamates inhibit synthesis and activity of prostaglandin and have an antagonistic effect on prostaglandin receptors. Ethanol and betamimetic agents, although tocolytic, are not highly effective in treating dysmenorrhea.

Premenstrual Tension Syndrome

The premenstrual tension syndrome is a symptom complex occurring in the days or week before menstruation. It comprises tension, irritability, or depression, sometimes associated with tenderness or fullness of the breasts, abdominal bloating, headache, and edema. The onset of the syndrome is usually in the fourth decade of life.

Premenstrual tension is almost always associated with ovulatory cycles. In its severe form it may cause psychic and physical incapacitation of the woman for one third of the month. It is temporally related to an increase in crimes committed by women, accidents, and suicides. It may be associated with secondary hyperaldosteronism, causing retention of sodium and water and resulting edema and headache. Treatment includes strong reassurance, antidepressant drugs, and diuretics. Spironolactone (p. 331) is another drug that has provided considerable relief. Severe emotional disturbances may require referral to a psychiatrist.

VII

Control of Reproduction

Contraception

The exponential increase in the populations of the nation and the world has placed family planning and population control in the forefront of medical and social problems. The justification for detailed discussion of this subject is thus obvious.

Contraception may be either temporary or permanent. Permanent contraception is often referred to as sterilization. The effectiveness of a contraceptive technique is determined by the pregnancy rate (P. R.), which is defined as follows:

$$P. R. = \frac{\text{Number of pregnancies} \times 1200}{\text{Patients observed} \times \text{months of exposure}}.$$

The pregnancy rate in a population that does not use contraception is about 80. The birth rate is the number of births per 1000 population. The fertility rate is the number of live births per 1000 female population between the ages of 15 and 44 years. The marriage rate is the number of marriages per 1000 population.

By 1987 the world's population had reached 5 billion. This is more than twice the number of people on earth at the end of World War II (1945). By the year 1850 the population of the world had reached one billion; the second billion were added in less than a century. With an annual birth rate of 29 and a death rate of 11, the current rate of growth is 1.8%.

The time required for doubling the world's population at its present rate of growth is only 38 years. Although the rate is smaller in highly developed countries, the life expectancy at birth is greater there. In the United States life expectancy is 74 years.

The crude birth rate, death rate, and natural increase (annual percentage) for the United States are 16, 9, and 0.7, respectively. These figures correspond to a doubling time of the population of 95 years. Thus, the projected population of the United States for the year 2000 is 268 million.

The effectiveness of a contraceptive is defined by its theoretical effectiveness and its use-effectiveness. Theoretical effectiveness is the antifertility action of any contraceptive method under ideal conditions with no omissions or errors in use. Use-effectiveness, or actual effectiveness, is the protection achieved under realistic conditions of life. It depends on motivation, cultural characteristics, and socioeconomic status of the population.

No ideal contraceptive is currently available. The characteristics of a perfect contraceptive include effectiveness, safety, low cost, esthetic qualities, ease of use, lack of relation to coitus, and absence of the requirement for repeated motivation.

Because patients are often receptive to discussions of contraception during pregnancy, it is wise to initiate these discussions at that time, immediately post partum, and again at the 4-week postpartum examination.

Folk Methods

Contraception may be divided into folk (primitive), conventional, modern, and experimental methods. The important primitive techniques include coitus interruptus (withdrawal), extravaginal intercourse, abstinence, prolonged lactation, and postcoital douches.

Coitus interruptus, or withdrawal, is still a common practice throughout the world. Its pregnancy rate is 15. The contraceptive effectiveness depends on prevention of ejaculation into the vagina. It requires, however, male control over ejaculation and the prevention of the preejaculatory dribble of spermatozoa-laden fluid. The technique is often unsatisfying to one or both partners.

The postcoital douche as a sole means of contraception is to be discouraged because it has a failure rate almost equal to that of unprotected intercourse. The lack of effectiveness results from the rapid entrance of the sperm into the cervical canal.

The failure rate of prolonged lactation as a contraceptive technique is unknown. The delay of ovulation post partum is highly variable and has been known to occur early during breastfeeding. The advantages of this technique are its lack of cost and ready availability.

Extravaginal intercourse is widely practiced, sometimes for purposes of contraception. Intertriginous, oral, and anal intercourse are effective only when not accompanied by vaginal intromission. Receptive anal intercourse, furthermore, carries the risk of AIDS when the active partner is infected with the virus.

Abstinence is time-honored and effective but obviously inapplicable to most couples.

The traditional contraceptive techniques include rhythm; intravaginal chemicals such as jellies, creams, and foams; and mechanical methods including the condom, diaphragm, and cervical cap.

Rhythm

Aside from abstinence, the rhythm method is the only means of contraception in compliance with all religious doctrines. It depends on the avoidance of coitus during the fertile period, which requires prediction of ovulation. Because of uncertainties in the duration of viability of the sperm and the egg, intercourse must be avoided for a week before and 3 days after ovulation. A clinically useful method of predicting ovulation that is independent of the length of the cycle is based on measurements of viscosity of cervical mucus. The pregnancy rate with this method is about 15.

Rhythm, or calendar, methods of predicting ovulation are dependent upon length of the prior cycle. Thus, historic data are needed to predict satisfactorily a future ovulation. The success of the method depends upon the regularity of the menses and requires strong motivation. For maximal safety, long periods of abstinence are required. Although menstruation occurs quite regularly at 14 days after ovulation, the length of the preovulatory phase is quite variable. A rise in basal body temperature of about 0.7° F during the luteal phase of the cycle can be used to detect ovulation, but it is necessarily a retrospective finding.

The symptothermal method of contraception combines features of the techniques that depend on detection of the rise in temperature and prediction of ovulation. The signs and symptoms of impending ovulation include thinning and flow of the cervical mucus, tenderness of the breasts, abdominal cramps, vaginal spotting, and changes in position and consistency of the cervix. This method requires abstention from intercourse from the time that vaginal wetness is first detected until the third day after the rise in temperature or the fourth day after the time of maximal production of mucus.

Spermicides

The use of spermicidal jellies, creams, and foams as the sole contraceptive technique is accompanied by a pregnancy rate of about 20, which is much higher than that of the most effective forms of contraception but only one quarter of the rate associated with the use of no contraception. These agents may be used to advantage in the woman who has infrequent intercourse, but are unesthetic, must be used just before coitus, and may taste objectionable to those who perform cunnilingus. Allergic reactions to certain components of the products may occur in one or both partners. Contraceptive preparations containing mercury may be teratogenic when used inadvertently in pregnancy, and antiseptic agents containing iodine may damage the conceptus. The Encare Oval tablet provides a foaming viscous barrier and contains the most commonly employed spermicide, nonoxynol-9. Rates of pregnancy with this preparation are similar to those with the older vaginal spermicides. Spermicidal agents are used most effectively in conjunction with the diaphragm. All of these products are available in the United States without prescription (over the counter).

Certain inhibitors of enzymes in spermatozoa are being tested as vaginal contraceptives. Among the more promising are the arylguanidinobenzoates that inhibit acrosin and the inhibitors of hyaluronidase. These substances may be used alone or in conjunction with spermicides.

Barrier Methods

The vaginal diaphragm is an occlusive device with a diameter of 65 to 90 mm. The pregnancy rate with the diaphragm alone is about 7, but it can be reduced by use in conjunction with a spermicidal agent. This form of contraception is inexpensive and it may render intercourse during menstrual periods more esthetic. The disadvantages of the diaphragm are the need for recurrent motivation, the association with coitus, and the requirement for fitting by a physician. For maximal effectiveness it is necessary to refit the diaphragm annually and post partum. Many women find the required vaginal manipulation unesthetic, but the sexual partner may be taught to insert the diaphragm. It may be inserted many hours before intercourse, but for maximal safety it should remain in place at least 8 hours after the last intercourse. This technique is not suitable with severe degrees of pelvic relaxation. Emphasis in the lay press on adverse effects of the oral and intrauterine contraceptives has resulted in increased utilization of the diaphragm in the last decade.

An occlusive technique that may be used in cases of vaginal relaxation is the cervical cap, which adheres by suction. The pregnancy rate with the cervical cap is about 7. Its principal disadvantage is the need for monthly removal, but it requires no manipulations during the cycle. Current experimental designs utilize one-way valves, which permit escape of menstrual efflux while excluding the entrance of spermatozoa into the cervix.

The condom, with a pregnancy rate of about 7, is still the most important traditional method of contraception throughout the world. It is also a mechanical device with an additional advantage of providing protection against sexually transmitted diseases. Its principal disadvantages are the relatively high cost, the need for interruption of the sexual act, and the requirement for high motivation. Failures with the condom are related to poor timing of its application, breaks or leaks, and spillage of semen during removal. Some condoms decrease penile sensitivity, an effect that is generally considered a disadvantage.

Intrauterine Devices

The intrauterine devices (IUDs) regained popularity as contraceptives during the 1960s and early 1970s. The newer varieties are made of inert plastics. The pregnancy rate is about 3. The theoretical effectiveness is about 99% and the use-effectiveness about 97%. The mechanism of action is incompletely known, although the most popular current hypothesis involves an antizygotic or antinidational effect produced by a subclinical endometritis. Advantages include the low cost and the lack of relation to coitus. For further safety the patient should feel for the string, which projects through the cervix into the vagina. Additional protection is provided by the use of a spermicidal agent at midcycle.

Quite recently the manufacturers of all but one of the popular IUDs have ceased distribution of their products within the United States. The decision was made for medicolegal rather than medical reasons. The inert loop (Lippes loop) was removed from the market in the autumn of 1985 and the major copper-containing devices (Copper-7 and Copper-T) were removed early in 1986. Because these devices are still available in Canada and elsewhere and because the ultimate fate of this form of contraception cannot be predicted, the following description of the method is included.

Intrauterine contraception is a reversible technique that involves only a single decision on the patient's part. It requires a physician or a physician's assistant to perform a pelvic examination to ascertain size and position of the uterus. The insertion is facilitated by application of a tenaculum to the anterior lip of the cervix. The larger devices have a lower rate of expulsion but generally cause more bleeding and cramps. The likelihood of uterine perforation is about 1 in 2000. Open (loop or coil) rather than closed (bow or ring) devices are used because perforation by the closed types is more likely to cause intestinal obstruction. An important advance in the field of intrauterine contraception was the addition of metallic copper to the plastic device. The ionization of the copper produces a spermicidal or antizygotic effect, which is in proportion to the amount of metal wrapped around the device. The Copper-7 and Copper-T require replacement every 3 years.

Another intrauterine contraceptive technique involves the impregnation of the device with a slowly released steroid. The Progestasert device releases progesterone and combines the action of an inert IUD with local effects of the steroid on the endometrium. It requires annual removal and replacement by a new device. The Progestasert has been associated with a higher rate of ectopic pregnancies than have some other IUDs, but it is currently the only intrauterine device distributed in the United States. Devices containing epsilon-aminocaproic acid are available in other countries; through inhibition of fibrinolysis they are designed to decrease the amount of blood lost.

Contraindications to the use of any IUD include pregnancy or suspicion of pregnancy; abnormalities of the uterus that cause distortion of the uterine cavity; acute pelvic inflammatory disease or a history of repeated bouts of pelvic inflammatory disease; postpartum endometritis or infected abortion in the preceding three months; known or suspected endometrial or cervical cancer and abnormal Papanicolaou smears without histologic confirmation; genital bleeding of unknown cause; and untreated acute cervicitis. In addition, copper-containing devices are contraindicated in patients with Wilson's disease or a known allergy to copper.

Insertion of an IUD should be performed, if possible, during or shortly after a menstrual period to avoid placement within a pregnant uterus. To reduce the risk of perforation or expulsion, insertion after delivery or abortion should be delayed until the uterus has returned to its normal size. The patient with an IUD in place should receive an annual pelvic examination and Papanicolaou smear, although it is not necessary to remove the inert device periodically. For maximal protection it may be desirable to use another form of contraception for the first few months that the device is in place.

Disadvantages of the IUD include difficulty of insertion and undesirability in the nullipara, and the possibility of uterine perforation, bleeding, and cramps, especially in the first few cycles. In addition, there is a rate of initial expulsion of about 10%. A major complication of the IUD is ectopic pregnancy, most likely a result of salpingitis. The risk of tubal infection is greatest during the first month after insertion or reinsertion of the device, although patients with IUDs are at higher risk for salpingitis up to 12 months after the device has been removed. Among users of IUDs about 1 pregnancy in 20 results in an ectopic implantation, in part because of the greater effectiveness of IUDs in preventing uterine as compared with ectopic pregnancies.

Unilateral nongonococcal adnexal abscesses, some of actinomycotic origin, have been described (Fig. VII-1). Because of the risks of infection and ectopic pregnancy it is inadvisable to prescribe the IUD for a nullipara to whom other contraceptive techniques are available, or for a patient who has already had one ectopic pregnancy.

When a woman becomes pregnant with an IUD in place and wishes to keep the pregnancy, the device should be removed if the strings are visi-

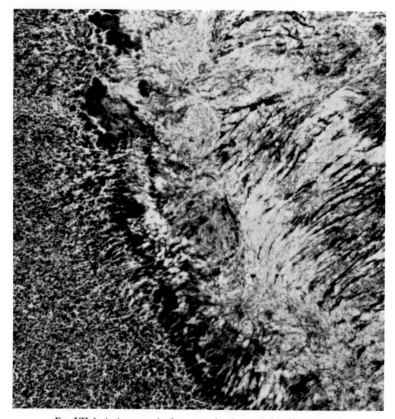

FIG. VII-1. Actinomyces in the ovary, showing typical "sulfur granule."

ble. If the strings are not visible and the device cannot be removed readily, the patient is asked whether she wishes to continue with the pregnancy. If she does, she is informed of the increased risks of spontaneous abortion, infection, and ectopic pregnancy. If she does not want to continue with the pregnancy, the IUD is removed and the pregnancy is terminated. Intrauterine infection demands termination of the pregnancy in any case.

If a closed or a medicated IUD perforates the uterus, it should be removed, by laparotomy or laparoscopy. An inert open device is generally innocuous, although it too should be removed to preclude perforation of an adjacent viscus.

Hormonal Contraception

Hormonal contraception is the most effective form of birth control presently available. For the most part these drugs are used orally (oral contraceptives), but they are also effective parenterally. Before any of these drugs is used a complete history and physical examination must be performed and pregnancy excluded. Particular attention must be paid to the breasts, the thyroid, and the blood pressure. A Papanicolaou smear should be obtained and the urine tested for protein and sugar. Young women should be examined at least annually and older women at even more frequent intervals.

The oral contraceptives are classified as either combined or sequential pills. The combined pills contain a synthetic estrogen and a progestin. The estrogen is either ethinyl estradiol or mestranol. Many standard preparations contain 35 μg of ethinyl estradiol. Pills with larger and smaller doses of estrogen are also on the market. A variety of progestins is available, the most commonly used of which are norethynodrel and norethindrone, both nortestosterones. One group of progestins is related to androgens (C-19 nortestosterone); a second group is related to progesterone; and the third group has some intrinsic estrogenic activity. The sequential pills were withdrawn from use in the United States in 1976.

The effects of the specific combined preparations depend on the doses and ratios of the estrogen and the progestin. All conventional combined oral contraceptives inhibit ovulation. They may also effect a change in cervical mucus, which results in decreased penetrability by spermatozoa. Furthermore, these drugs may affect the endometrium or tubal and uterine fluids. In the combined form of oral contraception a pill containing estrogen and progestin is taken every day for 20 or 21 days starting on Day 5 of the cycle. Bleeding normally occurs 3 or 4 days after the last pill is taken. In the 21-day regimen no pill is taken for 7 days. In the 28-day regimen a placebo is taken for 7 days after the last active pill.

With the traditional combined pills the amounts of estrogen and progestin in each pill remain unchanged during the cycle. With the newer biphasic and triphasic methods, only the amount of estrogen remains fairly constant; with the biphasic technique, the amount of progestin is increased shortly after midcycle; and with the triphasic technique, the amount of progestin is increased on about Day 12 and again on about Day 17. The lower steroid content of the triphasic oral contraceptive, as compared with the fixed-dose combination pill, ideally lessens systemic side effects and interference with normal hypothalamic-pituitary function without decreasing contraceptive efficacy.

In one of the popular biphasic preparations, tablets containing 0.5 mg of norethindrone and 35 μg of ethinyl estradiol are given for 10 days, and tablets containing 1 mg of norethindrone and 35 μg of ethinyl estradiol are given for the next 11 days. In one of the popular triphasic preparations, the dose of ethinyl estradiol is kept constant at 35 μg but that of norethindrone is raised from 0.5 mg in the first week, to 0.75 mg in the second week, to 1 mg in the third week. The biphasic and triphasic pills are available in 21-day and 28-day regimens.

A new hormonal agent described as an antiprogesterone and named RU-486 was introduced in France in 1982. This drug is capable of expelling from the uterus any ovum fertilized during that month. The conventional oral contraceptives must be taken for 3 weeks each month, whereas RU-486 is effective when taken only once a month in the form of a pill or an injection. The drug competes with and displaces progesterone from its endometrial receptors, renders the uterus deficient in progesterone, and causes progesterone-withdrawal bleeding. The dual potential action of RU-486 as both contraceptive and abortifacient has led to the designation of the drug as a "contragestive." Extensive testing of this compound is presently in progress, but it has not yet been approved by the Food and Drug Administration.

The advantages of all forms of oral contraception are their lack of relation to coitus and their extreme effectiveness. The disadvantages are their relatively high cost, the need for constant motivation, the mild common side effects, and the rare but serious hazard of thromboembolism and other cardiovascular complications.

Mild and inconstant complications of the pill include nausea and occasional vomiting, bloating, enlargement and tenderness of the breasts, chloasma (melasma, or irregular brownish discoloration of the skin of the face), weight gain, hypomenorrhea, benign cervical hyperplasia, post-pill amenorrhea (oversuppression syndrome), and altered metabolic functions, which may include increase in binding globulins, increase in Bromsulphalein retention, increase in triglycerides and total phospholipids, decrease in glucose tolerance, and possibly jaundice. The estrogen in the combined pill may lead to increase in high-density lipoprotein (HDL) cholesterol, whereas some progestins may cause the reverse. There is an increase in coronary occlusion, a disease that is ordinarily rare in women of reproductive age.

Additional possible complications include a reversible hypertension (perhaps of the renin-dependent variety), uncommon neurologic or ophthalmologic problems, a change in libido (increase or decrease), and occasional increase in vaginal discharge.

Less common complications include an increase in gallbladder disease and urinary tract infections, presumably as a result of hormonal effects similar to those of pregnancy. Unusual complications, associated particularly with mestranol-containing compounds, are focal nodular hyperplasia of the liver and hepatic adenomas. Although most of the hepatic adenomas related to the pill are benign, they may rupture and produce serious hemorrhage. The association of hepatic carcinoma with use of the pill has not been confirmed.

The most serious complication that has been documented is thromboembolism. The causes of the increased risk of deep venous thrombosis and thromboembolism are not well understood. Vascular intimal and medial lesions with occlusive thrombi have been described. In addition, use of combined estrogen-progestin pills may lead to acceleration of platelet aggregation and reduction in activity of both plasma antithrombin III and endothelial plasminogen activator. The incidence of thromboembolism associated with use of oral contraceptives is directly related to the dose of estrogen. Pills containing less than 50 μg of synthetic estrogen are associated with a low risk of thromboembolism and, in some studies, no increased risk at all in women not otherwise predisposed to these complications.

The FDA requires detailed information in the package labeling of oral contraceptives. All mortality and morbidity rates, however, must be compared with those associated with pregnancy itself. Furthermore, the seriousness of the cardiovascular complications is proportional to the prevalence of those diseases in the geographic area under consideration. The risks are therefore greater in western Europe and the United States than they are in most of Africa, for example, where the rate of thromboembolism is low.

Anterospective studies report that the cardiovascular effects of oral contraceptives are synergistic, rather than simply additive, with those of hyperlipidemia, diabetes mellitus, hypertension, obesity, and cigarette smoking. The date from these studies, furthermore, indicate that the increased risk of death from cardiovascular disease in women is greater than that suggested in prior retrospective studies and that it occurs at an age somewhat lower than previously reported. Women who have taken the pill for more than 5 years and who smoke are at particular risk. Again, diabetes, hypertension, and obesity add to the danger. These studies show that even if the pill is stopped, there is an increased likelihood of later death from cardiovascular disease. For women under the age of 35 there occurs only one death per year per 20,000 women on the pill. The risk rises sharply over this age. Between the ages of 35 and 44, the rate is one per 3000 women, and for women over the age of 45 the rate is one in 700. The overall annual rate is one death per 5000 women on the pill.

In addition to pulmonary embolism, myocardial infarction, and stroke, several other cardiovascular complications have been associated with the pill: subarachnoid hemorrhage, malignant hypertension, cardiomyopathy, mesenteric arterial thrombosis, and exacerbation of congenital and rheumatic cardiac diseases. Logical recommendations based on this new information are as follows. For women under the age of 30 there is no need to stop oral contraception, although cessation of smoking is advantageous. Between the ages of 30 and 35 the risk gradually increases. Some women in this group, for example those who have used oral contraceptives continuously for 5 years and smoke cigarettes, should reconsider the use of the pill. Nonsmokers could probably continue the pill. Women over the age of 35, particularly those who have used the pill continuously for 5 years or more or who smoke, would do well to consider other forms of contraception. Inasmuch as the pill takes several years to affect the cardiovascular system, there is no reason to stop it suddenly. The pill should not be stopped without an alternate temporary contraceptive method or sterilization.

Two factors associated with the use of oral contraceptives appear to increase the likelihood of venous thrombosis and thromboembolism: decreased activity of antithrombin III and lower levels of epithelial plasminogen activator. Among users of the pill, furthermore, those with blood types A, B, or AB have three times the likelihood of thromboembolic and other cardiovascular disease than do those with blood type O. This finding suggests a genetic predisposition to thromboembolism.

Except for a history of a thromboembolic disorder or actual thrombophlebitis, contraindications to the pill are relative. There are no data to support the relation of combined oral contraceptives to the development of carcinoma of the cervix. A prospective study, however, of women with dysplasia of the cervix showed an increase in severity of dysplasia and of conversion to carcinoma in situ in users of the contraceptive pill compared with users of other nonbarrier contraceptive methods, although factors such as age at first intercourse and number of sexual partners were more significant. The incidences of endometrial and ovarian carcinoma may, in fact, be decreased by use of the pill. The incidence of mammary carcinoma is neither increased nor decreased by use of the pill.

The oral contraceptives should not be used in a patient with undiagnosed uterine bleeding. Relative contraindications include hypertension, obesity, cardiovascular and venous diseases, hepatic disorders, a strong familial history of thromboembolism, diabetes mellitus, and possibly migraine headaches. Pills with a large dose of estrogen may cause myomas to increase in size. Use of steroidal contraception during lactation may, rarely, cause jaundice in the newborn.

The main cause of failure of oral contraception is irregular or incorrect use of the pills. With this form of birth control the use-effectiveness is considerably lower than the theoretical effectiveness. The pregnancy rate based on theoretical effectiveness of the standard combined pills is 0.1, which is equivalent to virtually complete effectiveness. The pregnancy rate based on use-effectiveness, however, is close to 1.0

The patient should not depend on the oral contraceptives for complete protection for the first 7 to 10 days of their use, but should use additional spermicidal agents or mechanical devices. If one pill is missed or if breakthrough bleeding occurs, the dosage should be doubled. If two pills are missed in sequence, some other form of contraception should be used for the remainder of that cycle. If no bleeding occurs by 7 days after the last pill, a new cycle of medication should be started as though bleeding had occurred. If two or more amenorrheic cycles occur in succession, the pill should be stopped and the possibility of pregnancy investigated.

The pill should be taken from the fifth to the twenty-eighth day of the cycle and begun again on the fifth day after the onset of bleeding, or on the fifth day of amenorrhea if no bleeding has occurred during that cycle. It is advisable to take the pill at the same time each day. If one pill is forgotten, it should be taken as soon as possible after the regular time and the next pill at the regular time. If two pills in succession are forgotten, two pills should be taken as soon as possible after remembering and two pills at the regular time on the next day. Another form of contraception should be used for the remainder of that cycle. If three pills in succession are missed, a different procedure is advised. No additional pills should be taken. The patient is advised to wait 4 days longer and resume the medication regardless of whether the absence of hormones for 7 days has resulted in uterine bleeding and even if the bleeding is still in progress. During the 7 days that no pills have been taken and during the first 10 days of the new cycle an additional form of contraception is required for maximal safety.

Slight spotting during the cycle, especially during the first 2 months of use, is not necessarily a contraindication to the pill. A tampon may be worn during the time of uterine spotting and a different pill prescribed. If the bleeding is equal in amount to a normal period, the pill should be stopped and a cycle of 21 pills begun on the fifth day, counting Day 1 as the first day of bleeding. If such heavy bleeding occurs twice, the patient should consult her physician. If a period is missed after proper use of 21 pills, it is most unlikely that pregnancy has occurred and the next cycle should be resumed on the eighth day after taking the last pill of the preceding cycle. If two periods in succession are missed, an examination is indicated to rule out pregnancy and possibly to switch medication.

Most of the side effects of the pill are mild, reversible, and related to the dosages of the steroids. The following less common but more serious complications require medical advice: cramps or swelling of the legs, chest pain, hemoptysis, dyspnea, sudden severe headache, dizziness, difficulty with vision or speech, and weakness or numbness of the extremities.

Many drugs in common use interfere with the action of oral contraceptives. The more important of these drugs include ampicillin, penicillin V, neomycin, phenobarbital, rifampicin, phenytoin, and phenylbutazone. Other drugs that may decrease the effectiveness of oral contraceptives include chloramphenicol, nitrofurantoin, phenacetin, meprobamate, clotrimazole, and kaolin in antidiarrheal preparations.

The "minipill" contains only a progestin (0.35 mg of norethindrone). Unlike other oral contraceptives it is administered continuously in a daily dosage throughout the year. Its effectiveness is lower than that of either the conventional combined or sequential pills. The pregnancy rate is approximately 3 per 100 woman-years, compared with less than 1 for estrogen-progestin combinations. The "minipill" has not achieved great popularity in the United States during the 1980s. The rate of dropout for minipills is higher than that for conventional oral contraceptives, presumably because of a significant incidence of unpredictable bleeding that may not follow any consistent pattern even after prolonged use.

The mode of action of the minipill is not clear, although it is known that it does not inhibit ovulation. For that reason the risk of ectopic pregnancy is increased. It may prevent the thinning at midcycle of the cervical mucus, preventing penetration by sperm, possibly affecting capacitation of sperm, or rendering the endometrium unfavorable for implantation.

Estrogen-progestin preparations with 20 to 30 μg of estrogen produce fewer estrogen-related complications, but are associated with a high incidence of breakthrough bleeding. Thus, after an initial period of popularity their use has declined.

Intramuscular contraception with long-acting progestins is used widely in many parts of the world (developed and developing), but the Food and Drug Administration continues to withhold its approval of medroxyprogesterone acetate for routine contraception, mainly because of the finding of mammary tumors in beagles that had received large doses of chlormadinone, a related drug. Furthermore, in rhesus monkeys that had received large doses of medroxyprogesterone, endometrial carcinoma was found, although animals that received the dose normally given to women were free of cancer. Medroxyprogesterone acetate, however, in doses of 50 to 100 mg I.M. has been used widely for treatment of endometriosis (p. 231). The drug, given as a monthly injection or possibly even as an injection every 3 months in doses of 150 mg, could provide contraception for mental defectives and other women who cannot be relied upon to take a pill daily. It could also provide a logical alternative to sterilization for those women.

Considerable effort in research and development is currently spent on delivery of long-acting contraceptive steroids that need not be taken orally on a daily basis. Among the most promising methods is an implant in which a continuous low dose of levonorgestrel is released into the woman's blood from six small silastic capsules placed under the skin on the inside of the arm. Because this formulation contains only a progestin, it may be suitable for women in whom estrogens are contraindicated. The most frequent side-effect is irregular uterine spotting, but the drug does not appear to influence blood pressure and does not have an unfavorable effect on plasma lipids.

Another promising technique is the vaginal ring, made of silastic containing levonorgestrel and estradiol. The ring, which is worn for 3 weeks out of 4, releases the two hormones into the vagina at a constant rate. A vaginal ring that contains only progestin and is worn continuously is under development.

A third technique is the injection of biodegradable polymeric microspheres containing norethisterone. These microspheres are injected intramuscularly as a suspension, a single dose providing contraception for 30, 90, or 180 days.

The differing proportions and dosages of the steroids in the conventional contraceptive formulations cause a variety of side effects. Fortunately, the drugs may be switched with ease, maintaining contraceptive effectiveness and minimizing the complications.

Signs of excess estrogen include nausea, edema, leg cramps, vertigo, leukorrhea, growth of myomas, chloasma, and uterine cramps. Estrogenic deficiency is manifested by irritability, nervousness, flushes, hot flashes, early and midcyclic bleeding, and decreased uterine bleeding.

Excess of progestins may be manifested by increased appetite and weight gain, fatigue, depression, acne, change in libido, jaundice, and hypomenorrhea. A deficiency of progestins may result in late breakthrough bleeding, heavy flow and clots, and delayed onset of the menses. The wide variety of combinations and dosages of estrogens and progestins usually permits the choice of a pill with minimal side effects and maximal effectiveness.

The "morning-after" pill is basically a large dose of an estrogen that is taken between 24 hours and 72 hours after unprotected intercourse. It is currently recommended in situations such as rape or other emergencies. It often causes nausea and vomiting. Diethylstilbestrol (DES) in doses of 25 mg b.i.d. for 5 days is a convenient estrogen to use as a postcoital contraceptive ("interceptive"), but its relation to reproductive losses in the offspring of mothers who took the drug during pregnancy raises doubts about the advisability of its use in any woman of reproductive age. Although the risk of clear cell adenocarcinoma is very small, the associated nonmalignant changes may affect fertility in daughters and possibly sons of DES-exposed mothers. The changes in the vagina and cervix include hoods, pseudopolyps, rims, and collars. An antiemetic medication may be given with the stilbestrol to minimize the nausea and vomiting. The availability of abortion in the event that the patient who takes these drugs is already pregnant reduces the hazard.

Several steroidal estrogens, none of which has yet been shown to be associated with vaginal or cervical carcinomas, also are effective. Suggested regimens include ethinyl estradiol, 2.5 mg twice a day; estrone, 5 mg twice a day; conjugated estrogens, 10 mg twice a day; and several combined estrogen-progestin oral contraceptive pills. The steroids have not yet been approved by the FDA for use as postcoital contraceptives. Pregnancy can be prevented also by the insertion of a copper intrauterine device within 5 days of coitus at midcycle. This method has the advantage of providing continued contraception but is currently unavailable in the United States (p. 346).

Nonstandard Methods

Among the experimental techniques, several antizygotic agents have been tested. These drugs are toxic, however, and the differences between abortifacient and teratogenic dosages are small. Again, perhaps the ready availability of abortion may lead to wider use of this class of drugs.

Male chemosterilants are also under investigation. These drugs may suppress spermatogenesis but they are generally toxic, resulting in a decrease in libido and in production of androgens. Some of these drugs have an antabuse effect.

Gossypol, a potential male contraceptive, appears to work by inhibiting lactate dehydrogenase, which is crucial in aerobic and anaerobic metabolism of sperm and sperm-generating cells. The drug has proved highly effective in parts of Asia and its contraceptive effects are apparently reversible. Its adverse effects include hypokalemia, nausea, weakness, gastric discomfort, changes in appetite, and rarely, paralysis. It also inhibits glutathione S-transferase, an enzyme that participates in the detoxification of certain potential carcinogens. Much more study is required before gossypol can be recommended for use as a male contraceptive in the United States.

Another approach to male contraception is through injection of large doses of testosterone, which reduces production of sperm. There are numerous undesirable side effects, however, and the obvious disadvantage of the required route of administration.

Preliminary data suggesting that prostaglandins may be effective contraceptives or early abortifacients have not been confirmed. The principal problem with the presently available prostaglandins is their widespread undesirable systemic effects.

A logical approach to contraception is the use of agonists and antagonists of gonadotropic releasing hormones. Unlike the oral contraceptives, these hormones have a highly localized site of action. An inhibitor of the gonadotropin releasing hormone (GnRH), for example, would specifically inhibit ovulation or spermatogenesis. These compounds are effective in nanogram doses. By controlling release of gonadotropins, GnRH plays a role in two critical events in the menstrual cycle: follicular development and production of progesterone by the corpus luteum. Subcutaneous injection of an agonist of luteinizing hormone releasing hormone induces a shortened luteal phase, with suboptimal concentrations of circulating estrogen and progesterone. Administration of these agonists for 3 successive days at the time of onset of the menstrual cycle thus appears to be a practical approach to control of fertility. Use of the analogs may be effective in men by suppressing spermatogenesis without interfering with production of LH and testosterone. It is thus necessary to produce a dissociated response of LH and FSH; current trials suggest that dissociation is possible.

The immunologic control of pregnancy has much to commend it theoretically, but has not yet reached the stage of clinical application to human reproduction. Antibodies to the β-subunit of hCG seem to provide a logical means of preventing pregnancy, but the dual problems of reversibility and adverse effects on tissues other than trophoblast remain to be overcome.

Several techniques that are theoretically promising have not yet reached the stage of clinical trials. Research is centering on new substances that are crucial to reproductive function. They include folliculostatin, which suppresses secretion of FSH; oocyte maturation inhibitor, which prevents the first meiotic division of the oocyte; inhibin, a testicular hormone that inhibits secretion of FSH without inhibiting LH; antibodies to estrogen receptors; an androgen-binding protein in the testis; an antigonadotropin of the pineal gland, which presumably blocks LH; and an agent that inhibits production of progesterone by the corpus luteum.

Sterilization

Sterilization, a permanent form of contraception, is an important adjunct to traditional contraception and abortion. It is now the most popular form of contraception in the United States, probably because of changing personal and societal values and the aging of the population. In about 1 of every 5 married white couples in the United States between the ages of 20 and 40, a sterilizing procedure has been performed on one of the partners. The pregnancy rate, depending on the technique employed, is between 0.1 and 0.5.

Because of recent changes in attitude, sterilization of the male has become much more acceptable. The possibility of sperm banking may have added further impetus to male sterilization. Men who consent to vasectomy only on the condition that their sperm may be banked are generally ambivalent about the procedure and should be discouraged from undergoing an operation that may be irreversible. The duration of viability of frozen human spermatozoa is unknown, furthermore, and the possibility of genetic defects in the resulting offspring must be considered. In general, ambivalence about any sterilizing procedure in the man or the woman is best managed by deferring permanent forms of contraception.

The major techniques of female sterilization involve destruction or resection of a portion of the oviduct. The principal techniques of tubal sterilization are immediate postpartum resection, laparoscopic cauterization or occlusion, and vaginal or abdominal tubal procedures in the nonpuerperal state.

There are several advantages to postpartum sterilization: the procedure can be performed in 10 to 20 minutes under the same anesthetic that is used for delivery; a small abdominal incision is sufficient; the cost to the patient and the length of hospitalization are not significantly increased; and the likelihood of failure and complications is small. The procedure must, however, be discussed with the patient before labor and the possibility that the child may not be of the desired sex or may not survive must be considered.

Laparoscopic sterilization involves induction of a pneumoperitoneum (p. 186) and occlusion or destruction of part of the tube. Its advantages include a short hospitalization (often in an ambulatory care facility), which varies from 8 to 24 hours, a very small point of entry into the abdomen, and relatively few complications. It is often, however, not quite so effective as sterilization through a formal laparotomy and it may involve injury to neighboring abdominal viscera. Several techniques have been devised recently to reduce the likelihood of thermal and electrical injuries during laparoscopy: the bipolar method, the Yoon (Falope) ring, and the Hulka clip. The rate of ectopic pregnancy after electrocoagulation is greater than that after other techniques. The reversibility of a technique, furthermore is usually inversely proportional to its effectiveness. Contraindications to laparoscopic sterilization include abdominal scars, adhesions, hernias, and peritonitis.

An alternative to laparoscopy is minilaparotomy. The tubal resection is carried out through a small suprapubic incision. Although the technique is inappropriate for obese women, it requires no elaborate equipment and is therefore more readily applicable to developing countries.

Nonpuerperal sterilization may be performed through the abdominal route (laparotomy) or through the vagina (colpotomy). Formal laparotomy provides excellent access and visualization with a very high rate of success, but it entails a stay in the hospital of three or more days, a relatively high cost, and a sizable abdominal scar. Vaginal tubal ligation or resection is performed through an incision in the posterior cul-de-sac. Its advantages are the absence of an abdominal scar and a shorter hospital stay. Disadvantages include increased difficulty in exposure and identification of the tubes. Postoperative complications including abscesses are somewhat more common than with abdominal procedures. A current or recent pregnancy is a contraindication to the vaginal route. Pelvic adhesions are a relative contraindication.

The major reasons for failure of tubal sterilization are : an early undetected pregnancy at the time of the operation, abnormalities of the tube or technical errors during the procedure, and postoperative opening of the tube.

Hysterectomy, abdominal or vaginal, provides virtually complete protection against subsequent pregnancy. It may be performed in conjunction with a cesarean section. It is a more extensive procedure than a tubal resection and is associated with a longer hospitalization and a higher incidence of postoperative complications such as hemorrhage, infection, and injury to the urinary tract. In addition to terminating fertility it removes a functionless organ and prevents carcinoma of the corpus or cervix.

Hysterectomy terminates menses, which may be an advantage or a disadvantage, depending on the patient's attitude. Despite the prophylactic value of hysterectomy it cannot be justified as a routine alternative to tubal sterilization. Federal regulations do not permit payment for hysterectomy for purposes of family planning when the operation is performed in programs funded by the federal government. Even though 10% of women may have gynecologic disease that requires surgical operation after tubal sterilization, the complications of hysterectomy justify the procedure only when there is a reason in addition to termination of childbearing potential, such as myomas or intraepithelial neoplasia of the cervix.

The most serious complications of tubal ligation or resection are pulmonary emboli and ectopic pregnancy. A principal technique of tubal resection is the Pomeroy operation, in which the tube is not crushed, an absorbable suture is used, and the knuckle of ligated tube is resected. The failure rate of a properly performed Pomeroy sterilization does not exceed 0.5%. The reversibility of tubal sterilization varies between 10 and 50%, depending on the procedure used. Techniques involving fimbriectomy and electrocoagulation are less amenable to reversal than are properly performed Pomeroy operations. Microsurgical techniques have increased the rate of success in certain types of tubal reconstructive procedures.

In techniques such as the Madlener operation the tube is crushed and ligated with a nonabsorbable suture and the knuckle is not resected. Because the failure rate of this procedure is considerably higher than that of the Pomeroy operation, the technique of ligation without resection is not recommended.

A somewhat more complicated technique with a very high rate of success is the Irving sterilization. In this operation the proximal end of the tube is buried in a tunnel within the myometrium and the distal end is often buried between the leaves of the broad ligament.

Hysteroscopy, a promising endoscopic technique, permits transvaginal cauterization of the uterine ostia of the fallopian tubes. A potentially reversible hysteroscopic technique involves delivery of a plug of methylcyanoacrylate (MCA) into the uterine ostia of the oviducts. The rapid polymerization of the compound prevents spillage into the peritoneal cavity. The use of MCA provides sterilization in not more than about 85% of cases and is therefore not likely to be popular in the United States. Metal devices inserted hysteroscopically into the uterine ostia of the oviducts and polymerized silicone plugs are additional methods of potentially reversible sterilization, but they too are currently associated with an unacceptably high rate of failure.

Ablation of the endometrium, by cryosurgery or the laser, is an additional technique under current investigation. Potentially reversible methods of female sterilization include the use of fimbrial hoods and drugs such as quinacrine, which can be delivered in the form of pellets or in an intrauterine device. The block caused by quinacrine may be reversed by estrogens.

The most popular form of male sterilization is vasectomy. This procedure involves bilateral scrotal incisions, or occasionally a single midline incision, and division of each ductus deferens. Its advantages are rapidity, inexpensiveness, and the possibility of accomplishment in the office with only local anesthesia. There is no demonstrable effect on production of androgens, libido, or sexual performance. Disadvantages are the fear of impotence by the male and the obvious but crucial fact that the female partner may still become pregnant. Several techniques of reversible male sterilization involving insertion of a removable device into the vas are currently under investigation.

The ejaculate must be shown to be free of spermatozoa on two successive occasions before reliance can be placed on the method for complete contraception. This procedure is reversible in fewer than 50% of cases. Granulomas that occasionally follow section of the ductus deferens have rarely caused serious clinical problems. Preliminary reports of autoimmune disease resulting from vasectomy have not been substantiated, although antibodies to sperm are found in over half of all vasectomized men. A small preliminary study showed that vasectomy exacerbates the development of atherosclerosis in monkeys fed a diet high in cholesterol but no association was found between vasectomy and atherosclerosis in human subjects.

The Department of Health and Human Services has promulgated regulations governing nontherapeutic sterilizations paid for by federal funds. It has imposed a moratorium on sterilization of minors and mentally incompetent men and women. Furthermore, it has required a greatly detailed informed consent that lists complications of sterilization and alternatives to the procedure. It also requires a mandatory 30-day period of delay between the signing of the consent and the performance of the sterilization, except in certain cases of premature labor or surgical operations performed as emergencies. In the case of premature labor, the informed consent must have been given at least 30 days before the expected date of delivery.

Patients whose sterilizations are financed by federal funds must be informed that they are free to withhold or withdraw their consent to the procedure without affecting their rights to future treatment and without loss of any federal benefits to which they are entitled. They must be given a description of other methods of birth control, advice that sterilization should be considered irreversible, and a thorough explanation of the specific procedure for sterilization that is to be performed. They must, furthermore, be given a full description of the benefits of sterilization and of the discomforts and risks (including those of anesthesia) that may be expected during and after the procedure. An interpreter must be provided for patients who do not understand English and suitable provisions made for those who are blind, deaf, or otherwise impaired. Consent for sterilization may not be obtained while the patient is seeking or undergoing an abortion.

Abortion

Although abortion is not recommended as a primary means of family planning or population control, it serves as a backup for failed contraception. Perhaps with ready availability of abortion, contraceptives can be developed that are less than 100% effective but are devoid of the complications of the currently available drugs and devices.

Until 1973 abortion was closely regulated by statute in most of the states to the extent that a serious medical problem was required to justify the procedure. Circumstances in which abortion is mandatory to save the life of the mother are most unusual. They may include advanced cardiac disease with prior decompensation, severe renal or vascular disease, and carcinoma of the cervix. Psychiatric indications for abortion and fetal indications such as prevention of the birth of an infant with structural or biochemical defects have been subject to wide differences of interpretation by various states. The most restrictive abortion laws allowed the procedure only to save the life of the mother. Other legislatures allowed the procedure to protect the life or health of the mother. The more liberal laws defined health, according to the interpretation of the World Health Organization, as including mental and social well-being. The abortion issue is still debated hotly, largely along religious lines, as a question of maternal versus fetal rights.

The status of abortion in the United States was drastically changed by the historic decision of the United States Supreme Court on January 22, 1973. That decision, which strengthened women's rights, was influenced by the finding that the fetus has no constitutional rights and that neither biologists, nor theologians, nor legal scholars could agree when life begins. All state laws must now be consistent with the ruling of the Supreme Court, which essentially leaves decisions about abortion in the first trimester of pregnancy to the patient and her doctor without any regulation or interference by the State. For the period from the end of the first trimester to approximately the end of the second trimester, the State, in promoting its interest in the health of the mother, may regulate but not prohibit abortion for the protection of maternal health. For the stage subsequent to viability, at approximately the beginning of the third trimester, the State, in promoting its interest in the potentiality of human life, may regulate or proscribe abortion, except where the physician reasonably believes an abortion based on physiologic or psychologic grounds to be necessary for the preservation of the life or health of the mother. To comply fully with the ruling of the Supreme Court the State cannot impose the requirement of a husband's signature or parental consent, for example, in first-trimester abortions. In 1977, however, the Supreme Court ruled that individual states are not required to pay for abortions with Medicaid funds. Although its legal basis is clear, the effect of this decision was to deny to poor women a medical service that is available to the wealthy. In 1986 the Supreme Court in a 5:4 decision reaffirmed its 1973 ruling.

More than one quarter of all pregnancies in the United States have been terminated by abortion in recent years. The medical justification, which is not necessarily an ethical justification, for liberalization of the laws relating to abortion is based on the following facts: first-trimester abortion is safer than any alternative available to pregnant women; the death-to-case ratio for legal abortion has been reduced from 6.2 per 100,000 procedures in 1970 to less than 0.5 in 1986; legal abortion has resulted in more abortions that are performed earlier in pregnancy and are associated with a lower maternal risk; the risk of death increases as pregnancy progresses and is greater in those women whose pregnancies are unwanted; legal abortion is responsible for a decline in out-of-wedlock births; the option of legal abortion after amniocentesis has resulted in 10% more pregnancies in the population at high risk of having genetically damaged offspring; and there is a positive correlation between increased legal abortion and an increasing proportion of women using contraceptives.

Techniques of abortion fall into several main categories: dilatation of the cervix followed by sharp curettage or evacuation by suction, instillation of solutions into the amniotic cavity, hysterotomy, and hysterectomy.

Medicinal induction of abortion is not considered further here. Oxytocin is not effective in the early stages of pregnancy and numerous herbal and folk remedies are insufficiently tested to be recommended as routine abortifacients. A long-acting prostaglandin analog, 15-methyl-prostaglandin $F_{2\alpha}$, which may be administered either intravaginally in a suppository or intramuscularly by injection, has been used as an early first-trimester abortifacient, although it has achieved greater popularity for cervical softening and effacement later in pregnancy.

The principal technique for evacuating the uterus under 12 weeks' gestational size is curettage, usually by suction. Because it is slightly less dangerous and can be performed on larger uteri, suction is more widely used today than is sharp curettage. Occasionally it is necessary to remove some products of conception by gentle sharp curettage after an attempt at evacuation by suction.

A modification of the suction technique applicable to very early pregnancy involves the insertion of a semirigid plastic catheter, with dimensions approximately equal to those of an ordinary drinking straw, through the virtually undilated cervix. Suction may then be applied and products of conception removed. Such techniques performed at the time of the first missed period or earlier have been termed "menstrual regulation" or "menstrual induction," but they are merely early abortions.

Dilatation and curettage or suction require a block or a general anesthetic, but may be performed as an outpatient procedure within a hospital or in a facility with immediate access to a hospital for the management of complications. The time required for the surgical procedure and recovery is short. Disadvantages of the procedure are the occasional perforation of the uterus, which may require laparotomy. Infection, hemorrhage, and the likelihood of perforation increase with the size of the uterus and decrease with the experience of the operator.

Injections of intraamniotic solutions are most effectively performed in a uterus of 16 weeks' gestational size or greater. Until the midseventies it was considered desirable to perform the abortion before 12 weeks' gestation, when a curettage can be performed with minimal danger, or to wait until 16 weeks, when intraamniotic solutions may be instilled. Successful results are now generally obtained with dilatation and evacuation of the uterus larger than 12 weeks' gestational size. The data show that in well-trained hands, midtrimester abortion (up to 20 gestational weeks) by suction may be safer than intraamniotic solutions. Before injection of intraamniotic solutions it is neccessary that the placenta be located by sonography to avoid fetomaternal hemorrhage. The amniocentesis is then performed, removing 100 to 200 ml of amniotic fluid, which is replaced very slowly by the abortifacient solution. The most commonly used solutions for this purpose are prostaglandins and hypertonic saline (20 to 23% NaCl). The current trend is away from intraamniotic solutions and toward dilatation and evacuation.

The insertion of laminaria tents into the cervical canal the night before abortion reduces the likelihood of damage to the cervix by forcible instrumental dilation or precipitous delivery through an undilated and uneffaced cervix. Variations in technique include simultaneous intraamniotic instillation of prostaglandin and urea, intraamniotic prostaglandin and intravenous oxytocin, and intraamniotic urea and intravenous oxytocin.

Certain studies suggest that there is no increase in risk of reproductive loss after one legally induced abortion but a twofold to threefold increase in the risk of first-trimester spontaneous abortion after two or more prior induced abortions. Other studies come to the perhaps more logical conclusion that the degree of damage to the reproductive tract with any particular abortion or abortions is more significant than the number of prior abortions.

Abortion through injection of intraamniotic solutions avoids instrumental dilatation of the cervix and laparotomy. Abortion usually follows injection of the solutions by 24 to 36 hours. The procedure is generally considered a failure if abortion has not occurred within 48 hours after injection. In cases of failure the procedure may be repeated, perhaps with the addition of oxytocin, or a dilatation and evacuation may be performed. Injection of hypertonic saline is contraindicated in the presence of cardiovascular or renal disease, and use of any intraamniotic solution is impossible in the presence of ruptured membranes.

The main complications of injection of saline result from inadvertent intravascular or intraperitoneal injection. They include hypernatremia, cardiac arrest, pulmonary edema, hemoglobinuria, encephalopathy, and necrosis of tissue. Additional complications include hemorrhage; infection; retained products of conception, which may require curettage; and coagulopathies, which very likely result from disseminated intravascular coagulation. Because of the high rates of these complications, saline is not commonly used today as an abortifacient. Prostaglandins, which are now the most commonly used agents, often result in incomplete abortions, which may require completion by curettage. In addition, their use occasionally results in delivery of a living fetus. Intraamniotic solutions have become less popular as techniques and instruments for midtrimester abortion have improved and as experience with the procedure has increased.

Ideally, abortions should be prevented by effective contraception; when unwanted pregnancy requires abortion, the procedure should be done as early in pregnancy as possible in the interests of maternal safety.

Hysterotomy is rarely performed for abortion today, and then only when the uterus is too large to empty by curettage or suction and when intraamniotic solutions are ineffective or medically contraindicated. Disadvantages of hysterotomy include the prolonged hospitalization (4 or more days) and the scars in the abdomen and uterus, which may require subsequent delivery by cesarean section.

Abortion may also be effected through hysterectomy, although the increased morbidity associated with this procedure precludes its wider use. The advantages of the procedure include the removal of a potentially or an actually diseased organ and permanent sterilization. Disadvantages include the increased morbidity associated with hysterectomy in general and with hysterectomy in pregnant patients in particular. The special example of carcinoma of the cervix complicating early pregnancy is best managed by abortion through simultaneous radical hysterectomy and pelvic lymph node dissection or complete radiotherapy.

The American College of Obstetricians and Gynecologists has described the ideal circumstances for performance of an elective abortion. Abortion should be regarded as a surgical procedure and its performance should require appropriate surgical, anesthetic, and resuscitative equipment. In addition, the diagnosis and duration of pregnancy should be verified. Laboratory procedures should include blood typing and identification of the Rh-type. Any factors or illness that might have a bearing on the anesthesia and any drug sensitivities should be recorded.

Rh immune globulin (p. 155) is often given after abortion to any Rh-negative patient when the father's Rh-type is positive or unknown. It is not necessary to give a full dose of 300 μg, especially in very early abortion, when the extent of fetomaternal hemorrhage is minimal. The small dose of 50 μg offers sufficient protection in very early abortion. Postoperative and contraceptive advice should be available. No physician should be required to perform an abortion and no patient should be forced to undergo the procedure. An informed consent should be obtained and the procedure should be performed only by physicians who are qualified to identify and manage the complications that may arise from the procedure. Attempts should be made to provide facilities where abortions can be performed with maximal safety but with minimal disruption of other hospital functions.

VIII

Human Sexuality

Scope of the Subject

Detailed discussions of human sexuality are beyond the scope of even large textbooks of gynecology, but awareness of the wide range of normal sexual behavior and recognition of common psychosexual problems are requisite to effective gynecologic diagnosis and therapy. The necessity for obtaining a complete factual history of sexual habits is discussed in Unit I. The same objectivity should be applied to this area of gynecology as to a discussion of cardiovascular or gastrointestinal function. The criteria of sexuality are enumerated on page 323.

The gynecologist is often the first physician to deal with female sexual inadequacies and is also required to exclude organic causes of sexual dysfunction in his patients. He or she must be competent to counsel young patients and avert psychiatric sexual problems. Control of conception is one important facet of sexual counseling, for fear of pregnancy may lead to sexual inadequacy.

The physician requires knowledge of sex-specific differences in the cycle of sexual response and the wide variations in psychologic attitudes and physical behavior in both sexes. The physician must differentiate sexual problems based on ignorance from true sexual psychiatric disorders and organic diseases. He must recognize the enormous variety of cultural mores and taboos and strive to prevent his own sexual inhibitions from interfering with effective rapport with the patient. He must expand his concept of normal sexual behavior, which is defined by some experts in the area as including any activity that mutually pleases two consenting adults without causing physical or psychologic harm.

Statistically, an act may be classified as normal if it is practiced without deleterious effects by large numbers of people. In this sense, orogenital activity, masturbation, and in some circumstances, homosexual relations between consenting adults are not classified by psychiatrists as aberrations. The physician must help destroy psychologically harmful sexual myths. In particular, he must assure his patient that some form of masturbation is almost universally practiced at certain times of life and that it serves a useful function in relieving tension. He must also dispel the myths about the value, or indeed the existence, of specific aphrodisiacs. It is important that he distinguish love from sex and explain the differences to his patients.

The physician should be familiar with the basic Freudian concepts and recognize the need for psychiatric referral. He should be aware of changing patterns of sexuality and the sexual readjustments by men and women that are created by female liberation, the abolition of the double sexual standard, and the active role assumed by women in sexual encounters. The physician must be able to explain to the patient the changes in sexual response after major gynecologic operations and during the prenatal course and post partum. He should discourage unnecessary restriction of sexual activity in pregnancy that is based on unfounded fears of injuring the fetus or inducing prematurity. He should explain that the woman's libido may be increased or decreased during her pregnancy, whereas the male's is often unchanged. The physician should understand that sexual activity and sexual problems may involve patients of advanced age.

Sexual counseling requires time and patience. The first visit is often devoted simply to establishing confidence of the patients in the physician. Successful treatment requires a careful sexual history obtained independently from each partner. Difficult problems should be referred to expert sexual counselors, often a team comprising a gynecologist and a psychologist. Deep-seated disorders should be referred to a psychiatrist.

The frequency of sexual activity varies enormously within any age group, although in general, frequency decreases with age. Libido in women increases between the early twenties and the middle thirties. In men libido is greatest in the late teens, decreasing notably in the late twenties. In both sexes libido may continue into advanced years. It is affected throughout life by general mental health, depression, and anxiety. It is influenced also by chronic alcoholism and by drugs such as morphine, heroin, and LSD. The physician must be sufficiently well informed about the current AIDS epidemic to advise his or her patients appropriately about safer sexual practices.

Human Sexual Response

Human sexual response is basically similar in both sexes. Sexual stimulation leads to vascular engorgement, muscular tension, and their physiologic consequences. The four phases of sexual response described by Masters and Johnson are excitement, plateau, orgasm, and resolution. The excitement phase is the longest. It may be induced by somatic or psychogenic stimuli and delayed or interrupted voluntarily.

Whereas the female may have multiple orgasms in rapid succession, the male undergoes a refractory period of 5 to 30 minutes, during which orgasm cannot be achieved by any means. Ordinarily orgasm in the male is reached faster and more directly than in the female, in whom physical contact appears to be a less significant erotogenic factor. The feeling that the female is desired may in itself lead to heightened sexual response. The intensity of the female reaction may depend upon amount and type of foreplay. The physician should advise against attempts to attain simultaneous orgasms in both partners, for such a result is neither common nor necessarily desirable. He should also refute the concept of the superiority of vaginal over clitoral orgasm, since, despite Freud's teaching, the two means of stimulation produce identical orgasms. Direct contact with the clitoris is not usually achieved during intercourse in the "missionary position" (man over woman), since the clitoris normally retracts under the symphysis. Effective stimulation of the clitoris is more directly achieved by digital manipulation.

Another myth concerns the advantage of the large over the small penis as an effective organ of copulation; nor does circumcision increase or decrease sensation or delay ejaculation. Most important, the physician should recognize that sexual incompatibilities are usually psychogenic rather than physical. He should identify serious psychosexual disorders and obtain psychiatric consultation at the first opportunity.

The details of human sexual response have been described in the writings of Masters and Johnson. In general, there is notable similarity in the genital and extragenital responses in both men and women during excitement, plateau, orgasm, and resolution.

During the excitement phase in women there is tumescence of the glans of the clitoris, vasocongestion, and increase in diameter and length of the shaft. The vagina provides lubrication within 10 to 30 seconds of stimulation and the vaginal tube expands and assumes a darker purplish hue. The uterus is partially elevated and the corpus becomes irritable. The labia majora in the nullipara undergo flattening, separation, and anterolateral elevation away from the vaginal outlet; in the multipara vasocongestion, increase in diameter, and slight movement away from the midline occur. The labia minora undergo slight thickening and expansion.

In the plateau phase the clitoris retracts under the symphysis. The vagina forms an orgasmic platform at its outer third and undergoes further increase in width and depth. Corpus and cervix are fully elevated and there is further increase in irritability of the corpus. The labia majora in the nullipara are severely engorged; in the multipara further vasocongestion occurs. The labia minora undergo a striking change in color from bright red to deep wine, indicating impending orgasm. At this stage Bartholin's glands secrete a drop or two of mucoid material.

At orgasm, contractions of the orgasmic platform in the vagina are noted at intervals of 0.8 seconds, recurring 6 to 12 times. The uterus undergoes contractions, the extent of which parallels the intensity of the orgasm. In the multipara there may be up to a 50% increase in uterine size.

During the phase of resolution the clitoris returns to its normal position. Five to 10 seconds after orgasm the platform ceases to contract and undergoes rapid detumescence. The vaginal walls relax and their normal color returns within 10 to 15 minutes. The uterus returns to its normal position, but the external os continues to gape for about 20 to 30 minutes. In the nullipara, the labia majora return to their normal thickness and midline position; in the multipara, the labial vasocongestion disappears. The labia minora change color from bright red to light pink within 15 seconds and their size decreases.

In addition, there are numerous extragenital reactions during the various phases of female sexual response. During excitement several changes occur in the breasts. The nipples become erect and increase in size; concomitant tumescence of the areolae occurs. A maculopapular rash (sex flush) develops late in the phase of excitement, beginning over the epigastrium and spreading over the breasts. Myotonia, both voluntary and involuntary, increases. Tachycardia parallels the degree of sexual tension.

During the plateau phase the nipples become turgid. The breasts increase further in size and the areolae undergo further erection. The sex flush is better developed and myotonia increases, accompanied by spastic contractions. Tachycardia increases to as high as 175/minute, accompanied by increases in systolic and diastolic blood pressures of 20 to 60 and 10 to 20 mm Hg, respectively.

At the time of orgasm the sex flush parallels the intensity of the reaction. Myotonia is maximal, with loss of voluntary control, accompanied by involuntary contractions of the rectal sphincter. The respiratory rate increases to as high as 40/minute and tachycardia increases to between 110 and 180/minute. Blood pressure rises about 30 to 50 mm Hg systolic and 20 to 40 mm Hg diastolic.

During resolution rapid detumescence of the nipples and areolae occurs. The decrease in volume of the breasts is slower. The sex flush disappears rapidly in the reverse order in which it appeared. Myotonia rarely continues for more than 5 minutes after orgasm. Hyperventilation and tachycardia return rapidly to normal. A widespread film of perspiration appears, unrelated to the extent of physical activity.

In the male, the genital and extragenital reactions are similar to those just described in the female. During excitement the most obvious event is the rapid erection of the penis. Erection may be lost and regained or inhibited by numerous stimuli during this phase. There is tensing and thickening of the scrotal skin and elevation of the sac. The testes are elevated as a result of shortening of the spermatic cords.

During the plateau phase the penis undergoes an increase in circumference at the coronal ridge and possibly a change in color of the corona. The testes are said to undergo an enlargement of 50% over their nonstimulated state. Full elevation of the testes indicates impending ejaculation. Cowper's glands provide a preejaculatory emission of a few drops of fluid containing numerous active spermatozoa.

At orgasm the penis undergoes contraction along the entire length of the penile urethra. The contractions start at intervals of 0.8 seconds. After the first three or four contractions, the expulsive force is reduced.

During resolution the penis undergoes detumescence in two stages, a rapid and a slow. The scrotum rapidly loses its congestion and its normal folds reappear. The testes return to normal size and position.

The male also undergoes certain extragenital reactions. In excitement there is occasional erection of the nipples, myotonia (including voluntary and involuntary components), and tachycardia and hypertension in proportion to the degree of sexual tension.

During the plateau phase, an inconsistent further increase in erection of the nipples occurs. A maculopapular rash develops late in this phase. The rash originates over the epigastrium and spreads to the chest wall, neck, forehead, and other locations. Myotonia is characterized by a further increase in voluntary and involuntary components. Hyperventilation occurs late in this phase, and tachycardia may range between 100 and 175/minute, with an increase in blood pressure from 20 to 80 mm Hg systolic and 10 to 40 diastolic.

At orgasm, a well-developed sex flush is seen in about 25% of men. Myotonia is characterized by loss of voluntary control and by involuntary contractions and spasm. The rectal sphincter undergoes contractions occurring at intervals of 0.8/second and the respiratory rate may rise to as high as 40/minute. Tachycardia ranges from 110 to 180, and a rise in blood pressure of 40 to 100 systolic and 20 to 50 diastolic occurs.

During resolution there is involution of erection of the nipples and rapid disappearance of the sex flush in reverse order of its appearance. Myotonia disappears within 5 minutes after the end of orgasm. The increased blood pressure, heart rate, and respiratory rate return to normal. Perspiration in the male is inconsistent and involuntary and is usually confined to the palms and soles.

Common Sexual Complaints

Sexual dysfunction may result from disorders of sexual desire or arousal. Education and counseling are of great benefit in simple cases of ignorance of sexual function. Disorders of female arousal are sometimes effectively treated by so-called sensate focus exercises. With this technique the male is asked to defer orgasm as he proceeds through three stages of sexual activity. The first stage avoids contact with either the female genitalia or breasts. In the second stage the breasts are stimulated. In the third stage coitus is permitted. The woman assumes a superior position, which increases her control of the coital act. She initiates intercourse and thrusts slowly while contracting her pubococcygeal muscles.

Orgasmic dysfunction may be treated by teaching the woman how to masturbate. If manual stimulation of the clitoris and breasts is ineffective, she may use a vibrator. Sexual reeducation in this disorder involves the woman's deferring coitus until she is close to orgasm, use of fantasy, contraction of the perineal and abdominal muscles, use of the stop-start technique, adjunctive stimulation of the clitoris during coitus, and rapid thrusting by the woman when she feels an impending orgasm.

Pelvic congestion is a vague syndrome that is thought to be of neurovascular origin. It may be a manifestation of psychosexual conflict, fear of pregnancy, inadequate sexual response, or failure of orgasm. The venous channels of the pelvis are congested and the uterosacral ligaments are indurated. Deep pelvic pain increases just before menses and dyspareunia is common. Diagnosis is suggested by multiple complaints in an unusually tense patient. The uterus is often retroverted and enlarged to the size of a 10 weeks' gestation. Differential diagnosis includes endometriosis (p. 228) and chronic pelvic inflammatory disease (p. 215). In the pelvic congestion syndrome, unlike endometriosis, the tense ligaments seem to disappear under anesthesia. Treatment may include tranquilizers, psychotherapy, and adrenergic blocking agents.

Dyspareunia, painful or otherwise unsatisfactory intercourse, may result from organic causes such as atrophy of the introitus, scars, or severe vaginitis. Additional common causes include endometriosis of the uterosacral ligaments, the pelvic congestion syndrome, and purely psychogenic factors.

Vaginismus is painful spasm of the vagina, sufficient to prevent satisfactory coitus. The pelvic muscles are spastic and penetration may be prevented. It may be caused by repugnance to the sexual act and is almost always psychogenic. Use of progressively larger dilators is occasionally effective. Psychologic counseling is more often helpful.

Frigidity, or sexual coldness, is lack of libido or desire for the sexual act. It should be differentiated from lack of orgasm. Permanent frigidity is psychosexual, perhaps representing subconscious repression. Women with frigidity may achieve orgasm by masturbation.

Nymphomania is defined as extreme eroticism or sexual desire in women. It corresponds to satyriasis in men. These are poor terms because eroticism is most difficult to quantitate.

Premature ejaculation is defined as failure to delay ejaculation for 30 seconds after penetration. It is a very common complaint, which only in its severe or chronic form may be termed a psychosexual disorder. A technique in which the penis is squeezed by the partner is frequently recommended to delay ejaculation.

Impotence is failure to achieve and maintain an erection during coitus. It is primarily a psychologic problem, in which fear of failure to perform well sexually may create a vicious cycle.

Index

Syndrome (*Continued*)
Hunter's, 89
Hurler's, 89
Klinefelter's, 85
Laurence-Moon-Biedl, 315
Lesch-Nyhan, 89
Morquio's, 89
Prader-Willi, 315
respiratory distress, 83
Sanfilippo's, 89
Sjögren's, 170
Stein-Leventhal, 280, 326
supine hypotensive, 110
transfusion, 157
Turner's, 85
Syphilis, 124, 194
congenital, 195
vulva, 236

TABOOS, sexual, 368
Tachycardia, fetal, 102
Tamoxifen, 308
Tay-Sachs disease, 89
Temperature, basal body, 333
Tenderness, rebound, 51
Tension, premenstrual, 5, 8, 339
Teratoma,
benign cystic, 280, 283
ovary, solid, 291
Terbutaline, 134
Term, 80
Test,
complement fixation, 196
Frei, 196
immunologic pregnancy, 58
nontreponemal, 195
Testicle, differentiation, 323
Testicular feminization, 315, 322
Testosterone,
male contraception, 356
Tetracaine, 114
Tetracycline, 93, 166, 196, 206
Thalassemia, 89
Thalidomide, 93
Thayer-Martin medium, 53, 199
Theca cell tumor, 328
Theca externa, 273
Theca interna, 69, 273
Theca lutein cyst, 129, 280
Thecoma, 288
Therapy, cyclic, 338
Thermography, 303

Thiazides, 93, 153
Thiopental, 113
Thrill, 162
Thromboembolism, oral contraceptive, 352
Thrombophlebitis, 171
breast, 300
pelvic, 171
puerperal, 171
Thrombosis, pregnancy, 65
Thromboxane, 154, 227
Thyroid, 91, 122
changes in pregnancy, 66
free hormone, 170
storm, 169
tests, 329
Thyroidectomy, 169
Thyrotropic releasing hormone, 116
Thyroxine, 63
free index, 170
T-mycoplasmas, 122
Tobramycin, 213
Toluidine blue, 184, 234
Tomography, computed, 314, 326
Tonus, 98
TORCH syndrome, 165
Toxic shock syndrome, 217
Toxoid, 92
Toxoplasmosis, 94, 122, 165
Tranquilizers, 111, 332
Transcortin, 67
Transcription, 311
Transfer, placental, 79
Transfusion,
anemia, 168
exchange, 118
intrauterine, 156
placental, 117
syndrome, 91, 148
Transglutaminase, 76
Translation, 311
Translocation, 87
Transposition, great vessels, 91
Transsexual, 324
Transudate, vaginal, 39
Transverse perineal muscles, 220
Transvestite, 324
Trauma, abortion, 124
Treponema pallidum immobilization, 194
T_3-resin uptake, 170
Triangle,
anal, 21
urogenital, 21, 24